T0329544

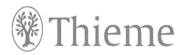

Imaging in Neurovascular Disease

A Case-Based Approach

Waleed Brinjikji, MD
Associate Professor
Radiology and Neurosurgery
Mayo Clinic Foundation
Rochester, Minnesota

Timo Krings, MD, PhD, FRCP (C)
Professor of Radiology and Surgery
Head of the Division
Diagnostic and Interventional Neuroradiology
Joint Department of Medical Imaging of the University Health Network
Chief of Radiology
Toronto Western Hospital
Chair of Interventional Neuroradiology
University of Toronto
Ontario, Canada

793 illustrations

Thieme
New York • Stuttgart • Delhi • Rio de Janeiro

Library of Congress Cataloging-in-Publication Data
is available from the Publisher

© 2020 Thieme. All right reserved.

Thieme Publishers New York
333 Seventh Avenue, New York, NY 10001 USA
+1 800 782 3488, customerservice@thieme.com

Thieme Publishers Stuttgart
Rüdigerstrasse 14, 70469 Stuttgart, Germany
+49 [0]711 8931 421, customerservice@thieme.de

Thieme Publishers Delhi
A-12, Second Floor, Sector-2, Noida-201301
Uttar Pradesh, India
+91 120 45 566 00, customerservice@thieme.in

Thieme Publishers Rio de Janeiro,
Thieme Publicações Ltda.
Edifício Rodolpho de Paoli, 25º andar
Av. Nilo Peçanha, 50 – Sala 2508
Rio de Janeiro 20020-906 Brasil
+55 21 3172 - 2297

Cover design: Thieme Publishing Group
Typesetting by DiTech Process Solutions, India

Printed in USA by King Printing Company, Inc.   5 4 3 2 1

ISBN 9781684200535

Also available as an e-book:
eISBN 9781684200542

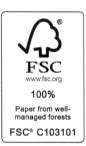

FSC
www.fsc.org
100%
Paper from well-managed forests
FSC® C103101

To our mentors…

Waleed Brinjikji
Timo Krings

Contents

Foreword

Imaging in Neurovascular Disease authored by Dr. Krings and Dr. Brinjikji represents the latest addition to a series of textbooks produced under the primary authorship of Dr. Timo Krings, which included *Case-Based Interventional Neuroradiology* and *Neurovascular Anatomy in Interventional Neuroradiology.* Both authors have contributed extensively to the neurovascular literature and their experience with neuroimaging and interventional techniques at the Toronto Western Hospital in Toronto and at Mayo Clinic in Rochester has resulted in an outstanding contribution highlighting the role of modern imaging in the management of neurovascular disorders.

Imaging in Neurovascular Disease addresses a need that has become apparent over the past few years as more and more neurointerventional therapists no longer possess a background training in diagnostic neuroradiology but rather entered the field with primary training in neurosurgery and neurology and become endovascular neurosurgeons and neurologists.

National and international professional organizations have accepted and promoted the concept that neurointerventional procedures can be performed by specialists having followed different training paths in neurosciences. Guidelines for such training routes have been published.

At the same time, noninvasive and invasive imaging techniques have become much more sophisticated compared to those 10 or 20 years ago and major advances have been made particularly in diagnostic neuroimaging, providing much improved information to guide modern neurointerventional treatment decisions and procedures. In fact, the imaging information that is currently available is often critical in making proper treatment decisions and neurovascular practitioners unfamiliar with these modern imaging techniques may make erroneous decisions leading to (preventable) poor outcome.

The authors have addressed this very important issue in a well-designed format and with high-quality state-of-the-art images. The description of the imaging findings is well done and clearly understandable. The critical imaging findings from a clinical point of view are highlighted at the end of each chapter and recent literature is provided to allow for further reading and understanding.

This book represents a very important and useful contribution to the field of neuroendovascular therapy and will be much appreciated by all neuroendovascular therapists, in particular by those with a background in neurosurgery and neurology.

Karel ter Brugge, MD, FRCP
Professor
Department of Radiology and Surgery
University of Toronto
Toronto, Canada

Preface

Cross-sectional imaging has become an integral component in the diagnosis and management of patients suffering from cerebrovascular and spinal vascular diseases. Over the past several decades, many vascular diseases which could only be diagnosed using conventional angiographic techniques earlier, are now evaluated with extensive cross-sectional imaging techniques such as CTA and MRA, with angiography being reserved for problem-solving purposes, in difficult cases, or for the purposes of treatment. With the increased utilization of MRI and "newer" sequences, such as perfusion imaging, susceptibility weighted imaging, and dynamic four-dimensional imaging, we are now able to better characterize the dynamic and functional aspects of many cerebrovascular diseases, and thus provide patients and physicians with better insight into the pathophysiology of many disease processes.

The purpose of this book is to help the readers, whether they be radiologists, surgeons, or neurologists, unlock the potential of cross-sectional imaging so as to (1) make more accurate diagnoses; (2) better characterize disease processes so as to guide treatment decisions; and (3) better understand the pathophysiological changes that are often staring us in the face on MRI or CT.

Both authors have trained in and currently practice diagnostic and interventional neuroradiology and, therefore, have a very solid background in the management of neurovascular diseases as well as imaging. Thus, in addition to providing a relatively detailed explanation of imaging findings in neurovascular diseases, the unique strength of this book is that it also provides background information on the pathophysiology of the disease processes, and review of various treatment options, and highlights how imaging findings can guide treatment decisions. We hope that the amount of clinical background provides enough context for readers to understand the significance of the various imaging findings.

A vast majority of the cases presented are routine diagnoses encountered in a standard neurovascular clinical or neuroradiological practice. However, we have also presented some exotic, bizarre, and exceptional cases out of necessity only to emphasize certain teaching points. Some of the entities discussed in this book are rare by nature and may only be encountered in supersubspecialized practices (e.g., vein of Galen malformations, pial arteriovenous fistulas, spinal arteriovenous malformations, etc.).

We believe that this book will fill a unique void in the field of diagnostic neuroradiology as it provides extensive information about the pathologic mechanisms involved in the diseases that we are asked to image and describes in detail the imaging findings and their significance. We hope that you and your patients find it beneficial!

Waleed Brinjikji, MD

Abbreviations

ABRA	Amyloid-beta related angiitis
ACA	Anterior cerebral artery
ADC	Apparent Diffusion Coefficient
ADEM	Acute disseminated encephalomyelitis
aSAH	Aneurysmal subarachnoid hemorrhage
ASITN/SIR	American Society of Interventional and Therapeutic Neuroradiology/Society of Interventional Radiology
ASL	Arterial spin labeling
ASPECTS	Alberta stroke program early CT score
AVMs	Arteriovenous Malformations
BCVI	Blunt cerebrovascular injury
BOLD	Blood oxygen level dependent
CAA	Cerebral amyloid angiopathy
CAA-RI	CAA-related inflammation
CAMS	Cerebral arterial metameric syndrome
CAS	Carotid artery stenting
CBF	Cerebral Blood Flow
CBV	Cerebral blood volume
CCA	Common carotid artery
CCF	Carotico-cavernous fistula
CEA	Carotid endarterectomy
CE-MRA	Contrast enhanced MR angiography
CEUS	Contrast enhanced ultrasound
CISS	Constructive interference steady state
CISS	Constructive Interference Steady State
CJD	Cruetzfeld Jacob disease
CM-AVM	Capillary malformation-arteriovenous malformation
CNS	Central nervous system
CoW	Circle of willis
CTA	CT angiography
CTP	CT Perfusion
CTV	CT venogram
CVR	Cerebral vascular reserve
CVT	Cortical vein thrombosis
DAVFs	Dural Arteriovenous Fistulas
DAWN	DWI or CTP Assessment with Clinical Mismatch in the Triage of Wake-Up and Late Presenting Strokes Undergoing Neurointervention with Trevo Trial
DCI	Delayed Cerebral Ischemia
DEFUSE	Endovascular therapy following imaging evaluation for ischemic stroke trial
DSA	Digital subtraction angiography
DSC	Dynamic susceptibility contrast
DSVT	Dural sinus venous thrombosis
DWI	Diffusion weighted imaging
ECA	External carotid artery
ELAPSS	Earlier subarachnoid hemorrhage, location, age, population, size, and shape
ESR	Erythrocyte sedimentation rate
EVD	External ventricular drain
FIESTA	Fast imaging employing steady-state acquisition
FLAIR	Fluid attenuation inversion recovery
FMD	Fibromuscular dysplasia
GCA	Giant Cell Arteritis
GCS	Glasgow coma scale
GRE	Gradient recall echo
IAD	Intracranial arterial dissection
ICH	Intracerebral hemorrhage
ICP	Intracranial pressure
IPH	Intraplaque hemorrhage
IVH	Intraventricular haemorrhage
LRNC	Lipid-rich necrotic core
MCA	Middle cerebral artery
MELAS	Mitochondrial encephalomyopathy, lactic acidosis, and stroke-like episodes
MIP	Maximum intensity projection
MIPs	Maximum intensity projections
MMA	Middle meningeal artery
MPR	Multiplanar reformat
MPRAGE	Magnetization prepared rapid gradient echo
MRV	MR venogram
MS	Multiple sclerosis
MTT	Mean transit time
NASCET	North American symptomatic carotid endarterectomy trial
NCCT	Non-contrast CT
NPV	Negative Predictive Value
PACNS	Primary angiitis of the central nervous system
PCA	Posterior cerebral artery
pc-ASPECTS	Posterior circulation ASPECTS
PCR	Polymerase chain reaction
PCR	Polymerase chain reaction
PHASES	Population, hypertension, age, size, earlier subarachnoid hemorrhage, site
PICA	Posterior inferior cerebellar artery
PPV	Positive Predictive Value
PRES	Posterior reversible encephalopathy syndrome
pSAH	Perimesencephalic Subarachnoid Hemorrhage
RCVS	Reversible Cerebral Vasoconstriction Syndrome
SAH	Subarachnoid hemorrhage
SAMS	Spinal arterial metameric syndrome
SDAF	Spinal Dural Arteriovenous Fistula
SEDAVFs	Spinal epidural AVFs
SOV	Superior ophthalmic vein
SPACE	Single slab 3D TSE sequence with slab selective, variable excitation pulse
sSAH	Sulcal Subarachnoid Hemorrhage
SSS	Subclavian steal syndrome
STA	Superficial temporal artery
SWI	Susceptibility weighted imaging
T1CE	T1 contrast enhanced
TA	Takayasu arteritis
TCA	Transverse cervical artery
TCD	Transcranial Doppler
TCD	Transcranial doppler
TIA	Transient ischemic attack
TICI	Thrombolysis in cerebral infarction
TOF	Time of flight
TTD	Time to drain
TTP	Time to peak
VNC	Virtual non-contrast
VOGM	Vein of GALEN malformation
VWI	Vessel wall imaging
VZV	Varicella zoster virus

Chapter 1

Acute Ischemic Stroke

1 Acute Ischemic Stroke

1.1 Hyperdense Vessel Sign

1.1.1 Clinical Case

A 23-year-old female, who woke up with aphasia and right-sided hemiparesis following a cardiac surgery (▶ Fig. 1.1).

1.1.2 Description of Imaging Findings and Diagnosis

Diagnosis

Left M1 occlusion with hyperdense artery sign.

1.1.3 Background

Non-contrast CT is the primary modality in acute ischemic stroke imaging at a vast majority of centers. Because of this, understanding the imaging manifestations of acute ischemic stroke is essential for radiologists, neurologists, and other neurovascular specialists. Because acute stroke, secondary to large vessel occlusion is the most devastating type of acute ischemic stroke, the prompt identification of imaging manifestations of large vessel occlusion is essential. The hyperdense artery sign is a well-described imaging manifestation of large vessel occlusion. In some centers, a hyperdense artery sign in the setting of a clinical severe stroke and a good Alberta stroke program early CT score (ASPECTS) will prompt endovascular intervention, even without a CT angiogram or CT perfusion study.

1.1.4 Imaging Findings

When evaluating the presence of a hyperdense vessel sign on non-contrast CT, the use of thin-slice (<2.5 mm) CT is strongly recommended. Many centers have shifted to using 1-mm slice thickness for all stroke protocols as it allows for the excellent delineation of the cerebral vasculature and has been shown to be substantially more sensitive and specific in identifying the hyperdense artery sign. The use of thicker slice CT (i.e., 3 mm or larger) will result in partial volume averaging of the horizontally traversing MCA branches due to their diameter being typically 3 mm or less (▶ Fig. 1.2). Thin-slice CT also allows for a more accurate evaluation of thrombus density, thrombus location, and thrombus length-variables, which have been shown to be correlated with angiographic outcomes after mechanical thrombectomy. It is particularly helpful in identifying distal MCA occlusions, particularly branches which course along the insula (▶ Fig. 1.3).

Studies examining the association between non-contrast CT findings and clot composition have been very consistent in demonstrating that the proportion of RBCs in a clot is strongly correlated with clot density. Meanwhile, fibrin-rich clots are known to be low density on non-contrast CT. Because roughly 70–80% of clots are RBC rich, in approximately 70–80% of large vessel occlusion cases, there will be a hyperdense artery sign. It is important to point out that the absence of a hyperdense artery sign does not mean the absence of intravascular thrombus or large vessel occlusion (▶ Fig. 1.4).

There are pitfalls of the hyperdense artery sign as an imaging marker of a large vessel occlusion. First, the density of blood in the vessels is strongly correlated with hematocrit. This explains why RBC-rich clots are more hyperdense than fibrin-rich clots. However, patients with a high hematocrit will have diffusely hyperdense arteries. Thus, looking for symmetry in vascular attenuation between the affected hemisphere and the non-affected hemisphere is important. When using thicker slices of CT, the partial volume averaging of vascular calcifications can result in the appearance of a hyperdense artery sign. This can be potentially mitigated by using a thinner-slice CT protocol. The hyperdense artery sign is not reliable in patients who have had recent contrast administration

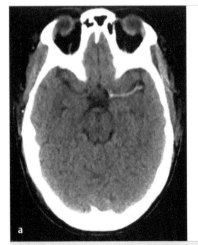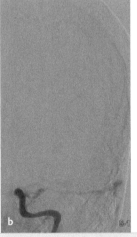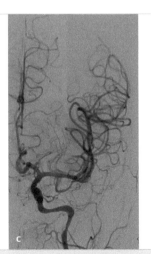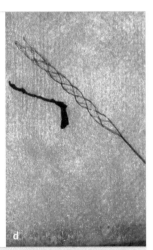

Fig. 1.1 A 23-year-old female who woke up with aphasia and right-sided hemiparesis following a cardiac surgery. (**a**) Non-contrast CT demonstrates a hyperdense left middle cerebral artery (MCA). Based on the presence of the hyperdense vessel and symptoms alone, the patient was brought directly to angio. (**b**) Left ICA cerebral angiogram demonstrates occlusion of the left ICA terminus. (**c**) Following one-pass with a solitaire stent retriever thrombolysis in cerebral infarction (TICI) 3 flow was achieved. (**d**) Gross and histopathological analysis of the clot demonstrated a thrombus rich in RBCs with minimal fibrin content.

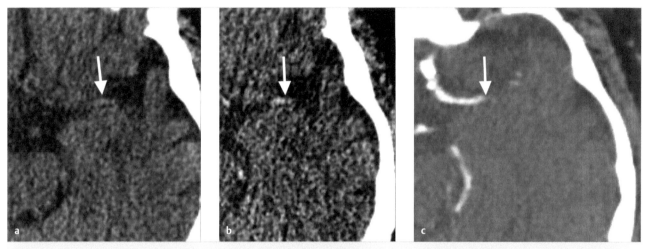

Fig. 1.2 Value of thin-cut non-contrast CT. (**a**) A 78-year old female who presented with sudden onset aphasia and right-sided weakness. Non-contrast CT with 3-mm slice thickness demonstrated no gray-white changes and no hyperdense vessel (*arrow*). (**b**) However, 0.5-mm thin cut CT source images demonstrated a hyperdense thrombus in the distal left M1 (*arrow*). (**c**) CT angiogram confirmed the occlusion (*arrow*).

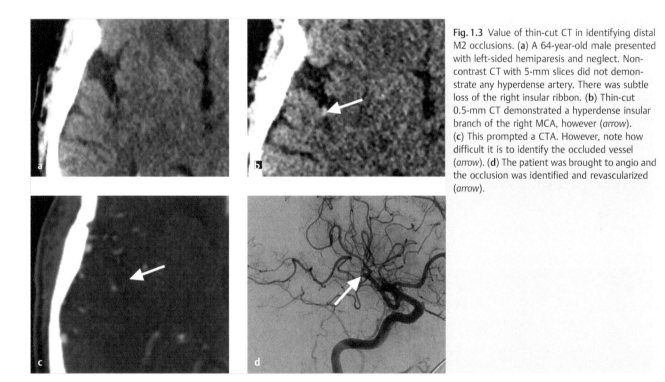

Fig. 1.3 Value of thin-cut CT in identifying distal M2 occlusions. (**a**) A 64-year-old male presented with left-sided hemiparesis and neglect. Non-contrast CT with 5-mm slices did not demonstrate any hyperdense artery. There was subtle loss of the right insular ribbon. (**b**) Thin-cut 0.5-mm CT demonstrated a hyperdense insular branch of the right MCA, however (*arrow*). (**c**) This prompted a CTA. However, note how difficult it is to identify the occluded vessel (*arrow*). (**d**) The patient was brought to angio and the occlusion was identified and revascularized (*arrow*).

(i.e., post-cardiac catheterization strokes). Lastly, it is essential to point out again that a fibrin-rich clot will not be dense on CT and these lesions make up roughly 20% of clots in the setting of large vessel occlusion.

CT angiography (also using thin-section CT) is very useful in clot imaging. Identification of a contrast gap between the proximal and distal end of the clot can help to assess clot length and thus aid in device choice, especially stent retriever length. Delayed-phase CTA is particularly useful in assessing clot burden and thrombus length as it can take time from contrast to make

it to the distal face of the clot. There has been growing interest in the assessment of clot perviousness/permeability to iodinated contrast as increasing density/enhancement of clot on CTA has been shown to be associated with revascularization outcomes.

1.1.5 What the Clinician Needs to Know

• Presence or absence of hyperdense artery sign
• Location and estimated length of the thrombus

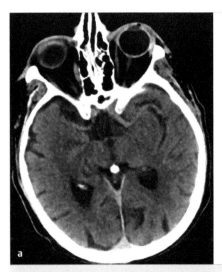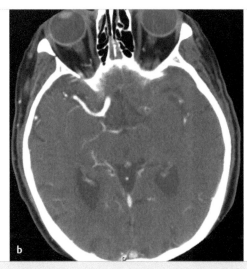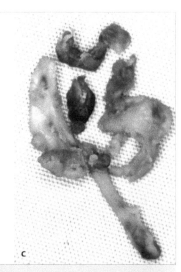

Fig. 1.4 Absence of hyperdense artery sign indicating fibrin-rich clot. (**a**) Non-contrast CT demonstrates early signs of ischemia in the left basal ganglia and insula. Note the symmetry in density of the bilateral MCAs. There was no hyperdense artery. (**b**) CTA demonstrates occlusion of the left ICA terminus and M1 segment. (**c**) After four passes with a stent-retriever, the vessel was revascularized. In this case, the clot was very fibrin rich with minimal RBC content.

1.1.6 High-Yield Facts

- The hyperdense artery sign is a sensitive and specific marker for large vessel occlusion in the setting of acute ischemic stroke.
- Pitfalls for the hyperdense artery sign include high hematocrit, recent contrast administration, and partial volume averaging in the setting of a calcified vessel.
- Thin-slice CTA with delayed phase imaging is an important tool in characterizing clot location and extent.

Further Reading

[1] Ahn SH, Choo IS, Hong R, et al. Hyperdense arterial sign reflects the proportion of red blood cells in the thromboemboli of acute stroke patients. Cerebrovasc Dis. 2012; 33:236

[2] Riedel CH, Zoubie J, Ulmer S, Gierthmuehlen J, Jansen O. Thin-slice reconstructions of nonenhanced CT images allow for detection of thrombus in acute stroke. Stroke. 2012; 43(9):2319–2323

[3] Borst J, Berkhemer OA, Santos EMM, et al. MR CLEAN investigators. Value of thrombus ct characteristics in patients with acute ischemic stroke. AJNR Am J Neuroradiol. 2017; 38(9):1758–1764

1.2 ASPECTS Score and CT Signs of Early Ischemia

1.2.1 Clinical Case

An 83-year-old male with acute onset right arm weakness, right facial droop, and aphasia (▶ Fig. 1.5).

1.2.2 Description of Imaging Findings and Diagnosis

Diagnosis

Left M1 occlusion with hyperdense artery sign. ASPECTS score of 7 with infarction affecting the left insula, lentiform nucleus, and caudate.

1.2.3 Background

As mentioned previously, non-contrast CT is the workhorse in acute stroke imaging. When patients present with stroke-like symptoms, the three most important tasks the radiologist must accomplish are: (1) rule out an intracranial hemorrhage or any other imaging findings that would contraindicate thrombolysis; (2) characterize the extent of infarction using the ASPECTS score; and (3) identify the presence or absence of a hyperdense artery sign.

The ASPECTS score has been shown to be a reproducible tool in assessing the extent of infarction in the setting of acute ischemic stroke affecting the internal carotid artery and middle cerebral artery territories, the locations for the vast majority of large vessel occlusions. It is important to note that it does not apply to the posterior circulation or the anterior cerebral artery (ACA) territory. Most of the recently published randomized controlled trials on mechanical thrombectomy for acute ischemic stroke used an ASPECTS score of ≥ 6 as the part of their inclusion criteria. In general, patients with ASPECTS scores of 5 or lower have been shown to have a very poor prognosis regardless of successful intervention; however, this issue is still up for debate. The data are clear however that the higher the ASPECTS score, the better the chance for a meaningful neurological recovery in the setting of successful revascularization.

There has been growing interest in developing reliable and reproducible tools for assessing infarct extent in the posterior circulation and correlating this to patient prognosis. To date, there is no tool that has been widely accepted. One reasonable imaging scale is the posterior circulation ASPECTS (pc-ASPECTS) that uses CT angiographic source images to assess infarct extent. A pc-ASPECTS on CTA source images of < 8 has been shown to be strongly correlated with poor functional outcomes.

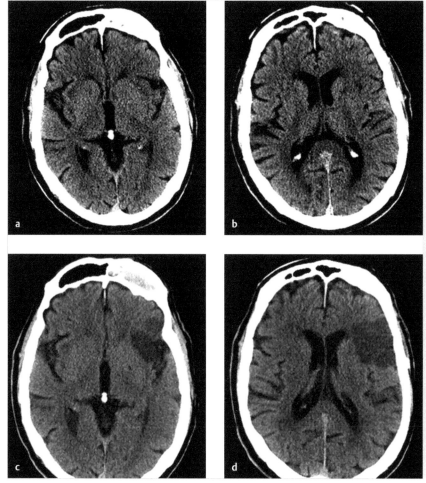

Fig. 1.5 A 78-year-old female with sudden onset aphasia and right-sided weakness. (a) Non-contrast CT shows loss of the left insular ribbon as well as subtle loss of the gray white junction in the left frontal operculum (a and b). CT images obtained 24 hours after successful thrombectomy (c and d) demonstrate completed infarcts in the left insular ribbon, anterior lentiform nucleus and left frontal operculum.

1.2.4 Imaging Findings

The ASPECTS score is a 10-point grading scale for identifying the extent of infarcted brain in the setting of acute ischemic stroke affecting the ICA and MCA territories. The territories of the ASPECTS score are shown in ▶ Fig. 1.6 and include the lentiform nucleus, caudate head/body/tail, internal capsule, and insula. At the level of the basal, ganglia are the M1-M3 territories, which include the anterior MCA cortex corresponding to the frontal operculum (M1), MCA cortex lateral to the insular ribbon corresponding to the anterior temporal lobe (M2), and posterior MCA cortex corresponding to the posterior temporal lobe (M3). At the level of the ventricles immediately above the basal, ganglia are the M4-M6 territories, which include the anterior MCA territory immediately superior to M1 (M4), lateral MCA territory immediately superior to M2 (M5), and posterior MCA territory immediately superior to M3 (M6). For each of the 10 above-listed territories, one point is subtracted, if the grey-white matter differentiation is attenuated in this territory. The ASPECTS score is thus scored as 10 (number of affected territories).

When assessing the ASPECTS score, it is important to narrow your windows width and levels to so-called "stroke windows." The ideal window width and levels vary by study and center; however, many neuroradiologists prefer reviewing acute stroke CTs using WW of 50 and WL of 30. Ultimately, the goal is to window and level the CT in order to maximize gray-white differentiation to allow for more easy identification of infarcted brain (▶ Fig. 1.7).

There are pitfalls to the assessment of ASPECTS score. Patient motion may severely affect the interpretation of ASPECTS, particularly in the MCA cortices. Old infarctions and leukoaraiosis should not be counted as part of the ASPECTS score; however, they can confound one's ability to properly assess gray-white differentiation and in such cases evaluating the presence or absence of parenchymal enhancement on CTA source images may be helpful.

There are a number of basic stroke imaging signs that the radiologist or other neurovascular specialist should be keenly aware of. In the setting of acute ischemic stroke, there is often gaze deviation toward the side of the stroke due to impairment of the frontal eye fields (▶ Fig. 1.8). Thus, a patient with a right MCA stroke often has gaze deviation to the right. Loss of the insular ribbon (Insular Ribbon Sign) is another common early finding and included in the ASPECTS score. The presence of hyperdense arteries or calcified emboli, as discussed in the previous Chapter (Chapter 1.1), is important imaging manifestations of stroke as well.

Non-contrast CT is not as reliable for the posterior circulation due to the presence of beam hardening artifact. Posterior circulation structures include the thalami, cerebellar hemispheres, posterior cerebral artery territories (occipital lobes and inferior/mesial temporal lobes), and midbrain and pons. In the pc-ASPECTS score, the midbrain and pons are each given 2 points, whereas all other structures are given 1 point. Because non-contrast CT is not as helpful due to artefactual findings, evaluating

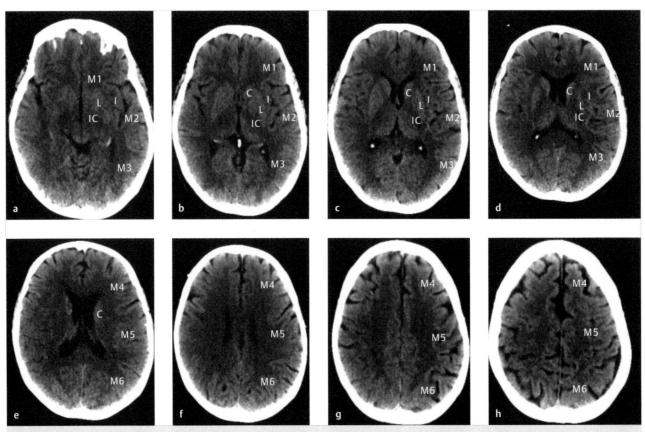

Fig. 1.6 Eight slice non-contrast CT demonstrating ASPECTS score regions.

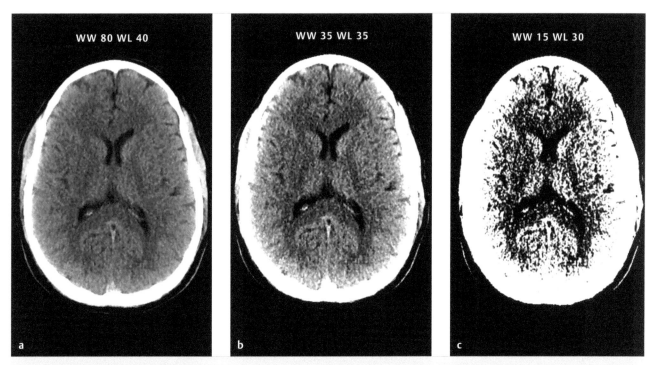

Fig. 1.7 Right lentiform nucleus and insular ribbon infarction at various window-width and window-levels. Note how the infarcted regions become more apparent as the window width and levels are narrowed.

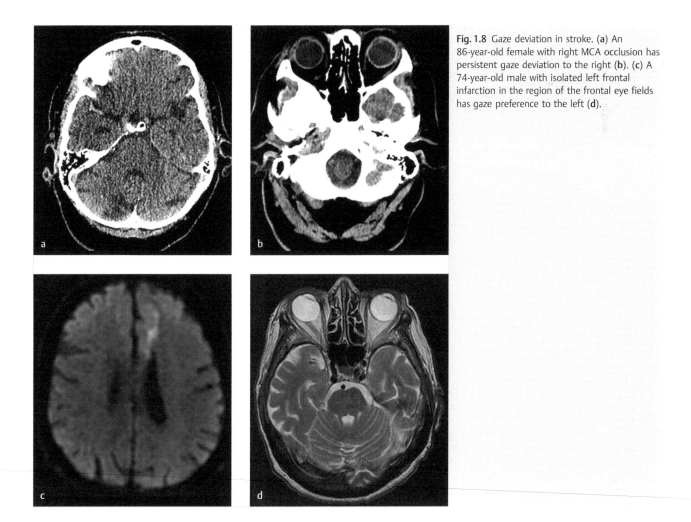

Fig. 1.8 Gaze deviation in stroke. (a) An 86-year-old female with right MCA occlusion has persistent gaze deviation to the right (b). (c) A 74-year-old male with isolated left frontal infarction in the region of the frontal eye fields has gaze preference to the left (d).

the presence or absence of diminished contrast enhancement in affected territories on CTA is recommended when assessing the extent of ischemia in basilar artery occlusions.

1.2.5 What the Clinician Needs to Know

- ASPECTS score including the location of all areas with affected ischemia
- Presence of hyperdense artery sign
- Other imaging manifestations of acute stroke including gaze deviation
- Presence or absence of intracranial hemorrhage

1.2.6 High-Yield Facts

- ASPECTS score is the gold standard in CT assessment of ischemic injury to the MCA territory.

- Pitfalls include motion artifact, old infarct, and chronic white matter ischemic changes. Using source images of CTA is helpful in assessing the extent of ischemia in such cases.
- Assessing the extent of ischemia in the posterior circulation is difficult due to beam hardening artifact from skull base structures.
- Using narrow window widths and levels (50/30) allows for improved assessment of ASPECTS score.

Further Reading

[1] Barber PA, Demchuk AM, Zhang J, Buchan AM. Validity and reliability of a quantitative computed tomography score in predicting outcome of hyperacute stroke before thrombolytic therapy. ASPECTS Study Group. Alberta Stroke Programme Early CT Score. Lancet. 2000; 355(9216):1670–1674

[2] Pexman JH, Barber PA, Hill MD, et al. Use of the Alberta Stroke Program Early CT Score (ASPECTS) for assessing CT scans in patients with acute stroke. AJNR Am J Neuroradiol. 2001; 22(8):1534–1542

1.3 CT Angiography in Acute Stroke including Imaging of Collateral Supply

1.3.1 Clinical Case

A 56-year-old male with acute onset left arm and leg weakness, dysarthria (▶ Fig. 1.9).

1.3.2 Description of Imaging Findings and Diagnosis

Diagnosis

Right M2 branch occlusion with hyperdense artery sign in the right insula. ASPECTS score is 9 with infarction affecting the right insula. Branch occlusion is best appreciated on coronal MPR. Excellent collaterals.

1.3.3 Background

CT angiography is the workhorse of intracranial and extracranial vascular imaging in the emergency setting. CT angiography is essential in the setting of acute ischemic stroke as it allows for evaluating the patency of the cervical and intracranial vasculature, aortic arch anatomy, and the presence of collaterals.

There has been much emphasis as of late on imaging of collateral artery supply in acute ischemic stroke. There are two types of collaterals, primary, and secondary. Primary collaterals include large vessels such as the anterior communicating and posterior communicating arteries. Secondary collaterals are primarily leptomeningeal collaterals. Leptomeningeal collaterals are pial anastomotic branches joining the terminal cortical branches of major cerebral arteries (i.e., middle, anterior, and posterior cerebral arteries) along the surface of the brain. These vessels are dormant under normal circumstances but can be recruited in the setting of a chronic or acute occlusion. Some degree of leptomeningeal collaterals can be seen in approximately 80% of patients. The longevity and robustness of these collaterals is however limited. There is also wide variability in the distribution, size, and number of collaterals between patients. The robustness of one's collaterals has been found to be strongly correlated with clinical outcomes.

1.3.4 Imaging Findings

CTA is invaluable in the setting of acute ischemic stroke. The most important information obtained on CTA for acute ischemic stroke is the presence or absence of a vascular occlusion

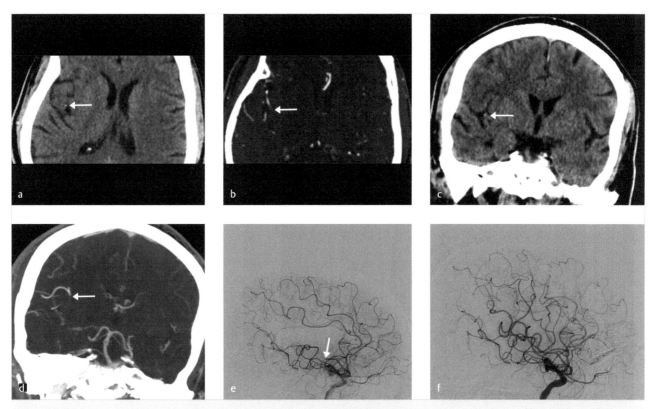

Fig. 1.9 Right M2 branch occlusion in a 56-year-old male. (**a**) Non-contrast CT demonstrates a hyperdense artery in the right sylvian fissure (*arrow*). There is also a loss of the right insular ribbon. (**b**) Axial CTA demonstrates the occlusion (*arrow*); however, it is difficult to identify without the assistance of the hyperdense artery sign in A and the coronal MPR in D. (**c**) Coronal MPR of a non-contrast CT demonstrates the hyperdense artery in the right insula (*arrow*). (**d**) On the coronal MPR of the CTA, it is clear that there is a cutoff in the distal M2 just before its bifurcation (*arrow*). Mid-basilar fenestration is incidentally noted. (**e**) Lateral projection cerebral angiogram shows the distal M2 occlusion (*arrow*). (**f**) Following one-pass with a stent-retriever, the M2 was revascularized.

that can be identified as a focal filling defect in the artery. There are a number of useful tips and techniques for maximizing one's ability to detect such an occlusion, particularly when the occlusion is located beyond the M1 segment.

When interpreting a CTA, it is important to look at both source images (thinner cuts) and the MIP images. Multiplanar reformats are constructed with maximum intensity projection images, which have a slice thickness of 6.5 mm, at every 2.5 mm. Source images are typically between 0.5 and 0.75 mm thick. In most cases, the axial MIP images are sufficient for identifying a large vessel occlusion. However, evaluating thin-cut images substantially increases the sensitivity and specificity for the detection of both proximal and distal branch occlusions. In fact, if MIP images are read in isolation, the sensitivity and specificity for the detection of a vascular abnormality are only 70 and 50%, respectively. These values increase to 90 and 80%, respectively, when axially reformatted source images are also interrogated. Multiplanar reformats in the coronal plane are extremely useful in identifying M2 branch occlusions as well as the patency of insular branches. Multiplanar reformats in the sagittal plane are helpful in identifying patency of distal M2/M3 branches as they course along the insula. When an occlusion is not obvious, a careful interrogation of sagittal and coronal reconstructed images is essential. Optimal window settings for interpreting a CTA are in the neighborhood of WW 600 and WL 200 (▶ Fig. 1.9).

When evaluating a CTA in the setting of acute ischemic stroke, there are a number of other important imaging findings one should report. Reporting the presence of a bovine arch, left vertebral artery origin directly from the arch or a complex Type 3 aortic arch is very helpful as it can influence the neurointerventionalist's choice or route of access. The presence of substantial arch atheromatous disease or an aortic dissection can provide clues regarding stroke origin (▶ Fig. 1.10). The patency and tortuosity of the cervical vasculature should also be evaluated. Large stenotic atheromatous plaques or dissections ipsilateral to the ischemic territory can alter endovascular management strategies and provide information regarding stroke origin. Substantial cervical vascular tortuosity may change management strategies as well.

The evaluation of cerebral blood flow using CT perfusion, single-phase CTA, and multiphase CTA have all been proposed as tools that can be used to identify collaterals in patient selection for acute ischemic stroke treatment. Examples of patients with good and poor collaterals is provided in ▶ Fig. 1.11. Grading scores using single phase and multiphase CTA are typically subjective with the assessment of collaterals being a rough estimate of the proportion of the affected vascular territory in which the distal vessels are opacified. These collateral grading scores are used primarily for research purposes but familiarity with their general concepts is important to refine patient selection for stroke thrombectomy. The Christoforidis and Miteff collateral scores use single phase CTA while the ASPECTS and

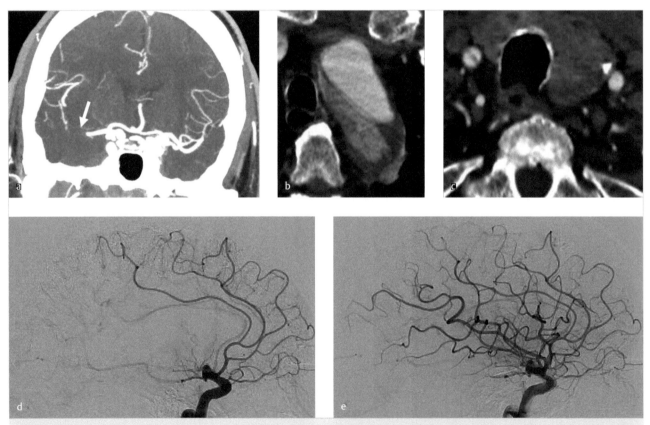

Fig. 1.10 Aortic arch dissection in M1 occlusion. **(a)** Coronal MPR CTA demonstrates an occlusion of the distal right M1 (*arrow*). **(b)** Axial CTA image at the top of the aortic arch demonstrates a large aortic dissection. The false lumen is poorly opacified, whereas the true lumen is densely opacified. **(c)** Axial CTA through the neck demonstrates extension of the dissection into the right common carotid artery (CCA). Such a finding will surely complicate thrombectomy approaches. **(d)** Lateral right ICA cerebral angiogram shows loss of the entire right MCA territory vascularization. **(e)** Following thrombectomy, the patient was revascularized.

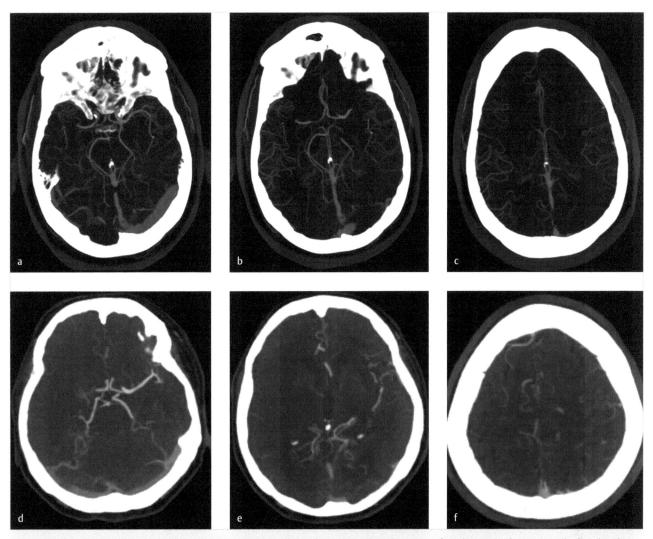

Fig. 1.11 Extremes of collaterals. (**a–c**) demonstrate a patient with excellent collaterals in the setting of a right MCA occlusion. Note the fact that there is symmetry in the number of pial MCA branches opacified when compared to the non-occluded left side. In addition, the vessels overlying the right hemisphere are actually slightly more opacified than those on the left due to a reduction in contrast washout in the setting of an MCA occlusion. (**d–f**) demonstrate just the opposite. This patient has a right M1 occlusion and there are visually no vessels opacified in the right MCA territory. This patient has a malignant collateral pattern.

modified American Society of Interventional and Therapeutic Neuroradiology/Society of Interventional Radiology (ASITN/ SIR) scores use multiphase CTA (▶ Table 1.1). In multiphase CTA, images are acquired during peak arterial, peak venous, and late venous phases. By acquiring temporal information at three time points, multiphase CTA allows for a dynamic assessment of pial collateral filling. Multiphase CTA has been shown to reliably predict clinical outcomes in patients with acute ischemic stroke. Delayed phases also allow for a more accurate assessment of thrombus length. Another advantage of multiphase CTA is the fact that it does not require any mathematical algorithms or complex post-processing tools like CT perfusion.

There are a number of pitfalls to both single-phase and multiphase CTA. For single-phase CTA, a common pitfall is the so-called pseudoocclusion (▶ Fig. 1.12). In the setting of an ICA

terminus occlusion, there is poor antegrade flow in the cervical ICA. Because of this, the cervical ICA is often not opacified or poorly opacified. This results in the appearance of a cervical ICA occlusion. Delayed phase imaging can be helpful in sorting out the presence or absence of a pseudoocclusion by allowing enough time for contrast to reach the mid and distal cervical ICA. The presence of a proximal flow limiting stenosis can affect contrast opacification on both single and multiphase CTA as can the presence of poor cardiac output.

1.3.5 What the Clinician Needs to Know

- Location and extent of intracranial vascular occlusion
- Collateral grade
- Challenges in access (vascular tortuosity, cervical vascular occlusion, difficult arch)

Table 1.1 Collateral Grading Scores

Scoring System and Points	Imaging Findings
ASPECTS MultiPhase CTA	
0	Compared to asymptomatic contralateral hemisphere there are no vessels visible in any phase within the occluded vascular territory
1	Compared to asymptomatic contralateral hemisphere there are just a few vessels visible in any phase within the occluded vascular territory
2	Compared to asymptomatic contralateral hemisphere there is a delay of two phases in filling in of peripheral vessels and decreased prominence and extent or a one-phase delay and some regions with no vessels in some part of the territory occluded
3	Compared to asymptomatic contralateral hemisphere there is a delay of two phases in filling in of peripheral vessels but prominence and extent is the same or there is a one-phase delay and decreased prominence (thinner vessels)/reduced number of vessels in some part of the territory occluded
4	Compared to asymptomatic contralateral hemisphere there is a delay of one phase in filling in of peripheral vessels but prominence and extent are the same
5	Compared to asymptomatic contralateral hemisphere there is no delay and normal or increased prominence of peripheral vessels/normal extent within the occluded arteries territory within the symptomatic hemisphere
Miteff Collateral Score	
1	Contrast opacification is merely seen in the distal superficial branches
2	Vessels can be seen at the Sylvian fissure
3	Vessels are reconstituted distal to the occlusion
Christoforidis Collateral Score	
1	Collaterals reconstituted the distal portion of the occluded vessel segment (i.e., if there was M1 segment occlusion the M1 segment distal to the occlusion reconstituted)
2	Collaterals reconstituted vessels in the proximal portion of the segment adjacent to the occluded vessel (i.e., if there was M1 segment occlusion with reconstitution to the proximal M2 vessel segments)
3	Collaterals reconstituted vessels in the distal portion of the segment adjacent to the occluded vessel (i.e., if there was M1 segment occlusion with reconstitution to the distal portion of the M2 vessel segments)
4	Collaterals reconstituted vessels two segments distal to the occluded vessel (i.e., if there was M1 segment occlusion with reconstitution up to the M3 segment branches)
5	Little or no significant reconstitution of the territory of the occluded vessel
Modified Version of ASITN/SIR Collateral Score for Dynamic CTA	
0	Non-existent or barely visible pial collaterals on the ischemic site during any point of time
1	Partial collateralization of the ischemic site until the late venous phase
2	Partial collateralization of the ischemic site before the venous phase
3	Complete collateralization of the ischemic site by the late venous phase
4	Complete collateralization of the ischemic site before the venous phase

Abbreviations: ASPECTS, Alberta Stroke Program Early CT Score; ASITN/SIR, American Society of Interventional and Therapeutic Neuroradiology/Society of Interventional Radiology; CTA, CT Angiography.

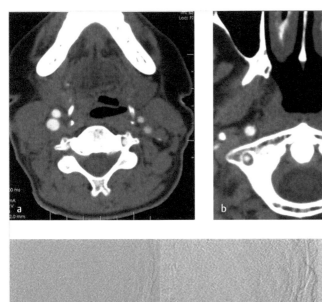
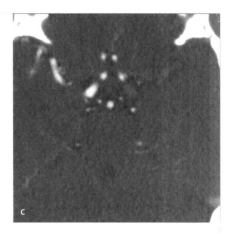

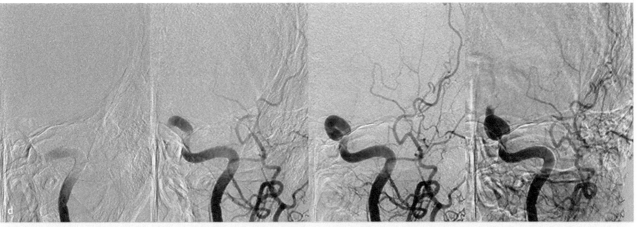

Fig. 1.12 Pseudoocclusion of the Left ICA. (**a**) Axial CTA through the carotid bifurcation demonstrates poor contrast opacification of the proximal right ICA; however, there is no obvious plaque. (**b**) At the level of C1, there is no opacification of the right ICA at all. (**c**) Intracranially, there is no opacification of the supraclinoid ICA or the MCA. This was called an ICA/MCA occlusion secondary to carotid dissection on non-invasive imaging. (**d**) Four frames of a diagnostic cerebral angiogram demonstrate slow progression of contrast to the level of the supraclinoid ICA. Indeed, there was no dissection or cervical carotid occlusion. Rather, the patient had a pseudo-occlusion due to a large amount of clot burden in the supraclinoid ICA.

1.3.6 High-Yield Facts

- The assessment of thin cuts in addition to multiplanar MIP images improves sensitivity and specificity for large vessel occlusion detection.
- Multiphase CTA can be extremely helpful in assessing collateral grade and improving patient selection for endovascular therapy.
- Pseudoocclusion of the cervical ICA can be seen in setting of ICA terminus occlusion. This can be mitigated by acquiring delayed phase images.
- Optimal window settings for interpreting a CTA are in the neighborhood of WW 600 and WL 200.

Further Reading

[1] Menon BK, d'Esterre CD, Qazi EM, et al. Multiphase CT Angiography: A New Tool for the Imaging Triage of Patients with Acute Ischemic Stroke. Radiology. 2015; 275(2):510–520

[2] García-Tornel A, Carvalho V, Boned S, et al. Improving the Evaluation of Collateral Circulation by Multiphase Computed Tomography Angiography in Acute Stroke Patients Treated with Endovascular Reperfusion Therapies. Intervent Neurol. 2016; 5(3–4):209–217

[3] de Lucas EM, Sánchez E, Gutiérrez A, et al. CT protocol for acute stroke: tips and tricks for general radiologists. Radiographics. 2008; 28(6):61673–1687

1.4 CT Perfusion in Acute Stroke

1.4.1 Clinical Case

A 56-year-old male with acute onset left arm and leg weakness, dysarthria (▶ Fig. 1.13).

1.4.2 Description of Imaging Findings and Diagnosis

Diagnosis

Right M1 occlusion with hyperdense artery sign; ASPECTS score of 10; excellent collaterals; large perfusion mismatch.

1.4.3 Background

CT perfusion imaging has become a mainstay in acute stroke imaging over the past 10 years. This imaging modality has been used in a number of randomized controlled trials for patient selection for mechanical thrombectomy. While there is some controversy as to whether CT perfusion is needed within 6 hours of presentation for acute ischemic stroke, it is highly recommended for patients presenting 6–24 hours following stroke onset given the results of the DWI (diffusion weighted imaging) or CTP assessment with clinical mismatch in the triage of wake-up and late presenting strokes undergoing neurointervention with trevo trial (DAWN) and endovascular therapy following imaging evaluation for ischemic stroke trial (DEFUSE) 3 trials.

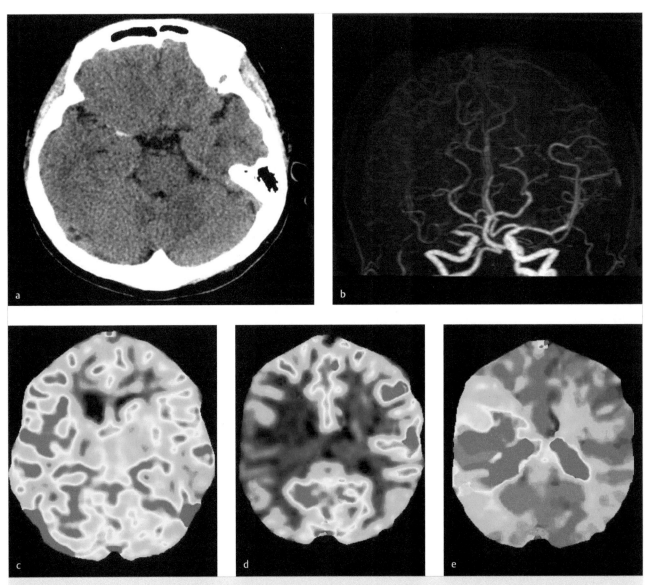

Fig. 1.13 CT Perfusion demonstrating small infarct core and large mismatch. (**a**) Non-contrast CT demonstrates a hyperdense right M1 with no CT evidence of infarct. (**b**) 4D-CTA demonstrates the right M1 occlusion and dilated leptomeningeal collaterals over the surface of the right cerebral hemisphere. (**c**) CBV map demonstrates *increased* perfusion in the right hemisphere due to vasodilatation of the leptomeningeal collaterals. This is called luxury perfusion. (**d**) CBF in the entirety of the right hemisphere is markedly reduced, however. (**e**) MTT is markedly increased.

Understanding basic core concepts of CT perfusion is essential to properly interpret CTP results. During a CT perfusion study, contrast is injected at a high rate (4–7 mL/sec). Multiple (dozens) scans are acquired over a given time period, which serve to visualize change in attenuation of the brain parenchyma over time. In general, parameters such as cerebral blood volume (CBV), cerebral blood flow (CBF), mean transit time (MTT), time to peak (TTP), and time to drain (TTD) are acquired automatically. Defining the CTP parameters is important. They are as follows:

- CBV: Volume of blood in the brain parenchyma (mL/100 g)
- CBF: Rate of flow into the brain parenchyma (mL/100 g/sec)
- MTT: Average of all transit times through the capillary network (seconds)
- TTP: Time from the start of contrast bolus to the peak attenuation of brain parenchyma (seconds)
- TTD: Time from maximum contrast attenuation to minimum contrast attenuation (seconds)

1.4.4 Imaging Findings

In the setting of ischemic stroke, we seek to understand the amount of irreversibly damaged brain tissue (the "core") and the amount of tissue at risk. The core is infarcted brain, which will not recover function even in the setting of revascularization. The tissue at risk is the ischemic territory which, while not yet infarcted, may progress to infarct unless the vessel is revascularized. Exact definitions of core and tissue at risk vary widely across CT perfusion software packages; thus, it is important to familiarize oneself to the software package available at her/his institution. One common technique is to use reduced CBV to measure infarct core while CBF, MTT, TTP, and TTD are suggested to be used to detect tissue at risk. Another common technique is to identify regions of reduced CBF (< 30–34% normal) to identify core and T_{max} to determine tissue at risk. This is a somewhat controversial topic so examples of both methods are presented in this chapter.

In the setting of an acute ischemic stroke from an arterial occlusion, CBF is usually prolonged due to the presence of a proximal blockage. TTP is always prolonged as it takes longer for blood to get to the affected area than the normal brain. Thus, TTP is more sensitive in detecting ischemic brain. MTT and TTD are also sensitive in detecting ischemic brain. CBV is not as intuitive. In general, completely infarcted brain parenchyma has a low CBV as well as a low CBF (▶ Fig. 1.14).

Many centers have moved toward the automatic calculation of core and penumbra infarct volumes using various software packages. These software packages all use different algorithms and thresholds for determining infarct core and penumbra and thus it is important to make sure that the software package being used has been validated. Without going into too much detail, there are a myriad of methods for calculating CTP maps including central volume theory, deconvolution, single value decomposition, inverse filter, box modulation transfer function and maximum slope. CBV calculations are the most stable and consistent across vendors while CBF, MTT, and TTP all display differences when the same source data are processed on different vendors software.

Because of the wide variability in autoprocessed results from CT perfusion studies, the direct visual evaluation of CTP studies by a radiologist is strongly recommended when deciding whether a patient is a candidate for endovascular therapy. Furthermore, the radiologist should be aware of the exact clinical deficit to determine if the clinical picture matches the findings on CTP. Colored CBV and CBF maps should be inspected to determine areas of low CBV or CBF corresponding to infarct core. Simultaneous study of CBF, MTT, TTP, and TTD maps should be performed to determine the extent of ischemic brain. The mismatch between the core and ischemic brain is sometimes called the penumbra. However, many radiologists have shied away from using this term in their reports. It is preferable to describe defects as matched defects or mismatched defects as mismatched defects do not always indicate the presence of a penumbra (▶ Fig. 1.15). In general however, patients with matched defects will have no salvageable brain tissue and will likely not benefit from revascularization. In addition to identifying the presence or absence of mismatch, the radiologist should comment on what functional area is at risk.

There are a number of important pitfalls to be aware of in interpreting CTP studies. First, it is important to review the time-density curves, which are being used to reconstruct the CTP maps to make sure they are similar to those seen in ▶ Fig. 1.16. If the curves do not look like ▶ Fig. 1.16, there may be an error in determining the arterial input function and venous outflow function. CTP is not sensitive in detecting smaller infarcts. Areas of microvascular ischemia (i.e., deep white matter leukoaraiosis) can have reduced CBF or CBV, thus, a careful inspection of these areas on NCCT is recommended. Patients with severe flow limiting intracranial or extracranial stenosis can have reduced perfusion and sometimes even reduced CBF in an entire hemisphere that can make the appearance of a large perfusion defect, even if there is no large vessel occlusion per se (▶ Fig. 1.17). There are a number of stroke mimics, which can result in altered CTP parameters as well (▶ Fig. 1.18). Typical findings for such mimics are provided in ▶ Table 1.2.

1.4.5 What the Clinician Needs to Know

- Size and location of infarct core
- Size and location of penumbra

1.4.6 High-Yield Facts

- CBV and CBF maps are generally reliable indicators of infarct core, whereas MTT, TTP, CBF, and TTD maps can be used to identify ischemic brain. Mismatch between infarct and ischemia is called the penumbra.
- CBV values are generally consistent across vendors and software packages. However, MTT, TTP, CBF, and TTD can vary widely across vendors.
- A careful review of input curves, when interpreting CTP studies, is needed to ensure that the perfusion maps are accurate.
- There are a number of important stroke mimics, which can result in altered CTP maps.

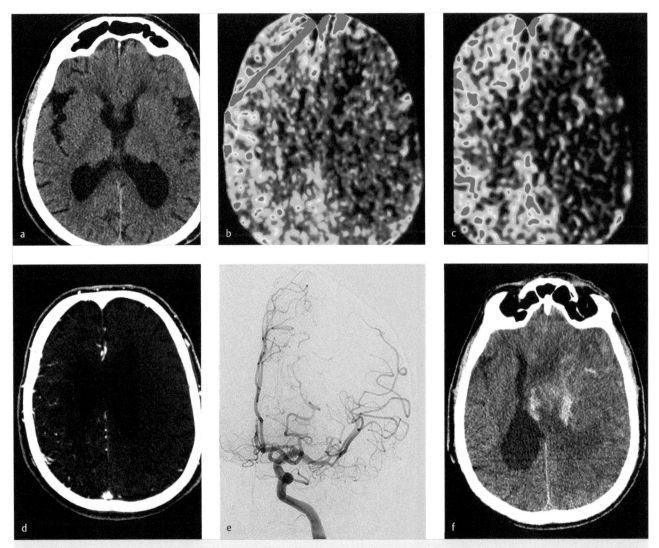

Fig. 1.14 CT perfusion demonstrating matched defect indicating absence of salvageable tissue. (**a**) Non-contrast CT demonstrates very subtle loss of gray white differentiation in the left basal ganglia and insula. (**b**) CBV map in this patient with an ICA terminus occlusion demonstrates marked decrease in CBV over the entirety of the left cerebral hemisphere, which is matched on the CBF map in (**c**). (**d**) CTA in this patient demonstrates a malignant collateral pattern with the total absence of leptomeningeal collaterals over the left cerebral hemisphere. (**e**) The patient was revascularized promptly. (**f**) However, the patient suffered a massive left cerebral hemisphere infarct with hemorrhagic conversion, the distribution of which matched the perfusion defects in (**b**) and (**c**).

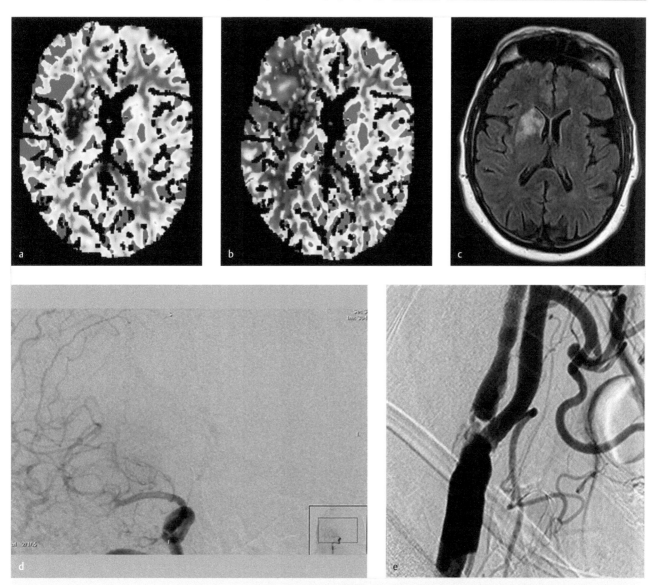

Fig. 1.15 CT perfusion demonstrating how mismatch is not penumbra. An 80-year-old male. NIHSS is 3, notable for left facial weakness and dysarthria, although he also has mild distal left upper extremity weakness. (**a**) CBV map demonstrates decreased CBV in the right basal ganglia. (**b**) CBF map demonstrates decreased CBF of the entire right MCA territory. CTA (not shown) demonstrated subocclusive clot in the right M1. There is obvious gross mismatch. If mismatch was the same as penumbra then the area of mismatch will go on to infarct if the patient was not recanalized. In this case, the team opted for conservative therapy because his NIHSS was low. (**c**) T2/FLAIR (fluid attenuation inversion recovery) MRI, the next day, demonstrates infarct in the right basal ganglia but nowhere else. (**d**) One might think the easiest explanation is that the patient recanalized; however, a right ICA angiogram the following day demonstrated persistent right MCA thrombus. (**e**) The patient had a severe stenosis of the right ICA. It is likely that a combination of a severe ICA stenosis and subocclusive thrombus resulted in the marked perfusion deficit. This case highlight the importance of correlating perfusion imaging findings with the clinical exam.

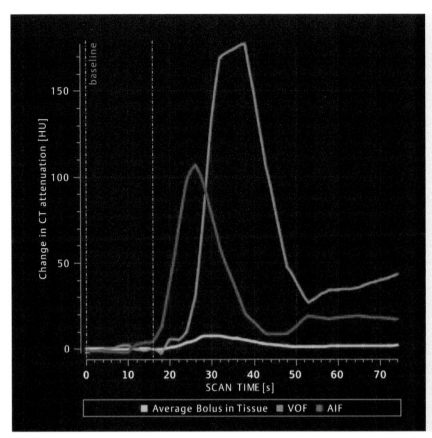

Fig. 1.16 Normal time-density curves with arterial attenuation (red) increasing prior to tissue attenuation (green), which increases prior to venous outflow attenuation (blue). Change in attenuation is highest for the VOF and lowest for average bolus in tissue.

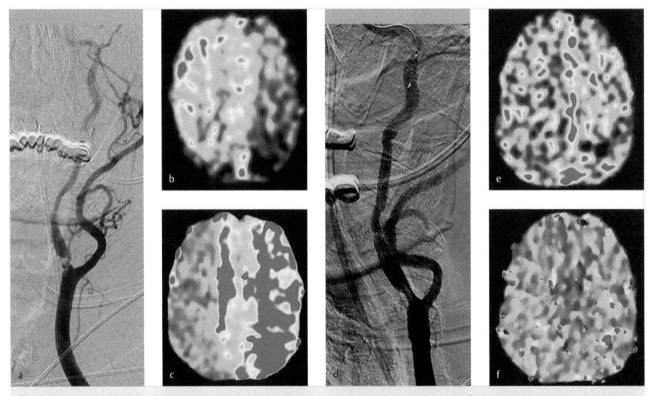

Fig. 1.17 CT perfusion demonstrating perfusion abnormalities in severe symptomatic carotid stenosis. (a) Left CCA cervical angiogram demonstrates a severe stenosis of the left carotid bulb. (b) CBF map demonstrates decreased CBF in the entire left cerebral hemisphere. (c) T_{max} map shows increased T_{max} in the entire hemisphere. This looks like a matched defect. (d) Following carotid stent placement, repeat CBF map (e) shows the normalization of CBF and (f) repeat T_{max} map shows normalization of T_{max}.

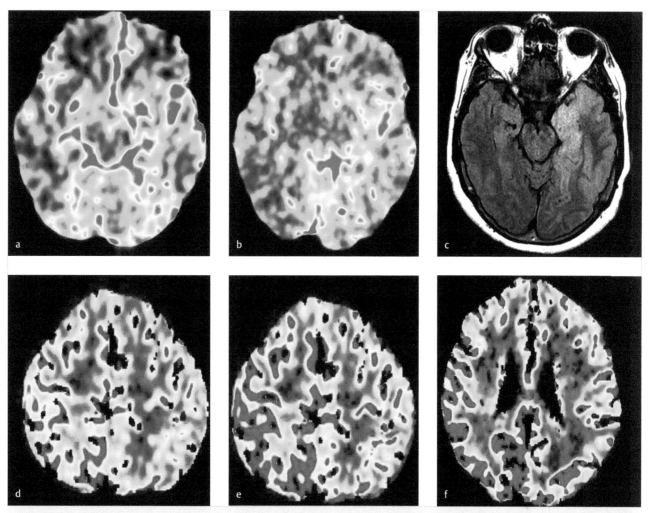

Fig. 1.18 CT perfusion findings in common stroke mimics. (a-c) are herpes encephalitis and (d-f) is Todd's paralysis. (a) CBV map shows increased CBV in the left temporooccipital lobe. (b) CBF is increased as well. (c) Fluid Attenuation Inversion Recovery (FLAIR) shows increased signal in the gray matter of the entire temporal lobe, most marked mesially. CSF confirmed a diagnosis of herpes encephalitis. (d) CBV map in a patient with Todd's paralysis shows increased CBV in the right hemisphere. (e-f) CBF is increased as well.

Table 1.2 Imaging Appearance of Common Stroke Mimics

Disease Process	CBV	CBF
Herpes encephalitis	↑	↑ ↑ ↑
PRES	↓	↓
Intra-ictal seizure	↑ ↑ ↑	↑ ↑ ↑
		↓
Post-ictal seizure	↓	↓
	↓	↓
Todd's Paralysis	↓	↓
Low Grade Glioma	↑	↑ ↑
Glioblastoma Multiforme	↑ ↑	↑ ↑ ↑

Abbreviations: CBV, Cerebral blood volume; CBF, Cerebral Blood Flow; PRES, Posterior Reversible Encephalopathy Syndrome.

Further Reading

[1] Lui YW, Tang ER, Allmendinger AM, Spektor V. Evaluation of CT perfusion in the setting of cerebral ischemia: patterns and pitfalls. AJNR Am J Neuroradiol. 2010; 31(9):1552–1563

[2] Allmendinger AM, Tang ER, Lui YW, Spektor V. Imaging of stroke: Part 1, Perfusion CT–overview of imaging technique, interpretation pearls, and common pitfalls. AJR Am J Roentgenol. 2012; 198(1):52–62

[3] de Lucas EM, Sánchez E, Gutiérrez A, et al. CT protocol for acute stroke: tips and tricks for general radiologists. Radiographics. 2008; 28(6):1673–1687

1.5 MRI in Acute Ischemic Stroke

1.5.1 Clinical Case

A 56-year-old male with acute onset left arm and leg weakness and neglect (▶ Fig. 1.19).

1.5.2 Description of Imaging Findings and Diagnosis

Diagnosis

Blooming artifact in an M3 branch in the right insula. Diffusion imaging shows mild restricted diffusion in the deep white matter. The arterial spin labeling (ASL) technique perfusion map shows decreased perfusion in the deep white matter and Rolandic cortex.

1.5.3 Background

CT is generally the imaging modality of choice at most institutions for acute stroke. This is due to the fact that CT is more widely available, allows for more rapid imaging evaluation and has fewer contraindications. However, some institutions prefer to use MRI in acute ischemic stroke patients. In general, such centers have ready access to an MRI scanner and, in some cases, the scanner is in the emergency room itself and established, fast protocols to screen for MR contraindications are in place. In centers which prefer CT, there are a few cases in which MRI may be preferable; namely, cases in which patients have a contrast allergy, in certain cases of posterior circulation stroke, or in children presenting with acute ischemic stroke symptoms where radiation is to be avoided. Limitations to widespread use of MRI include: (1) inability to determine if patients have any devices or metal in their body which may not be MRI compatible; (2) the lack of 24/7 availability of an MRI scanner; and (3) prolonged imaging times.

1.5.4 Imaging Findings

For those who are pursuing routine MRI in setting of acute ischemic stroke, a comprehensive protocol may include sagittal T1 FSE, axial T2 FSE, axial T2 FLAIR, axial DWI (B = 0, B = 1000, and ADC [apparent diffusion coefficient]), SWI, TOF MRA, and gadolinium bolus MR perfusion. Each of these sequences should be reviewed for the following findings:

- *Sagittal T1 FSE.* Provide an anatomic evaluation and can identify hemorrhage/cortical laminar necrosis as T1 hyperintensity.
- *Axial T2 FSE.* After 6–12 hours, infarcted tissue develops a high signal. Sulcal effacement and mass effect can develop within the first few days. In the setting of large vessel occlusion, T2 FSE images can show the loss of flow voids in large arteries.
- *Axial T2/FLAIR.* After 6–12 hours, infarcted tissue becomes hyperintense. Sulcal effacement and mass effect can develop within the first few days (▶ Fig. 1.20). An "Ivy sign" can determine whether distal slow flow is present (▶ Fig. 1.21).
- *Axial SWI/T2*.* High sensitivity for detection of hemorrhage (blooming artifact). In addition, RBC-rich thrombus can bloom in the MRI equivalent of the hyperdense artery sign. Blooming artifact in leptomeningeal vessels can be present due to slow flow and deoxyhemoglobin (▶ Fig. 1.22).
- *Axial DWI.* Early identification of ischemic stroke/infarct core as restricted diffusion is seen within minutes of ischemia.
- *3D TOF MRA.* Identification of large vessel occlusion.
- *MR Perfusion.* Evaluation of impaired cerebral blood flow and associated perfusion-diffusion mismatch.

There has been growing interest in DWI:FLAIR mismatch as a means to age infarction in the setting of acute ischemic stroke (▶ Fig. 1.22). Because many patients with stroke are precluded from thrombolysis treatment because the time from onset of their symptoms is unclear, an imaging biomarker to identify patients who are presenting within a 4.5 hour time window is particularly important. A number of studies have shown that

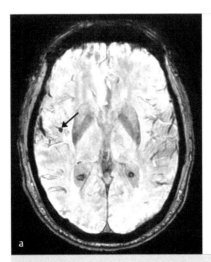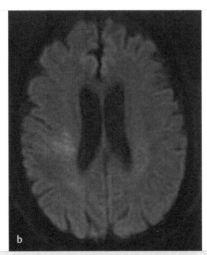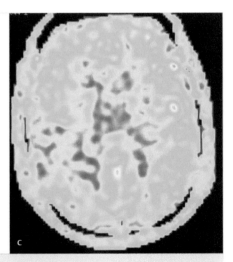

Fig. 1.19 Diffusion perfusion imaging in MRI in a 56-year-old male with acute onset left arm and leg weakness and neglect. (**a**) Axial SWI demonstrates blooming artifact in an M3 branch in the right insula (*arrow*). (**b**) Axial DWI shows faint restricted diffusion in the deep white matter of the right frontoparietal region. (**c**) Axial ASL perfusion map shows decreased perfusion involving both cortical and deep white matter territories consistent with a perfusion-diffusion mismatch.

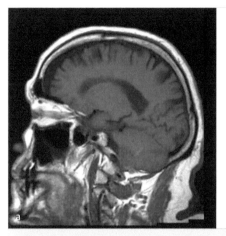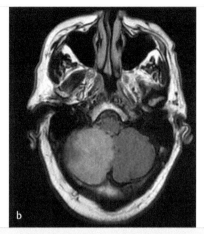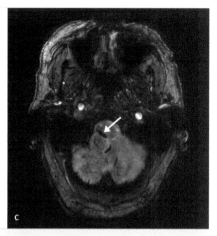

Fig. 1.20 Blooming artifact of clot in patient with 30 hours of dizziness from right posterior inferior cerebellar artery (PICA) infarction. (a) Sagittal T1 weighted image shows hypointensity of the entire inferior right cerebellar hemisphere. (b) Axial FLAIR shows FLAIR hyperintensity of the inferior right cerebellar hemisphere. (c) Axial SWI shows blooming artifact in the right PICA consistent with clot (*arrow*). There is also petechial hemorrhage in the right cerebellar hemisphere.

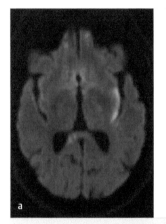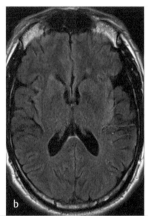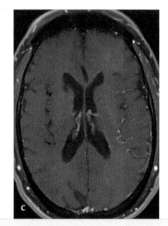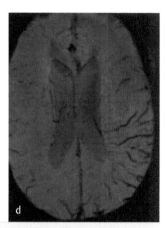

Fig. 1.21 SWI showing slow flow in setting of acute ischemic stroke. (a) Axial DWI shows infarct in the left insula. (b) Axial FLAIR shows a corresponding FLAIR hyperintensity of the left insula as well as high intravascular signal from slow flow. (c) Axial post-gad T1 shows dilatation and contrast enhancement of leptomeningeal collaterals over the left cerebral hemisphere. (d) Axial SWI shows increased T2* artifact in the leptomeningeal vessels overlying the left cerebral hemisphere due to slow flow and increased deoxyhemoglobin. These findings suggest that the penumbral region is still marginal around the infarction.

patients with an ischemic lesion detected with DWI but not with FLAIR are likely to be within a time window for which thrombolysis is safe and effective. Studies have now demonstrated that diffusion weighted imaging (DWI):FLAIR mismatch is indeed a biomarker for safe and effected thrombolysis.

MR perfusion in acute ischemic stroke is generally performed using a technique called dynamic susceptibility contrast imaging (DSC). In this technique, susceptibility sensitive echo planar imaging images are acquired dynamically during passage of a gadolinium based contrast agent through the brain. Gadolinium results in increased T2* artifact and as gadolinium progresses through the normal brain parenchyma, the parenchyma becomes darker. This is the inverse of CT perfusion where the parenchyma becomes brighter over time. Another MR perfusion

technique that is growing in popularity is ASL technique (▶ Fig. 1.19). This technique does not require contrast but rather uses endogenous proton spins as the tracer. Arterial blood flowing upstream is tagged using a short radiofrequency pulse and perfusion parameters are obtained by subtracting control, nonlabeled spin images from spin-labeled images. Currently, the major drawback of this technique is the significant time to acquire these images.

With both ASL and DSC, normalized curves can be obtained allowing us to calculate same parameters that we see on CT perfusion including CBV, CBF, MTT, and $T_{max.}$ Unlike a CTP however, the CBV map is not needed to assess infarct core as the area of restricted diffusion constitutes the core. Many centers primarily employ TTP and MTT as markers for at-risk tissue.

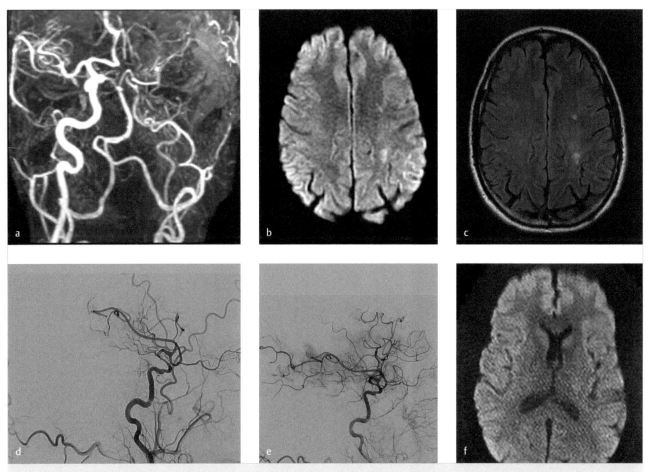

Fig. 1.22 A 56-year-old male with left terminal ICA occlusion and clot in the left M1 with DWI: FLAIR Mismatch. (a) MRA demonstrates the absence of flow related signal in the left cerebral hemisphere. (b) DWI image demonstrates cortical restricted diffusion in the left fronto-parietal region as well as in the deep white matter. (c) FLAIR shows T2 hyperintensity of the deep white matter infarct but no FLAIR signal in the area of cortical restricted diffusion. This indicates a DWI FLAIR Mismatch. (d) Lateral left ICA cerebral angiogram shows paucity of filling in the left MCA territory. (e) Postrevascularization angiogram shows the restoration of flow in most of the left MCA territory. (f) Post-op DWI shows no restricted diffusion.

1.5.5 What the Clinician Needs to Know

- Size and location of infarct core
- Size and location of penumbra
- Presence of hemorrhage as seen on T2* weighted imaging
- Intravascular blooming artifact (i.e., thrombus location)

1.5.6 High-Yield Facts

- DWI:FLAIR mismatch can be used to age infarcts. Lesions bright on DWI but not FLAIR are generally within the tPA window.
- DWI and MR perfusion can be used to assess infarct core and at-risk tissue, respectively. DSC perfusion is the imaging modality of choice.

Further Reading

[1] Allen LM, Hasso AN, Handwerker J, Farid H. Sequence-specific MR imaging findings that are useful in dating ischemic stroke. Radiographics. 2012; 32 (5):1285–1297, discussion 1297–1299

[2] Srinivasan A, Goyal M, Al Azri F, Lum C. State-of-the-art imaging of acute stroke. Radiographics. 2006; 26 Suppl 1:S75–S95

[3] Wolman DN, Iv M, Wintermark M, et al. Can diffusion- and perfusion-weighted imaging alone accurately triage anterior circulation acute ischemic stroke patients to endovascular therapy? J Neurointerv Surg. 2018; 10(12): 1132–1136

1.6 Post-Stroke Imaging with CT

1.6.1 Clinical Case

A 74-year-old female. Status post-endovascular revascularization of right ICA terminus occlusion. Patient is obtunded (▶ Fig. 1.23).

1.6.2 Description of Imaging Findings and Diagnosis

Diagnosis

Large right hemispheric infarct with gyriform hyperdensity in the right frontal lobe. Differential diagnosis of gyriform hyperdensity includes petechial hemorrhage (laminar necrosis) or contrast staining. Dual energy CT was performed. Post-iodine subtraction, diagnosis of contrast staining is made.

1.6.3 Background

Standard of care in management of acute ischemic stroke patients is to perform neuroimaging of the patient 24 hours following presentation with the aim of determining whether there is hemorrhagic conversion of the infarct and to evaluate final infarct size. The presence and size of hemorrhage will often dictate how aggressive the neurology team will be in using antiaggregation and anticoagulation therapy. At many centers, dual energy CT has emerged as the imaging modality of choice for evaluating patients who have undergone endovascular revascularization as dual energy CT allows for differentiation of acute hemorrhage and iodinated contrast, both of which are bright on CT and both of which have overlapping attenuation values.

With dual energy CT, patients are imaged simultaneously using two different x-ray energies (typically, 80 and 140 kVP). At 140 kVP, iodine and hemorrhage have similar densities. However, at 80 kVP, iodine is closer to its k-edge and attenuation is increased when compared to hemorrhage. With DECT, the 80kVP map can be subtracted from the 140kVP map

to calculate a VNC map and an iodine map thus allowing for differentiation between contrast and hemorrhage.

It is also important to have a conceptual understanding of what goes on pathologically to an area of infarcted tissue in order to understand what we are seeing on both CT and MR imaging. Histopathologic findings in ischemic stroke at various time points are as follows:

- *Early Hyperacute.* Oligemia in infarcted tissue. Early neuronal damage with cytotoxic edema affecting neurons.
- *Acute.* Early neuronal damage results in the necrosis of neurons and gross swelling of parenchyma. Pathologically, there is blurring of the grey-white junction.
- *Subacute.* Gross necrotic tissue is soft to touch, and usually pale. However, it may be congested if blood has permeated the tissue due to either luxury perfusion or hemorrhage. Organization of infarct begins with macrophages appearing and capillary sprouting. Edema diminishing.
- *Chronic.* Demolition and scarring. Shrinking of scarred area with ex vacuo dilation of the ventricle. Organization of scar tissue well established. Neurons disappear. Numerous macrophages. Gliosis.

1.6.4 Imaging Findings

The most important imaging outcomes that need to be reported on a 24-hour CT or MRI scan include extent of infarct, degree of edema/mass effect, and presence of intracranial hemorrhage. When performing post-thrombectomy imaging, dual energy CT is strongly recommended to differentiate between iodine staining and hemorrhage. Review of iodine maps and virtual non-contrast CT will make this differentiation very simple as all iodinated contrast will be subtracted out on the VNC. If there is hemorrhage, the radiologist must distinguish between petechial hemorrhage, parenchymal hematoma within the infarcted tissue, hematoma with mass effect and IVH, subarachnoid hemorrhage (SAH), and SDH.

Infarcts have a fairly standard evolution pattern on noncontrast CT as outlined below.

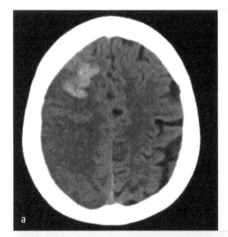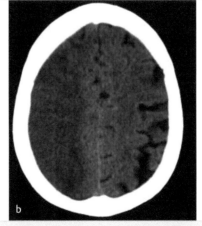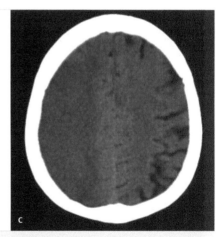

Fig. 1.23 A 74-year-old female. Status post-endovascular revascularization of right ICA terminus occlusion. Dual energy CT. (**a**) Axial non-contrast CT performed at 140 kVP shows a large infarct in the right hemisphere with an area of gyriform hyperdensity in the right frontal lobe. (**b**) The iodine map shows that this area of gyriform hyperdensity is, in fact, contrast (red). (**c**) Virtual non-contrast (VNC) map with iodine subtraction shows that there was no hemorrhage.

- *Early Hyperacute.* The loss of gray-white differentiation with cortical hypodensity, mild parenchymal swelling, and sulcal effacement.
- *Acute.* Progression of hypoattenuation and swelling. Increased sulcal effacement. May develop mass effect.
- *Subacute.* Swelling starts to subside. Petechial hemorrhage present in cortex resulting in increased cortical attenuation (CT fogging phenomenon) (▶ Fig. 1.24).
- *Chronic.* Gliosis, low-density tissue. Ex vacuo dilatation of ventricular system. Cortical calcification can occur but is rare.

Infarcts also have a fairly standard evolution pattern on MRI as outlined below:

- *Early Hyperacute.* Increased signal on DWI and reduced ADC values.
- *Late Hyperacute.* Restricted diffusion. High T2 signal on FLAIR and FSE T1. T1 hypointensity at 16 hours.
- *Acute.* High DWI signal. ADC values beginning to increase. Infarct hyperintense on FLAIR and T2. Some cortical intrinsic T1 hyperintensity from cortical laminar necrosis. Cortex demonstrates enhancement at 5 days.
- *Subacute.* Pseudonormalization of ADC within 10–15 days. T2-shine through on DWI. High T2/FLAIR signal. T2 fogging can occur around the 2nd week. Cortical T1 hyperintensity due to cortical laminar necrosis. Infarct enhancement.
- *Chronic.* Low T1 signal, high T2 signal. Cortical contrast enhancement for 2–4 months. ADC high.

1.6.5 What the Clinician Needs to Know

- Presence or absence of hemorrhage, hemorrhage extent, and hemorrhage type
- Mass effect from post-infarct edema. Herniation syndromes.
- Estimated age of infarct if time of onset or day of onset is unclear

1.6.6 High-Yield Facts

- Cortical petechial hemorrhage is a relatively common finding in the subacute phase of acute ischemic stroke. This is not the same as hemorrhagic transformation as it does not result in mass effect.
- CT fogging can occur at about 1 week post-stroke due to luxury perfusion and subtle petechial hemorrhage.
- Dual energy CT with iodine subtraction should be strongly considered in cases in which an endovascular revascularization procedure was performed.
- Infarctions have a stereotypical aging process on MRI.

Further Reading

[1] Robbins SL, Kumar V, Abbas AK, et al. Robbins and Cotran Pathologic Basis of Disease. W.B. Saunders Company; 2010
[2] Nakano S, Iseda T, Kawano H, Yoneyama T, Ikeda T, Wakisaka S. Correlation of early CT signs in the deep middle cerebral artery territories with angiographically confirmed site of arterial occlusion. AJNR Am J Neuroradiol. 2001; 22(4):654–659
[3] Postma AA, Das M, Stadler AAR, Wildberger JE. Dual-Energy CT: What the Neuroradiologist Should Know. Curr Radiol Rep. 2015; 3(5):16

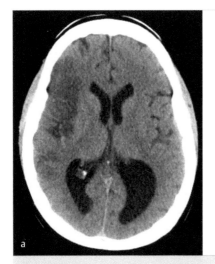 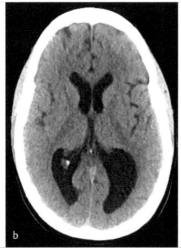 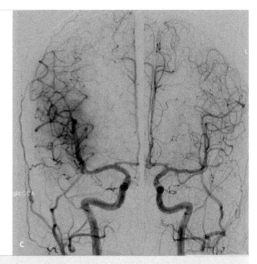

Fig. 1.24 Fogging effect 8 days after initial infarct. **(a)** Non-contrast CT obtained 2 days following presentation shows an established stroke in the right insula. **(b)** Follow-up non-contrast CT was performed in the preparation of carotid stenting. This demonstrates restoration of normal gray-white differentiation. However, this is a result of the fogging effect whereby there is luxury hyperperfusion to the infarcted territory. **(c)** Cerebral angiogram performed on day 9 shows marked parenchymal blush in the region of the right insula. This is the cause of the fogging effect! The normal left ICA injection is provided as reference. Note the absence of the dense parenchymal blush on the left ICA injection.

Chapter 2

Cervical Vascular Disease

2 Cervical Vascular Disease

2.1 Carotid Artery Atherosclerosis: CTA and Ultrasound

2.1.1 Clinical Case

A 56-year-old male with recurrent episodes of left-sided upper extremity weakness which resolve spontaneously over 10 minutes (▶ Fig. 2.1).

2.1.2 Description of Imaging Findings and Diagnosis

Diagnosis

Hypoechoic carotid plaque which is hypodense on CT. On ultrasound, there is a mobile thrombus on the surface of the plaque. Degree of stenosis by North American Symptomatic Carotid Endarterectomy Trial (NASCET) criteria is 45%.

2.1.3 Background

Carotid artery stenosis is a well-established risk factor of ischemic stroke contributing to up to 10–20% of strokes or transient ischemic attacks. Many clinical trials over the past 20 years have used measurements of carotid artery stenosis as a means to risk stratify patients. However, with improvements in vascular imaging techniques, such as CTA, MRA, ultrasound and PET/CT, we are now able to risk stratify patients not only on the degree

of carotid artery stenosis, but also on biological phenomena, such as plaque composition that can determine how vulnerable the plaque is to rupture and thus ischemic stroke. These imaging techniques are resulting in an emerging paradigm shift that allows for risk stratifications based on the presence of imaging features such as intraplaque hemorrhage (IPH), plaque ulceration, plaque neovascularity, fibrous cap thickness, and the presence of a lipid-rich necrotic core (LRNC).

It is important for the neurovascular specialist to be aware of these newer imaging techniques as they will allow for improved patient risk stratification and outcomes. For example, a patient with a low-grade stenosis, but an ulcerated plaque, may benefit more from a revascularization procedure or aggressive medical management than a patient with a stable 70% asymptomatic stenosis with a thick fibrous cap. In this chapter, we will discuss CTA and US techniques for the assessment of carotid atherosclerotic disease (▶ Table 2.1).

2.1.4 Imaging Findings

Prior studies characterizing components of unstable plaques have demonstrated that CT Hounsfield density can be used to distinguish between LRNC, connective tissue, IPH, and calcifications. Calcifications are easily identified by their high density (mean HU~250). However, there is considerable overlap between the CT densities of LRNC (mean HU~30-50), connective tissue (mean HU~45), and IPH (mean HU~20-30). Macroscopic changes, such as large hemorrhage and large low-density lipid cores, can be easily

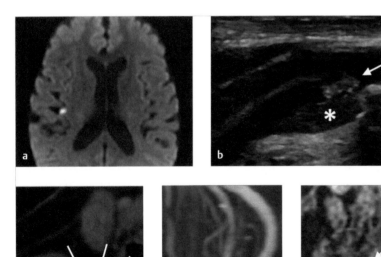

Fig. 2.1 Hypoechoic and hypodense plaque with intraluminal thrombus. **(a)** DWI (diffusion weighted imaging) MRI demonstrates a focal infarct in the right insula. **(b)** B-mode ultrasound demonstrates a hypoechoic plaque at the right carotid bulb (*). There is also a piece of intraluminal thrombus on the surface of the plaque (*arrow*). The patient later experienced another transient ischemic attack (TIA). **(c)** Repeat CTA shows no intraluminal thrombus but a large plaque with positive remodeling (*arrows*). The plaque's density was 33HU. Because it is a low-density and hypoechoic plaque, this indicates the presence of plaque hemorrhage or lipid rich necrotic core (LRNC). **(d)** MRA shows only a 45% narrowing. **(e)** Coronal magnetization prepared rapid gradient echo (MPRAGE) black blood imaging shows a large IPH, which is T1 bright (*arrows*). This case highlights how non-stenotic plaques can be symptomatic.

Table 2.1 Plaque Imaging Features on CT and Ultrasound

Plaque Characteristic	MDCTA	B-Mode US	*CEUS
IPH	Mean HU~20-30	Echolucent	Echolucent
LRNC	Mean HU~30-50	Echolucent	Echolucent
Neovascularity	Plaque enhancement	Not detectable	Plaque enhancement
Inflammation	Plaque enhancement	Not detectable	Plaque enhancement
Ulceration	Surface irregularity of plaque on multiplanar imaging	Surface irregularity	Surface irregularity
Calcification	Mean HU~250	Hyperechoic, posterior accoustic shadowing	Hyperechoic, posterior accoustic shadowing

Abbreviations: MDCTA, Multidetector computed tomographic angiography; CEUS, Contrast enhanced ultrasound; IPH, Intraplaque hemorrhage; LRNC, Lipid-rich necrotic core.

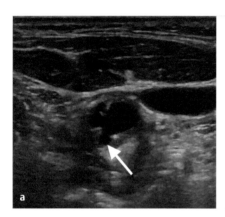
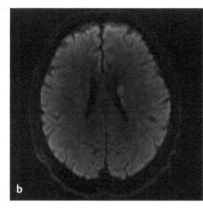

Fig. 2.2 Plaque ulceration on ultrasound. (**a**) Axial US of the left carotid bulb shows multiple crevices in the surface of a relatively hypodense carotid plaque (*arrow*). (**b**) DWI in this patient shows an infarct in the left caudate.

recognized on MDCT with high interobserver agreement. As a general rule, the lower the density of the plaque, the more likely it is to be vulnerable. MDCT is also very effective at detecting plaque ulcerations, which are defined as crevices within the plaque measuring 2 × 2 mm at minimum.

A strong correlation has been demonstrated between sonographic and histopathologic features of carotid plaques using B-mode ultrasound. B-mode carotid ultrasound has high specificity but only moderate sensitivity in identifying ulceration of the plaque surface. Large plaque ulcerations are easily identified as obvious craters within the plaque with reversed or stagnated flow. Determining the presence of ulceration in moderate stenosis patients is important due to the potential for changing the therapeutic approach. Conventional criteria require a size of the concavity greater than 2 × 2 mm and a color Doppler flow signal within the concavity to call something an ulceration (▶ Fig. 2.2).

Plaque echolucency is another strong marker of plaque vulnerability. This is the sonographic equivalent of a LRNC. Plaque echolucency is seen in up to 50% of recently symptomatic plaques compared to less than 5% of asymptomatic plaques. Furthermore, the risk of stroke among patients with echolucent plaques, regardless of the degree of stenosis. In addition, the size of the juxtaluminal hypoechoic area of the carotid plaque is strongly associated with stroke risk.

One critical imaging finding during conventional imaging of carotid disease is examining for the presence of mobile thrombus on the plaque surface. Mobile thrombus is an immediate risk factor for acute ischemic stroke. On ultrasound, it can be identified easily as a piece of plaque or clot that is extending into the lumen and waving in the breeze so to speak. On CTA, it is often seen as a thin hypodensity extending into the internal carotid artery (▶ Fig. 2.3).

Contrast enhanced ultrasound (CEUS) is used primarily to identify neovascularization within carotid plaques. Histologic examinations have demonstrated that plaque enhancement is strongly associated with plaque neovascularity and inflammation. Plaque enhancement is markedly increased in patients with symptomatic plaque and is associated with a higher rate of cardiovascular events in general. Retention of microbubbles on the plaque surface on delayed images has been shown to correlate with plaque disruption and inflammation as macrophages are known to phagocytose this contrast agent. Contrast bubble agents are also used in characterizing the plaque surface. Disruptions in the plaque-lumen border are easily characterized using CEUS. When compared with B-mode and color Doppler ultrasound, along with improved interobserver agreement, CEUS has higher sensitivity, specificity, and accuracy in identifying plaque ulceration.

2.1.5 What the Clinician Needs to Know

- Plaque characteristics including hypoechoic plaque on US or hypodense plaque on CT
- Presence or absence of plaque ulceration
- Presence of free-floating thrombus
- Degree of stenosis

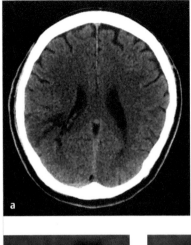
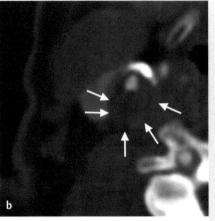
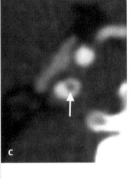
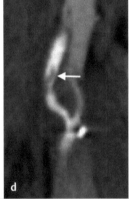
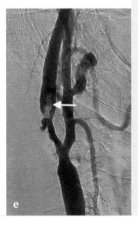

Fig. 2.3 A 76-year-old male with symptomatic right carotid stenosis and intraluminal thrombus. (a) Non-contrast CT shows an infarct in the right parietal lobe. (b) Axial CTA shows a low-density plaque with an average attenuation of 44HU (*arrows*). (c) At the level of the proximal ICA, there is a focal filling defect in the middle of the lumen (*arrow*). (d) Sagittal reconstruction shows the intraluminal thrombus which is attached to the plaque but floating distally in the right ICA (*arrow*). (e) Lateral cervical angiogram shows the floating filling defect which was very mobile (*arrow*).

2.1.6 High-Yield Facts

- Both hypodense plaque (CTA) and hypoechoic plaque (US) are associated with an increased risk of acute ischemic stroke.
- CEUS is an emerging tool in the assessment of carotid plaque vulnerability.
- Plaque ulcerations are independent risk factors for future ischemic events and can be easily identified on both US and CTA.

Further Reading

[1] Brinjikji W, Huston J, III, Rabinstein AA, Kim GM, Lerman A, Lanzino G. Contemporary carotid imaging: from degree of stenosis to plaque vulnerability. J Neurosurg. 2016; 124(1):27–42

[2] Gupta A, Gialdini G, Lerario MP, et al. Magnetic resonance angiography detection of abnormal carotid artery plaque in patients with cryptogenic stroke. J Am Heart Assoc. 2015; 4(6):e002012

[3] Gupta A, Baradaran H, Schweitzer AD, et al. Carotid plaque MRI and stroke risk: a systematic review and meta-analysis. Stroke. 2013; 44(11):3071–3077

2.2 Carotid Vessel Wall Imaging for Atherosclerosis

2.2.1 Clinical Case

A 76-year-old male with recurrent episodes of left-sided upper extremity weakness, which resolved spontaneously.

2.2.2 Description of Imaging Findings and Diagnosis

Diagnosis

Carotid atherosclerotic disease with T1 hyperintense plaque suggesting IPH (▶ Fig. 2.4).

2.2.3 Background

Plaque characterization with MRI has been shown to be a valuable tool in predicting subsequent ischemic events. In a systematic review of nine studies and 779 subjects, one group found that IPH, LRNC, and thinning/rupture of the fibrous cap were associated with hazards ratios of 4.59, 3.00, and 5.93, respectively, for subsequent TIA or stroke. In fact, MRI plaque characteristics have been found to have a stronger association with patient symptomatic status than the degree of stenosis. One large cross-sectional study of 97 patients with 50–99% stenosis found that the presence of a LRNC and thin or ruptured fibrous cap were associated with symptomatic events, whereas the degree of stenosis was not. Size of LRNC and the presence of ulceration have been found to be independent predictors of symptomatic events.

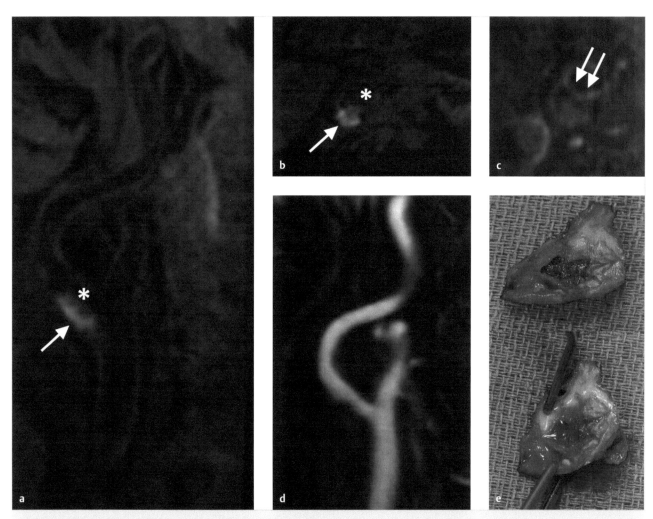

Fig. 2.4 A 76-year-old male with recurrent episodes of left-sided upper extremity weakness which resolved spontaneously. (**a**) Reformatted image from 3D MPRAGE acquisition of the neck with black blood demonstrates an eccentric focus of intrinsic T1 hyperintensity at the carotid bulb (*arrow*) (* indicates lumen). (**b**) Axial reformatted image shows the eccentric T1 hyperintense plaque with wall thickening and positive arterial wall remodeling (*arrow*) (* indicates lumen). (**c**) Gadolinium bolus MRA of the neck demonstrates an approximately 20% stenosis at the carotid bulb. (**d**) Post-contrast T1 weighted black blood image shows areas in which the fibrous cap enhancement is interrupted, suggesting rupture or fissure. (**e**) Endarterectomy specimen from the patient demonstrates a complicated carotid plaque with IPH and a thin/ruptured fibrous cap.

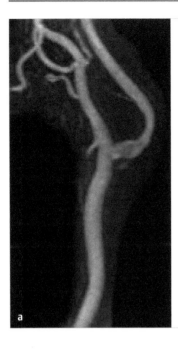
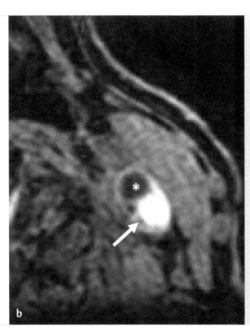

Fig. 2.5 Cryptogenic stroke secondary to hemorrhagic plaque with positive remodeling. (a) Gadolinium bolus MRA of the left internal carotid artery in a patient who has had multiple recurrent left hemispheric TIAs demonstrates no stenosis. (b) Black blood carotid vessel wall imaging (VWI) using a standard neurovascular coil and an MPRAGE sequence demonstrates a positively remodeled plaque which is markedly T1 bright consistent with IPH (*arrow*) (* indicates lumen).

Plaque imaging is also useful in the evaluation of patients with cryptogenic stroke. A number of studies have demonstrated that up to 20–30% of patients with cryptogenic stroke (i.e., stroke of unknown etiology) have a hemorrhagic plaque ipsilateral to the site of the ischemic stroke/TIA. Identifying such lesions early on is important as it can obviate an extensive work-up for other causes of ischemic stroke including arrhythmia and hypercoaguability (▶ Fig. 2.5).

MRI plaque imaging has also been used to identify surgical candidates. Yoshida et al. found that patients with low-grade carotid stenosis with IPH on MRI had high recurrence rates when placed on antithrombotics and statins. Because these patients with IPH were refractory to medical therapy, they elected to proceed with endarterectomy and found that surgery was associated with marked reductions in subsequent ischemic events. MRI plaque imaging has also been found to be useful in identifying revascularization candidates that would be better candidates for carotid endarterectomy (CEA) than carotid artery stenting (CAS) as high intraplaque signal on time of flight (TOF) imaging has been shown to be associated with vulnerable plaque and increased rates of adverse events in patients undergoing CAS, but not CEA.

2.2.4 Imaging Findings

MRI with carotid surface coils is the gold standard in carotid plaque imaging. Multiple contrast weightings are typically performed including fat-saturated T1 pre- and post-contrast, fat-saturated T2, Magnetization Prepared Rapid Gradient Echo, 3D TOF, and gadolinium bolus MRA. Suppression of blood flow signal using a fast spin echo (FSE) sequence with double inversion recovery preparation pulses can result in high contrast between the dark lumen and vessel wall. Pitfalls of surface coil imaging in carotid atherosclerotic disease include improper

coil positioning, long scan times, and motion artifact. More recently, some groups have proposed performing carotid plaque imaging with standard neurovascular (or, Head & Neck) coils acquiring plaque imaging with a larger field of view and shorter scan time at the expense of decreased spatial resolution. The images obtained in ▶ Fig. 2.4 were performed using a neurovascular coil and a 5-minute MPRAGE sequence.

IPH is the easiest plaque feature to characterize on MRI VWI. Plaque hemorrhage is invariably bright on MPRAGE and T1 weighted sequences with fat suppression. LRNC is characterized by peripheral plaque enhancement with low internal/non-enhancing signal on T1 fat-saturated post-gadolinium imaging (▶ Fig. 2.6). Fibrous cap assessment is often difficult to assess with larger field of view exams; however, surface coil MRI provides an exquisite assessment of fibrous cap status. In cases where there is thick and continuous enhancement of the lumen-plaque interface, the fibrous cap is considered to be intact/thick, whereas in cases where there is discontinuous or disruption of enhancement, the cap is considered to be thin or ruptured (▶ Fig. 2.7). Plaque ulceration is typically defined as a crevice in the plaque of 2 mm or larger and is often indicative of ruptured plaque. A summary of imaging findings of various carotid plaque features on MRI is provided in ▶ Table 2.2.

One of the most commonly asked questions about carotid plaque imaging is related to distinguish plaque hemorrhage from dissection. Both will present with high intramural T1 signal. One common means of distinguishing these lesions is location. Carotid plaques are typically located at the carotid bulb, a location that is not typical for dissection. Furthermore, demographically, carotid atherosclerotic disease typically affects older adults, whereas dissections are typically seen in younger patients. Last, carotid atherosclerotic disease is typically associated with disease in the same and other vessels including calcifications, findings which are not typical in acute dissection.

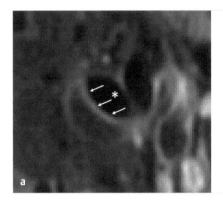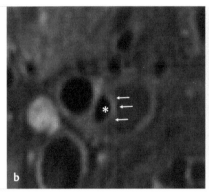

Fig. 2.6 Example of LRNC and thick fibrous cap in a 50-year-old gentleman with hypercholesterolemia. (**a**) and (**b**) Post-gadolinium T1 QIR image with black blood performed using a surface coil demonstrates thick peripherally enhancing plaque of the bilateral proximal internal carotid arteries consistent with LRNC (*). Note the thick enhancing fibrous cap at the interface between the low-signal plaque and vessel lumen (*arrows*).

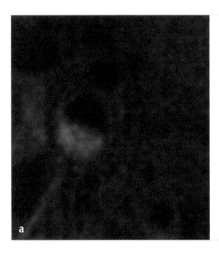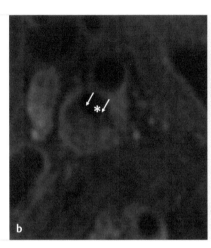

Fig. 2.7 Example of a thin and ruptured fibrous cap. (**a**) Pre-contrast T1 CUBE and (**b**). Post-contrast T1 CUBE images demonstrate a hemorrhagic plaque (*) with no enhancement at the vessel-plaque interface (*arrows*). This suggests presence of a thin or ruptured fibrous cap.

Table 2.2 MRI Findings in Vulnerable Plaque

Plaque Characteristic	T1	T2	PD	CEMRA
IPH	Hyperintense	Variable	Variable	Hyperintense
LRNC	Iso/Hyperintense	Variable	Iso/Hyperintense	Iso/Hyperintense
Neovascularity	Not detectable	Not detectable	Not detectable	Plaque enhancement
Inflammation	Not detectable	Not detectable	Not detectable	Plaque enhancement
Ulceration	Surface irregularity	Surface irregularity	Surface irregularity	Surface irregularity
Calcification	Hypointense	Hypointense	Hypointense	Hypointense

Abbreviation: CEMRA, Contrast-Enhanced Magnetic Resonance Angiography.

2.2.5 What the Clinician Needs to Know

- Plaque characteristics including IPH, lipid-rich core, and thin-ruptured fibrous cap
- Whether IPH is juxtaluminal
- Presence of free-floating thrombus
- Degree of stenosis

2.2.6 High-Yield Facts

- IPH is associated with a 5–7 × increased risk of acute ischemic stroke.
- LRNC and thin-ruptured fibrous cap are also associated with a 3–5 × risk of future ischemic stroke.
- Plaque characteristics are independent risk factors for acute ischemic stroke-even when controlling for degree of stenosis.

- Including a T1 hemorrhage sensitive protocol such as an MPRAGE or 3D-TOF allows for the detection of most hemorrhagic plaques.

Further Reading

[1] Brinjikji W, Huston J, III, Rabinstein AA, Kim GM, Lerman A, Lanzino G. Contemporary carotid imaging: from degree of stenosis to plaque vulnerability. J Neurosurg. 2016; 124(1):27–42

[2] Gupta A, Gialdini G, Lerario MP, et al. Magnetic resonance angiography detection of abnormal carotid artery plaque in patients with cryptogenic stroke. J Am Heart Assoc. 2015; 4(6):e002012

[3] Gupta A, Baradaran H, Schweitzer AD, et al. Carotid plaque MRI and stroke risk: a systematic review and meta-analysis. Stroke. 2013; 44(11): 3071–3077

2.3 Spontaneous Carotid Artery Dissection

2.3.1 Clinical Case

A 58-year-old male in a motor vehicle accident 10 days ago. Now presents with slight right-sided weakness (▶ Fig. 2.8).

2.3.2 Description of Imaging Findings and Diagnosis

Diagnosis

Watershed infarcts in the left hemisphere. Narrowing of the distal cervical ICA secondary to acute carotid dissection.

2.3.3 Background

Cervical carotid artery dissections are a leading cause of ischemic stroke in patients aged 45 years or younger accounting for 20% of all cases in this age group. The incidence of cervical carotid dissection is estimated to be 3/100,000/year. Dissections can be traumatic, or spontaneous. Traumatic dissections, which will be discussed in more details in the blunt cerebrovascular injury (BCVI) chapter, occur from direct injury to the arterial wall from strangulation, direct shock, or motor vehicle accidents. Spontaneous carotid artery dissections occur in the absence of any trauma or minor trauma such as neck manipulation or hyperextension and are often associated with underlying collagenopathies, such as fibromuscular dysplasia (FMD) or Marfan's syndrome. Typical treatments for non-flow limiting dissections include antiplatelet agents or anticoagulation.

Up to 50% of patients with cervical carotid dissections have histological abnormalities of the collagen tissue in the vessel wall. It is thought that aberrations in collagen III structure are responsible for the arterial wall weakness in these cases. In some cases, it is thought that carotid dissections could be related to an inflammatory etiology, particularly when multiple dissections occur simultaneously. This occurs in the setting of segmental arterial mediolysis.

Pathophysiologically dissections are characterized by a proximal endothelial tear and a further distal intramural hematoma. These hematomas can cleave the arterial wall for a distance. The intramural hematoma can compress the arterial lumen that can result in stenosis or occlusion and subsequent embolic or hemodynamic ischemic stroke. Dilatation can occur when the dissection extends to the subadventitial space and result in pain and cranial nerve compression syndromes including Horner's syndrome and hypoglossal nerve palsy. Most cervical carotid dissections affect the distal cervical ICA – i.e., where the mobile cervical segment of the ICA enters the foramen lacerum (and thus is immobilized). Usually, the hematoma spares the bulb. Cervical carotid dissections can result in cerebral ischemia through two principal mechanisms: (1) hypoperfusion due to a critical stenosis resulting in watershed distribution infarcts or holohemispheric infarcts in the case of an isolated hemisphere and (2) embolism related to local thrombus formation at the dissection flap/extrusion of intramural clot into the lumen (▶ Fig. 2.9, ▶ Fig. 2.10).

2.3.4 Imaging Findings

MRI and CT are the ideal imaging modalities for evaluating both the luminal and mural components of the dissection. The luminal imaging appearances of cervical carotid artery dissections are fairly standard. MRA/CTA should be performed from the aortic arch to the skull base. The typical appearance is a long and progressive stenosis, which spares the carotid artery bulb. A dissection flap is sometimes seen, but this is not typical. In the chronic phase, a pseudoaneurysm or fusiform dilation can be apparent, sometimes with a proximal stenosis.

MRI/MRA should be performed with the addition of axial fat-saturated T1-weighted imaging in order to better visualize the hematoma. The mural hematoma is typically T1 hyperintense with an eccentric and crescentic shape. The intramural hematoma ages similarly to an intraparenchymal hematoma of the brain. Within the first 72 hours, the hematoma is isointense on T1, whereas after 72 hours, the hematoma is hyperintense on T1. Thus, the sensitivity of T1-fat-saturated MRI is increased 72 hours post-presentation (▶ Fig. 2.11).

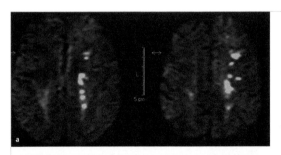
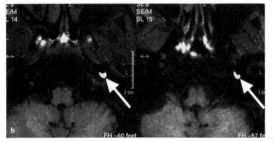
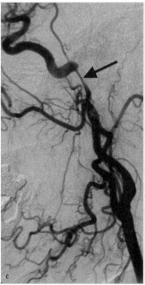

Fig. 2.8 A 58-year-old male with watershed infarct from carotid dissection. (a) Axial DWI MRI shows acute punctate infarcts in the internal watershed distribution. (b) Axial T1 fat-saturated MRI through the skull base shows T1 hyperintense intramural hematoma of the distal cervical ICA on the left (arrows). (c) Lateral cervical carotid angiogram shows a long-segment dissection of the left internal carotid artery (arrow). The patient's symptoms in this case were due to poor flow in the watershed territory rather than embolism.

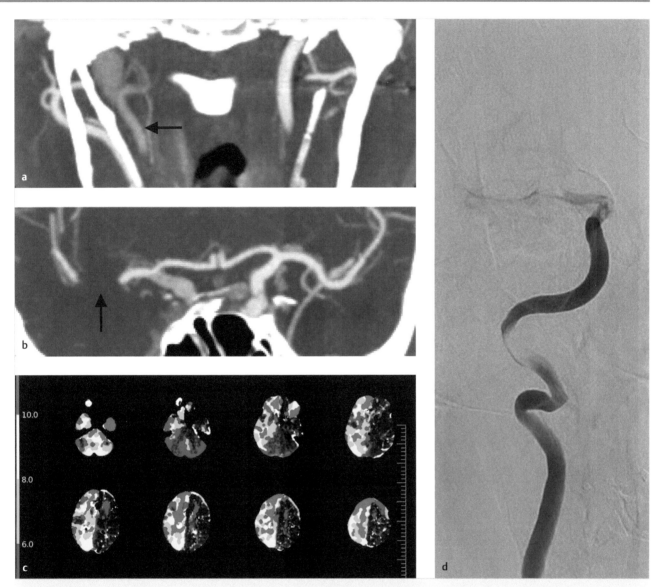

Fig. 2.9 Cerebral embolism from an acute right carotid dissection. (**a**) Coronal CTA demonstrates slow flow in the mid to distal cervical right ICA, which was secondary to dissection (*arrow*). (**b**) Coronal CTA of the head demonstrates occlusion of the right MCA from dissection related embolism (*arrow*). (**c**) CT perfusion shows reduced perfusion in the entire right hemisphere, which is due to a combination of a flow limiting dissection and the right MCA occlusion. (**d**) Conventional angiogram demonstrates the dissection of the right ICA and the intracranial occlusion.

CT/CTA can also be used to demonstrate the intramural hematoma, but it is usually not as apparent as on an MRI/MRA due to the lack of contrast resolution. CT/CTA will demonstrate non-specific asymmetric eccentric crescent-shaped wall thickening at the site of maximum stenosis. Soft tissue windows are best for identifying these findings.

It is important to understand the natural history of cervical carotid artery dissections. In general, the prognosis of a spontaneous cervical carotid dissection is good with no neurological sequelae in 90% of patients. In 80% of cases, there is regression of the dissection and mural hematoma (▶ Fig. 2.12). During regression, there may be some mild residual stenosis or a focal dilatation/pseudoaneurysm. Regression usually occurs within months. Dissecting aneurysms however rarely regress. Also, the arterial lumen does not

seem to change after 1 year (▶ Fig. 2.13). Relapse of the dissection can occur in 10% of cases – usually, within 2 months of the initial dissection. This is especially common in patients with tortuous vessels and connective tissue diseases (▶ Fig. 2.14).

2.3.5 What the Clinician Needs to Know

- Proximal and distal extent of the dissection as well as maximum degree of stenosis
- Presence of free-floating thrombus
- Presence of additional dissections (contralateral vessel) or stigmata indicating underlying collagenopathy (such as FMD)
- Regression of mural hematoma over time
- Presence of dissecting pseudoaneurysm

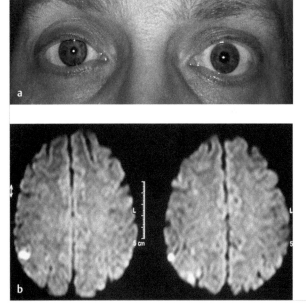

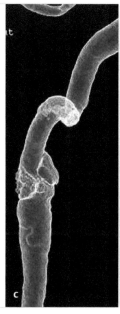

Fig. 2.10 A 53-year-old male with the Horner's syndrome and left upper extremity weakness. (a) Photograph demonstrates constriction of the right pupil. (b) Axial DWI demonstrates punctate infarcts in the right motor strip. (c) 3DRA reconstruction shows narrowing of the distal cervical ICA and a small pseudoaneurysm.

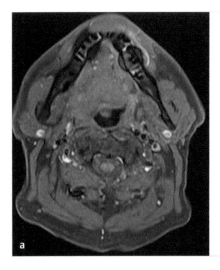

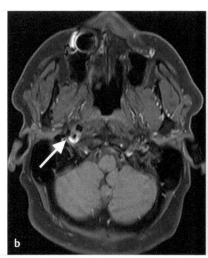

Fig. 2.11 Hypoglossal palsy secondary to carotid dissection. (a) Axial T1 fat-saturated MRI demonstrates right lateral deviation of the tongue and increased fullness in the right side of the oropharynx. (b) Axial T1 fat-saturated MRI demonstrates crescentic intramural hemorrhage secondary to dissection (arrow).

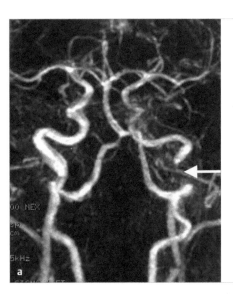

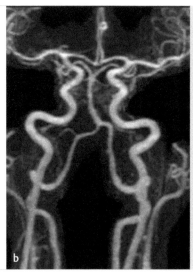

Fig. 2.12 Remodeling of a dissection over 4 years. (a) Coronal post-contrast MRA shows interruption of flow in the distal cervical ICA (arrow). (b) Follow-up post contrast MRA 4 years later shows spontaneous remodeling of the left internal carotid artery.

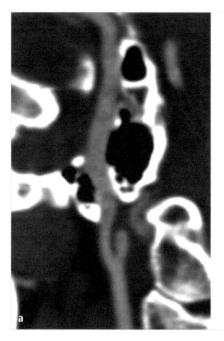
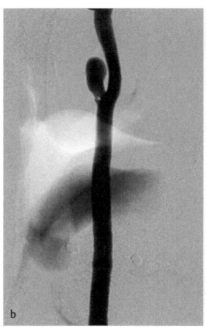

Fig. 2.13 Chronic dissection pseudoaneurysm of the right cervical ICA seen on CTA (**a**) and digital subtraction angiography (DSA) (**b**).

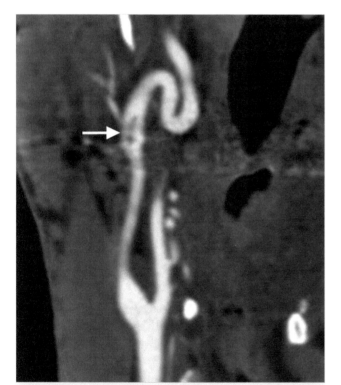

Fig. 2.14 Carotid dissection flap in a patient with a carotid loop (*arrow*).

2.3.6 High-Yield Facts

- Cervical carotid dissection comprises formation of a mural hematoma and can result in pseudoaneurysm or stenosis/occlusion of the ICA.
- Most dissections are subpetrous and spare the bulb.
- Carotid dissections have variable presentations including neck pain, headache, stroke, and cranial neuropathy.
- Mean time for normalization of the arterial lumen is 3 months.
- T1-fat-saturated imaging of the neck at 72 hours post-presentation is most sensitive for detecting intramural hematoma.

Further Reading

[1] Schievink WI. Spontaneous dissection of the carotid and vertebral arteries. N Engl J Med. 2001; 344(12):898–906

[2] Ben Hassen W, Machet A, Edjlali-Goujon M, et al. Imaging of cervical artery dissection. Diagn Interv Imaging. 2014; 95(12):1151–1161

[3] Debette S, Leys D. Cervical-artery dissections: predisposing factors, diagnosis, and outcome. Lancet Neurol. 2009; 8(7):668–678

2.4 Connective Tissue Diseases

2.4.1 Clinical Case

A 25-year-old female with pulsatile neck mass that has been slowly growing over the past 5 months (▶ Fig. 2.15).

2.4.2 Description of Imaging Findings and Diagnosis

Diagnosis

Carotid artery pseudoaneurysm secondary to chronic dissection.

2.4.3 Background

Patients with connective tissue diseases are at a higher risk for a number of cerebrovascular diseases including dissection, aneurysms, and acute ischemic stroke. The association between connective tissue diseases and arteriopathies is due to mutations in collagen and proteoglycans, which comprise the extracellular vessel wall matrix and therefore alterations in these structures weaken the vessel wall. The most commonly encountered connective tissue diseases include FMD, Marfan's syndrome, Ehlers-Danlos's syndrome (particularly, Type IV), Neurofibromatosis Type 1, and Loeys-Diez syndrome. In addition, as of yet unclassified collagenopathies may be present. In general, the cervical manifestations of these connective tissue diseases are similar. However, they each have different systemic manifestations. One key point is that patients with connective tissue diseases are prone to develop aneurysms, stenosis, and dissections in other vascular beds. Thus, the importance of aortic aneurysm screening (in cases of Marfan's, Ehlers-Danlos, and Loeys Dietz) and renal artery screening (in cases of FMD) has to be highlighted.

2.4.4 Imaging Findings

Cervical carotid dissections and their imaging appearance were described in Chapter 1. Cervical carotid dissections can be isolated to the cervical vasculature, extend to the intracranial vasculature, or be the result of extension of a Stanford Type A thoracic aortic dissection. Dissections which extend for thoracic aortic dissections are more likely to have an intimal flap and a clearly defined true and false lumen than those which are spontaneous and isolated to the cervical internal carotid artery (▶ Fig. 2.16).

Cervical pseudoaneurysms arise from disruption of the arterial wall, which allows blood to stream into the surrounding tissue to form a sac, which communicates with the arterial lumen (▶ Fig. 2.15). These are the result of dissections, neck trauma, or iatrogenic vascular injury. The (transmural) rupture risk of these lesions into the neck soft tissues is low. They can be

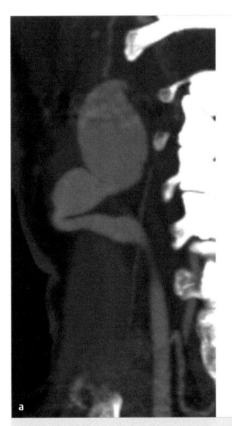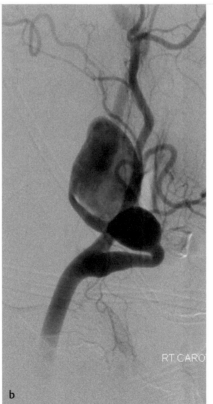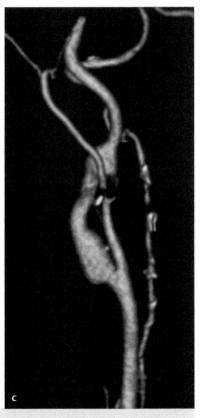

Fig. 2.15 A 25-year-old female with the Marfan's syndrome and chronic cervical carotid dissecting pseudoaneurysm. **(a)** Sagittal CTA demonstrates tortuosity and kinking of the left cervical ICA with two large aneurysmal dilatations. **(b)** Left common carotid artery (CCA) cervical angiogram demonstrates tortuosity of the proximal left ICA with two distinct pseudoaneurysms and evidence of slow flow distal to the largest pseudoaneurysm with poor contrast opacification. **(c)** Post-surgical CTA shows resolution of the lesions. The patient was treated with a saphenous vein reconstruction.

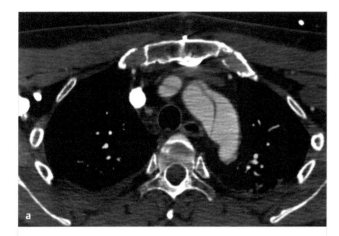

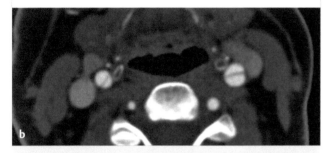

Fig. 2.16 Stanford type A dissection and bilateral CCA dissections in a patient with the Ehlers-Danlos's syndrome. (**a**) CTA of the thoracic aorta demonstrates a dissection involving the ascending thoracic aorta and aortic arch. (**b**) The dissection extended into the bilateral CCAs. Note the large dissection flaps bilaterally.

associated with ischemic stroke (either hemodynamic, related to perforator occlusion, or embolic) and cranial nerve mass effect (i.e., Horners's syndrome and hypoglossal nerve palsy).

A "string-of-beads" appearance is pathognomonic for FMD. Typically, this is multifocal and affects the bilateral cervical internal carotid arteries and bilateral vertebral arteries. It typically involves the mid-to-distal segments of the arteries. Medial FMD results in a "string-of-beads" appearance in which the diameter of the beading is larger than the artery diameter. Perimedial fibroplasia results in beading in which the beads are smaller than the diameter of the artery. Meanwhile, intimal FMD results in long, smooth narrowing.

An interesting variant of FMD is the so-called "carotid web" (▶ Fig. 2.17). Carotid webs are an increasingly recognized cause of acute ischemic stroke, particularly in younger adult patients. These lesions are defined as endoluminal shelf-like projections at the origin of the internal carotid artery just beyond its bifurcation. Carotid webs have also been described as atypical FMD, septal FMD, pseudo-valvular folds, and carotid diaphragms. The typical CTA appearance of these lesions is a thin intraluminal filling defect along the posterior wall of the carotid bulb just beyond the carotid bifurcation. On axial CTA images, there is often a septum visible. Examination of these lesions with MR VWI shows focal vessel wall thickening with a thin fibrous band and no enhancement, plaque hemorrhage, or other atherosclerosis-type characteristics.

Loeys-Dietz's syndrome has a very stereotypical appearance on cervico-vascular imaging. There is a high prevalence of marked cervical vertebral artery tortuosity and ectasia in Loeys-Dietz's syndrome. However, this is not found in other connective tissue diseases such as Marfan's syndrome or

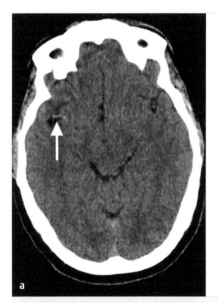
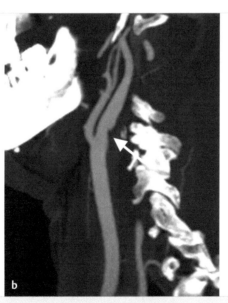
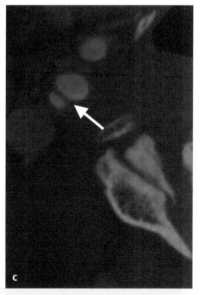

Fig. 2.17 Right MCA occlusion secondary to carotid web. (**a**) Non-contrast CT demonstrates a dense right MCA (*arrow*). CTA (not shown) confirmed the occlusion. (**b**) Sagittal reconstruction of a CTA demonstrates a shelf-like projection along the posterior wall of the right carotid bulb ICA (*arrow*). (**c**) Axial angiogram shows a small web in the posterior aspect of the right carotid bulb. Dissections typically do not involve the carotid bulb so, when one sees a "dissecting flap" isolated to the carotid bulb, the lesion is most likely a carotid web (*arrow*).

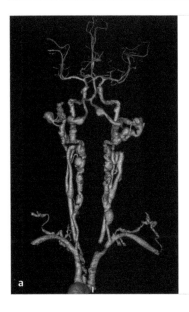
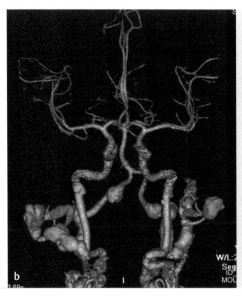

Fig. 2.18 Vertebral artery findings pathognomonic for the Loeys-Dietz's syndrome. Bilateral vertebral artery tortuosity with multifocal cervical vertebral artery dissecting aneurysms (a) and bilateral intradural vertebral artery dissecting aneurysms in the setting of the Loeys-Dietz's syndrome (b).

Ehlers Danlos. Another interesting finding that is specific to Loeys-Dietz is the presence of a very dilated and ectatic carotid bifurcation (▶ Fig. 2.18).

2.4.5 What the Clinician Needs to Know

- Connective tissue diseases often associated with arterial abnormalities in other vascular beds. Role of screening for other vascular pathologies should be discussed.
- Differentiation between spontaneous cervical carotid dissection and dissection extension from aortic dissection should be discussed.
- In some cases, the vascular findings are pathognomonic for a specific disease; this should be discussed.

2.4.6 High-Yield Facts

- "String-of-beads" appearance is pathognomonic for FMD.

- Marked cervical vertebral artery tortuosity and ectasia is common and pathognomonic for Loeys-Dietz's syndrome.
- Stanford Type A dissections, which are common in Marfan's syndrome, Ehlers-Danlos's syndrome, and Loeys-Dietz syndrome, can extend to the cervical carotid arteries.
- Carotid webs, defined as endoluminal shelf-like projections at the origin of the internal carotid artery just beyond its bifurcation, are an increasingly recognized cause of recurrent ischemic stroke in the absence of stenosis in young patients.

Further Reading

[1] Kim ST, Brinjikji W, Lanzino G, Kallmes DF. Neurovascular manifestations of connective-tissue diseases: A review. Interv Neuroradiol. 2016; 22(6): 624–637

[2] Touzé E, Oppenheim C, Trystram D, et al. Fibromuscular dysplasia of cervical and intracranial arteries. Int J Stroke. 2010; 5(4):296–305

[3] Kono AK, Higashi M, Morisaki H, et al. High prevalence of vertebral artery tortuosity of Loeys-Dietz syndrome in comparison with Marfan syndrome. Jpn J Radiol. 2010; 28(4):273–277

2.5 Blunt Cerebrovascular Injury

2.5.1 Clinical Case

A 37-year-old female status post-motor vehicle accident. Cervical spine trauma (▶ Fig. 2.19).

2.5.2 Description of Imaging Findings and Diagnosis

Diagnosis

Vertebral artery dissection secondary to foramen transversarium fractures, consistent with BCVI.

2.5.3 Background

BCVI is the term used to describe blunt force injuries to the cervical vertebral and carotid arteries. These injuries result from high-energy mechanisms to the thorax, neck, and head. These injuries are a rare, but highly significant, cause of morbidity and mortality following blunt force trauma. Cervical spine fractures have the highest association with BCVI with markedly higher rates among patients with C1-C3 fractures than C4-C7 fractures.

BCVI can result in intimal injuries or adventitiomedial injuries. Intimal injuries result in exposure of intravascular blood to the subendothelial extracellular matrix and carry a high risk of downstream embolization and stroke. Adventitiomedial injuries, which spare the intima, result in intramural hematoma, which can result in luminal stenosis or occlusion. Traumatic pseudoaneurysms can result when all layers of the vessel wall are disrupted and are kept from bleeding out by surrounding soft tissues and thrombus formation. Arterial transection is the most severe BCVI and often results in rapid exsanguination or death.

There is currently some controversy as to whether routine screening CTA is needed in evaluating patients following blunt force trauma. ▶ Table 2.3 provides a summary of clinical circumstances in which screening may be indicated in BCVI.

2.5.4 Imaging Findings

There is a wide spectrum in the severity of BCVI. The most widely accepted scale for grading BCVI is the Biffl scale, which is summarized in ▶ Table 2.4. This section will focus primarily on CTA as it is the most widely used imaging modality for the assessment of BCVI. Typical imaging manifestations of BCVI are as follows:

- Minimal intimal injury is the lowest grade of BCVI. On CT angiography, there is minimal non-stenotic luminal irregularity with subtle vessel wall thickening and undulation.
- Intramural hematoma is manifested as long-segments of mural thickening in a circumferential or eccentric distribution. This can be associated with mild, moderate, or severe stenosis.
- Dissection with raised intimal flap is classically seen as a double lumen sign. The true lumen has more contrast opacification than the false lumen.
- Intraluminal thrombus can occur as a complication of intimal injury or dissection. This is manifested as an intraluminal filling defect at the site of injury (▶ Fig. 2.19).
- Pseudoaneurysm results from partial or contained rupture of the vessel with focal ballooning of the arterial wall. These

Table 2.3 Screening Recommendations for BCVI

Signs/Symptoms

Arterial hemorrhage from neck, nose or mouth

Expanding cervical hematoma

Focal neurological deficit or ischemic stroke

Risk Factors

High-energy mechanism with Le Fort II or III fracture, basilar skull fracture or carotid canal involvement

DAI

Low GCS

Cervical spine fracture or dislocation involving body, transverse foramen, ligamentous injury

Any C1-C3 fracture

Near hanging

Clothesline injury

Mandible fracture

Complex skull base fracture

Degloving injury of scalp or face

Thoracic vascular injury

Abbreviations: BCVI, Blunt cerebrovascular injury; GCS, Glasgow coma scale.

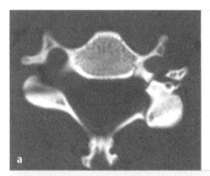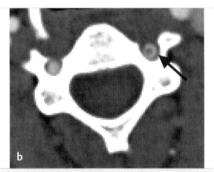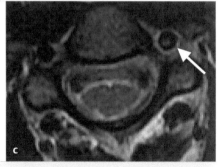

Fig. 2.19 Vertebral artery dissection from trauma. (a) Non-contrast CT demonstrates a comminuted fracture involving the left foramen transversarium. (b) CTA was performed which demonstrates a focal filling defect in the left vertebral artery secondary to a dissection related thrombus (*arrow*). (c) MRI performed to examine for the presence of cord injury demonstrates loss of the normal flow void in the left vertebral artery (*arrow*).

cases should be evaluated to determine the extent of the intramural hematoma, dissection, and pseudoaneurysm margins (▶ Fig. 2.20, ▶ Fig. 2.21).

- Arterial occlusions constitute grade IV injuries and typically have some degree of tapering before complete occlusion when in the ICA and an abrupt cutoff when affecting the vertebral artery.

- Arterial transection is a grade V injury. In these cases, delayed imaging will show the dispersion of contrast material consistent with active extravasation and possible occlusion of the vessel distal to the transection.
- Arteriovenous fistula is also a grade V injury. These are easily identified as a connection between the disrupted artery and the draining vein, sinus, or venous plexus. Arterialization of the vein is present in that it has a similar contrast density as the artery. There can also be enlargement of the draining vein.

2.5.5 What the Clinician Needs to Know

- Grade of BCVI and vascular territory that can be affected by the vascular injury.
- Presence of other associated injuries such as vertebral body fractures, ligamentous injury, upper mediastinal injury, soft tissue hematoma, and risk factors for airway compromise.
- In presence of severe fractures or lesions described in ▶ Table 2.3, screening CTA for BCVI may be indicated.

Table 2.4 BCVI Grading Scale

Grade	Description
I	Vessel wall irregularity, dissection or intramural hematoma with < 25% luminal stenosis
II	Any raised intimal flap, intraluminal thrombus or dissection/intramural hematoma with > 25% stenosis
III	Arterial pseudoaneurysm
IV	Arterial occlusion
V	Arterial transection and/or AVF

Abbreviation: BCVI, Blunt cerebrovascular injury.

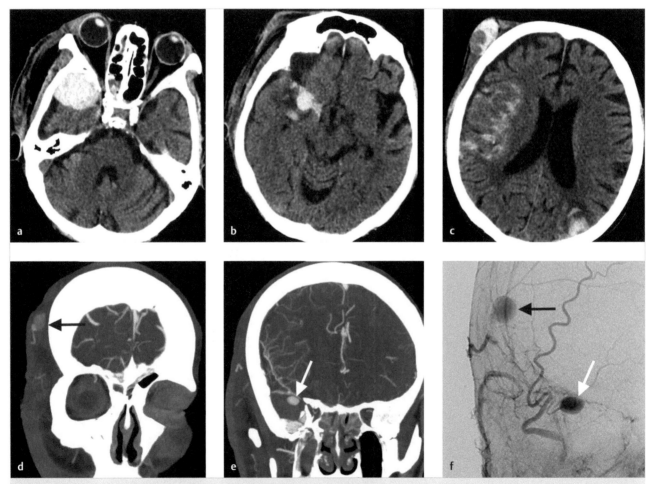

Fig. 2.20 Middle meningeal artery (MMA) and superficial temporal artery (STA) pseudoaneurysm. (**a–c**) Non-contrast CTs demonstrate an epidural hematoma in the right temporal fossa, a soft tissue hematoma in the right frontal region and intraparenchymal and subarachnoid hemorrhage (SAH). (**d**) CTA demonstrates a slow filling pseudoaneurysm of the right STA (*black arrow*). (**e**) There is also a pseudoaneurysm of the right MMA (*white arrow*). (**f**) Right external carotid artery (ECA) cerebral angiogram better demonstrates the right STA and MMA pseudoaneurysms (*arrows*).

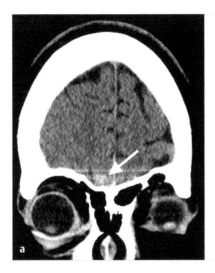 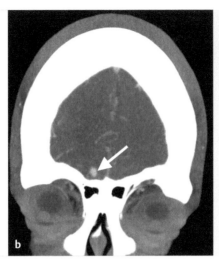

Fig. 2.21 Frontopolar artery pseudoaneurysm in a patient 4 weeks post-trauma. (**a**) Non-contrast CT demonstrates a focal hyperdensity in the right frontal region (*arrow*). (**b**) CTA was performed which demonstrates a focal pseudoaneurysm of the right frontopolar artery (*arrow*).

2.5.6 High-Yield Facts

- Upper cervical spine fractures are strongly associated with BCVI. In setting of upper C-spine fracture, screening CTA should be considered.
- CTA is the first-line imaging modality for the assessment of BCVI.
- The Biffl scale is a useful tool for grading BCVI and can be used to guide management of BCVIs.

Further Reading

[1] Rutman AM, Vranic JE, Mossa-Basha M. Imaging and Management of Blunt Cerebrovascular Injury. Radiographics. 2018; 38(2):542–563

[2] Mutze S, Rademacher G, Matthes G, Hosten N, Stengel D. Blunt cerebrovascular injury in patients with blunt multiple trauma: diagnostic accuracy of duplex Doppler US and early CT angiography. Radiology. 2005; 237(3):884–892

[3] Biffl WL, Cothren CC, Moore EE, et al. Western Trauma Association critical decisions in trauma: screening for and treatment of blunt cerebrovascular injuries. J Trauma. 2009; 67(6):1150–1153

[4] Krings T, Geibprasert S, Lasjaunias PL. Cerebrovascular trauma. Eur Radiol. 2008; 18(8):1531–1545

2.6 Inflammatory Carotid Arteriopathies

2.6.1 Clinical Case

A 37-year-old female with syncope in setting of malaise, fever, night sweats, weight loss, and fatigue (▶ Fig. 2.22).

2.6.2 Description of Imaging Findings and Diagnosis

Diagnosis

Occlusion of the bilateral common carotid arteries in the setting of mural inflammation of the aorta. Findings most consistent with Takayasus Arteritis.

2.6.3 Background

Although there are a number of inflammatory arteritis that can affect the cervical vasculature, the two most common ones are takayasu arteritis (TA) and giant cell arteritis (GCA). TA is a chronic, large-vessel vasculitis of unknown etiology that typically affects young women. Granulomatous inflammation of the aorta and its main branches gradually lead to stenosis and symptomatology related to end-organ ischemia. The clinical presentation of TA patients varies greatly and depends on the degree and location of disease progression. Cerebral ischemia can give rise to neurologic symptoms such as headache, seizure, stroke, syncope, and visual disturbances. These neurologic manifestations have been estimated to affect between 42 and 80% of TA patients and are usually secondary to large vessel involvement of the disease. The diagnostic criteria of Takayasu arteritis are summarized in ▶ Table 2.5.

GCA is a medium-to-large vessel arteritis, which typically affects elderly females. This entity is typically diagnosed on temporal artery biopsy. The rate of ischemic cerebrovascular events from GCA is 3–4%. Ischemia is usually the result of high-grade stenosis or occlusion of the cervical vertebral or carotid arteries and there is typically sparing of the intracranial cerebrovascular. Intracranial involvement can be seen however typically affecting the distal ICAs and V4 segments of the vertebral arteries.

2.6.4 Imaging Findings

Extracranial vascular abnormalities are the most common cause of ischemic neurologic symptoms in the setting of TA. In a vast majority of cases, smooth tapered narrowing of the subclavian arteries, brachiocephalic artery, or common carotid arteries can be seen (▶ Fig. 2.23). This is usually contiguous with disease affecting the aortic arch. Cervical internal carotid artery involvement is less common, but always occurs in the presence of CCA involvement. The rate of CCA stenosis has been reported to be 21–65%, compared to 16–18% in the internal carotid arteries, and 12–33% in the vertebral arteries. As opposed to stenotic disease secondary to atherosclerosis, in TA there is concentric vessel wall thickening as opposed to eccentric wall thickening as the cause of the stenosis. On MRA,

Table 2.5 Diagnostic Criteria for Takayasu Arteritis

Obligatory criterion:	
	Age less than or equal to 40 years
Major criteria:	
	Lesion of the left mid subclavian artery
	Lesion of the right mid subclavian artery
Minor criteria:	
	High ESR
	Common carotid artery tenderness
	Hypertension
	Aortic regurgitation or annulo-aortic ectasia
	Lesions of the pulmonary artery
	Lesions of the left mid common carotid artery
	Lesions of the distal brachiocephalic trunk
	Lesions of the thoracic aorta
	Lesions of the abdominal aorta

In addition to the presence of the obligatory criterion, the presence of 2 major, 4 minor, or 1 major plus 2 minor criteria suggests a high probability of Takayasu disease with 84% sensitivity.

Abbreviation: ESR, Erythrocyte sedimentation rate.

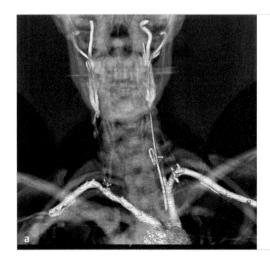 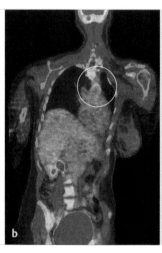

Fig. 2.22 A 37-year-old female with Takayasu's arteritis. **(a)** 3D reconstructed image from CTA demonstrates occlusion of the bilateral common carotid arteries. **(b)** PET CT coronal reconstruction shows circumferential area of increased FDG uptake in the wall of the aortic arch, (*circle*) a classic imaging finding in Takayasu's arteritis.

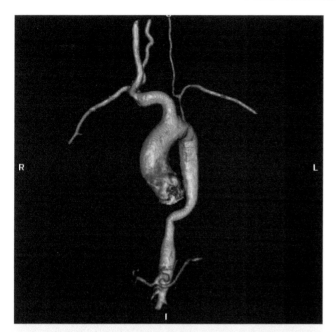

Fig. 2.23 Takayasu arteritis aorta. 3D reconstructed CTA image shows smooth narrowing of the bilateral vertebral arteries and occlusion of the left CCA. There is also smooth narrowing of the descending thoracic and abdominal aorta.

Interestingly, cases of intracranial vasculitis demonstrate a similar pattern of inflammation pathologically to that of the aorta and major cervical arteries in TA.

The typical MR and CT findings of GCA include arterial wall thickening with mural enhancement. Involvement of the internal carotid arteries is very rare. Several case reports have demonstrated narrowing of the cavernous internal carotid arteries and distal intradural vertebral arteries with high-grade stenosis and concentric wall enhancement and thickening on VWI MRI (▶ Fig. 2.25). Cervical internal carotid artery involvement can be seen and has a similar imaging appearance to that of TA with concentric wall thickening and enhancement on VWI.

The most useful imaging modality for evaluation of GA is high resolution CTA (to identify areas of vascular narrowing in the CTA). In evaluating such lesions, multiplanar reformatted imaging is necessary to get the STA in a plane to allow for more accurate imaging evaluation (▶ Fig. 2.26). VWI of the superficial temporal arteries can be performed with T1-SPACE or PD-SPACE techniques with and without gadolinium enhancement. Evaluation criteria should include mural thickening and mural contrast enhancement with close attention paid to both the frontal and parietal branches of the STAs and occipital arteries bilaterally. On T2 TSE weighted scans, fat-stranding surrounding the affected artery can be seen (▶ Fig. 2.25). Such an imaging can be useful to target biopsies.

2.6.5 What the Clinician Needs to Know

• Distribution and extent of vascular narrowing as well as maximum degree of stenosis.
• In absence of a known diagnosis, if TA is suspected, the radiologist should recommend additional vascular imaging of the thoracic and abdominal aorta.
• Exact location of vessel wall narrowing and/or enhancement of the STA should be relayed to the treating physician so that biopsy can be targeted in patients with suspected GCA.

the best way to identify this wall thickening is by using black blood VWI protocols. In patients with the aforementioned pattern of involvement, the radiologist should recommend imaging of the entire aorta to look for distal abdominal aortic narrowing.

It is important to point out that TA can have intracranial involvement as well (▶ Fig. 2.24). Intracranial stenoses in TA could be secondary to inflammatory vasculitis or a result of prior emboli. One recently published series identified a subset of TA patients with multifocal stenoses in a vasculitic pattern.

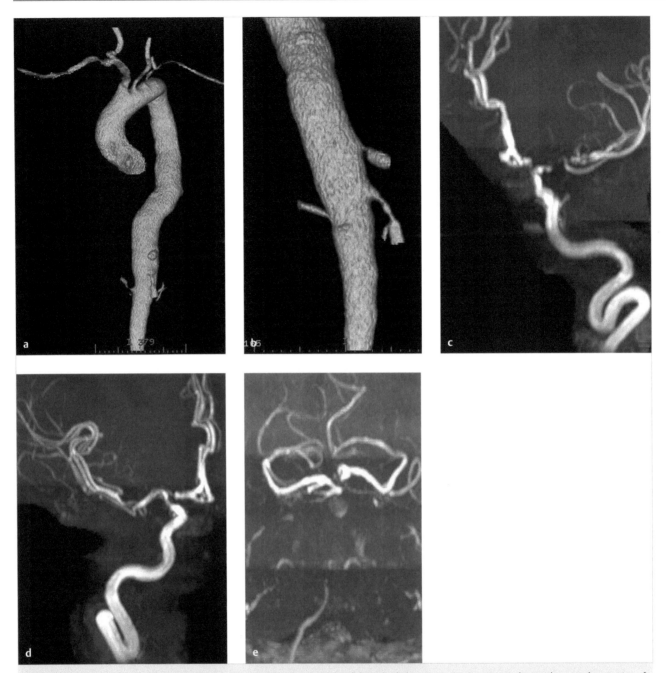

Fig. 2.24 Intracranial involvement of Takayasu's arteritis (**a**) Thoracic aorta has bilateral subclavian artery narrowing and smooth tapered narrowing of the abdominal aorta. (**b**) Abdominal aorta has narrowing at the origins of the celiac trunk and superior mesenteric artery. (**c-e**). MIP images from 3D-TOF MRA demonstrate narrowing of the bilateral ICA terminuses as well as occlusion of the basilar artery. This patient had biopsy proven Takayasu's arteritis.

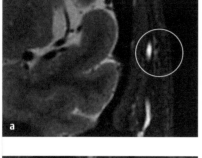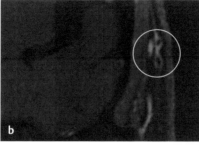
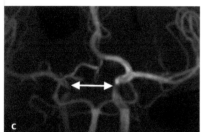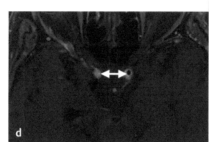

Fig. 2.25 VWI in giant cell arteritis. (**a**) High-resolution T2 image shows fat-stranding surrounding the left STA (*circle*). (**b**) High-resolution post-contrast VWI shows circumferential wall enhancement surrounding the left STA (*circle*). (**c**) MIP image from an MRA shows narrowing of the bilateral cavernous ICAs (*arrows*). (**d**) VWI shows circumferential and robust enhancement of the bilateral cavernous ICAs (*arrows*).

2.6.6 High-Yield Facts

- TA can only be diagnosed in patients who are < 40 years old.
- In GCA, age at disease onset is typically 50 years or older.
- Concentric wall thickening of the common and internal carotid arteries should prompt consideration of an inflammatory etiology such as TA or GCA.
- Unlike atherosclerosis, patients with TA do not develop skip lesions.

Further Reading

[1] Klink T, Geiger J, Both M, et al. Giant cell arteritis: diagnostic accuracy of MR imaging of superficial cranial arteries in initial diagnosis-results from a multicenter trial. Radiology. 2014; 273(3):844–852

[2] Bond KM, Nasr D, Lehman V, Lanzino G, Cloft HJ, Brinjikji W. Intracranial and Extracranial Neurovascular Manifestations of Takayasu Arteritis. AJNR Am J Neuroradiol. 2017; 38(4):766–772

Mpr (1)
MIP:5.8

Fig. 2.26 CTA in giant cell arteritis. When examining CTA images for giant cell arteritis, it is important to make MPRs of the STA. In this case, the MPR showed narrowing of the STA (*inset image*). This site was targeted for biopsy yielding a diagnosis of temporal arteritis.

2.7 Cervical Vascular Causes of Posterior Circulation Ischemia

2.7.1 Clinical Case

A 56-year-old male with recurrent strokes affecting the posterior circulation (▶ Fig. 2.27).

2.7.2 Description of Imaging Findings and Diagnosis

Diagnosis

Focal atherosclerotic narrowing of the left vertebral artery origin with perfusion defect in the posteroinferior left cerebellum.

2.7.3 Background

Atherosclerosis of the vertebral artery is a major cause of ischemic stroke affecting the posterior circulation. The origin of the vertebral artery is the second most common site for atherosclerotic narrowing involving the cerebral vasculature, after the carotid bifurcation. The risk of posterior circulation stroke in patients with vertebral artery stenosis is approximately 0.5% per year, and higher for patients with prior ischemic stroke.

One of the main differential considerations when evaluating steno-occlusive disease of the cervical vertebral artery is cervical vertebral artery dissection. Spontaneous vertebral artery dissections can affect any segment of the cervical vertebral arteries but have a propensity to affect the V3 segment of the vertebral arteries, where the artery is transitioning from a mobile segment into the immobile Atlantal Loop. Epidemiologic factors can be used to differentiate vertebral artery dissection from atherosclerotic disease as dissection patients tend to be younger.

Another cause of posterior circulation ischemia from vertebral artery occlusive disease is Bowhunter's syndrome. Bowhunter's syndrome is also known as rotational occlusion of the vertebral artery resulting in posterior circulation occlusion. In general, Bowhunter's syndrome is due to compression of the dominant vertebral artery by a hypertrophic osteophyte arising from the uncovertebral joint. These patients must have a hypoplastic contralateral vertebral artery and reproducible symptoms during stereotypical movements.

Subclavian steal syndrome is a rare cause of vertebrobasilar insufficiency. Subclavian steal is defined as steno-occlusive disease of the proximal subclavian artery with resultant retrograde flow in the ipsilateral vertebral artery with associated cerebral ischemia. The typical clinical presentation is weak or absent pulse, decreased blood pressure, and arm claudication in the ipsilateral upper limb and posterior circulation ischemic symptoms including dizziness, syncope, ataxia, visual changes, dysparthria, and motor/sensory deficits exacerbated by arm exercise. The most common cause of subclavian steal is atherosclerosis followed by vasculitis and dissection.

2.7.4 Imaging Findings

CT angiography and MR angiography are the two most commonly used noninvasive imaging techniques for the evaluation of vertebral artery origin atherosclerosis and stenosis. However, these studies suffer from substantial limitations. Owing to streak artifact from the clavicles and subclavian veins, it is often difficult to clearly resolve the origin of the vertebral artery on CTA. In general, CTA will overestimate the degree of stenosis and measurements are confounded by the presence of tortuosity at the vertebral artery origin. CE-MRA is probably the imaging modality of choice for the evaluation of vertebral artery stenosis due to the lack of streak artifact and the high contrast resolution, but it suffers from artifacts related to vertebral artery tortuosity. There is currently no reliable technique for plaque characterization of vertebral artery plaques; however, it is generally thought that non-calcified low-density plaques are more dangerous than those which are calcified.

Regarding vertebral artery dissection, the imaging modality of choice is the same as that for carotid dissections: Axial T1 weighted fat-saturated MRI of the neck. This type of imaging allows for clear delineation of the intramural hematoma (▶ Fig. 2.28). CTA is also helpful and can identify imaging signs including a double lumen, mural thickening, or focal narrowing. On CTA, the dissected vertebral artery will often have an irregular, serrated appearance.

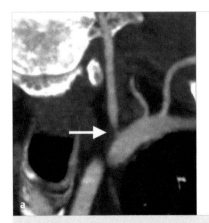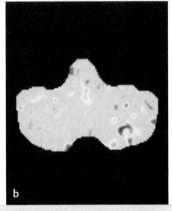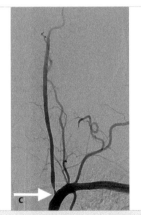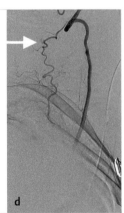

Fig. 2.27 A 56-year-old male with atherosclerotic origin stenosis of the left vertebral artery. (a) Coronal CTA demonstrates a focal atherosclerotic narrowing of the left vertebral artery (*arrow*). (b) CT perfusion mean transit time (MTT) map demonstrates an increased mean transit time in the inferior left cerebellar hemisphere. (c) Left subclavian artery angiogram demonstrates the atherosclerotic narrowing (*arrow*). (d) Lateral projection shows that flow is so slow through the origin stenosis that muscular collaterals from the deep cervical artery are necessary to allow antegrade flow through the left vertebral artery (*arrow*).

Bowhunter's syndrome can be easily diagnosed on noninvasive imaging by performing CTA at resting position and with the head turned toward the position which causes the symptoms. When performing the provocative maneuver, one can often appreciate focal narrowing of the vertebral artery at the site of a large osteophyte or prominent uncovertebral joint. It is key to point out that Bowhunter patients need to have a hypoplastic contralateral vertebral artery in order to develop symptoms. If CTA fails to demonstrate the causal lesion, DSA can be considered (▶ Fig. 2.29).

The subclavian steal syndrome has a very characteristic imaging appearance on noninvasive imaging. When there is a severe stenosis proximal to the origin of the vertebral artery, there is reversal of

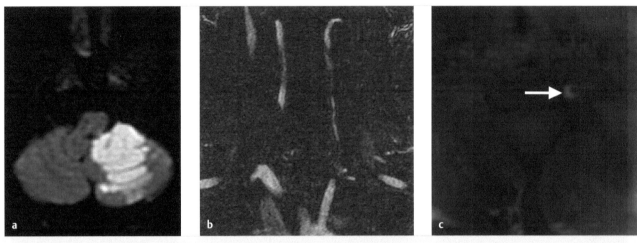

Fig. 2.28 Vertebral dissection after golf swing. (a) DWI MRI shows an infarct in the left posterior inferior cerebellar artery (PICA) territory. (b) Coronal gadolinium bolus MRA shows a string sign of the cervical left vertebral artery. Differential considerations at this point included dissection versus atherosclerosis. (c) Axial T1 fat sat non-contrast MRI of the neck shows a crescentic intramural hematoma consisted with dissection (*arrow*).

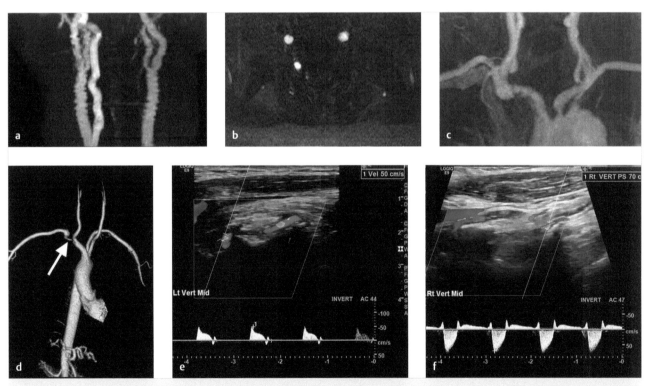

Fig. 2.29 Two patients with subclavian steal. (a) 2D-TOF MRA shows a normal right vertebral artery but absent flow related signal in the left vertebral artery. (b) Axial 2D-TOF MRA again shows normal flow related signal in the right, but not the left, vertebral arteries. (c) Gadolinium bolus MRA performed at the same time as the 2D-TOF MRA shows a stenosis at the origin of the left subclavian artery and a widely patient left vertebral artery. The loss of flow-related signal on the 2D TOF was due to reversal of flow. (d) A second patient with subclavian steal involving the right arm. CTA shows a severe stenosis at the origin of the right subclavian artery (*arrow*). (e) Ultrasound of the left vertebral artery shows normal antegrade flow while (f) ultrasound of the right vertebral artery shows reversal of flow.

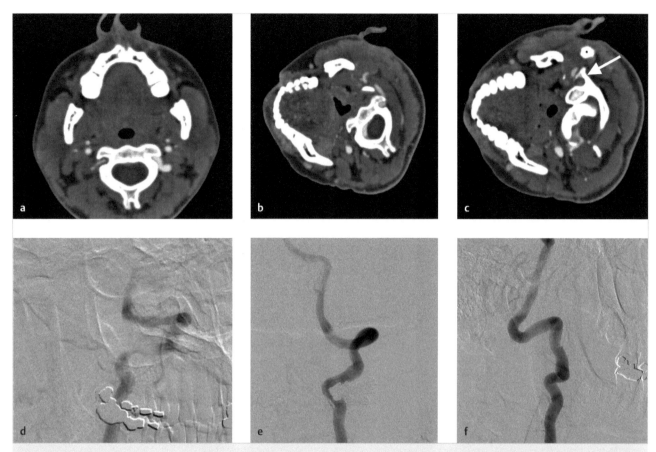

Fig. 2.30 Bowhunter's syndrome in a patient with dizziness and ataxia when turning his head to the right. (**a**) Axial CTA shows a hypoplastic right vertebral artery and large left vertebral artery. (**b**) When turning head to the right there is compression of the left vertebral artery by a small osteophyte. (**c**) One slice above the compression demonstrates no contrast opacification of the left vertebral artery within the foramen transversarium (*arrow*). (**d**) The patient was brought to angiography. With the head turned to the right there was slow flow in the vertebral artery and a focal kink at C2. Head in neutral position (**e**) and turned to the left (**f**) demonstrate a widely patent artery.

vertebral artery flow, which steals blood from the posterior circulation. On ultrasound, this is identified by the reversal of flow in the vertebral artery origin. The diagnosis can be confirmed using a combination of 2D-TOF and gadolinium bolus MRA of the aortic arch and neck. When performing cervical vascular imaging, 2D-TOF protocols are set to detect flow going superiorly (i.e., arterial flow). Thus, the vertebral artery that has retrograde flow will not be bright. However, on gadolinium bolus MRA, the vertebral artery will have a bright signal as long as it is patent. Thus, in the setting of a subclavian stenosis proximal to the vertebral artery, the presence of a vertebral artery on gadolinium bolus MRA along with its absence on 2D-TOF suggests a diagnosis of subclavian steal (▶ Fig. 2.30).

2.7.5 What the Clinician Needs to Know

- Distribution and extent of vascular narrowing as well as maximum degree of stenosis.
- In atherosclerotic lesions, careful examination of the adjacent subclavian artery is needed to identify any atherosclerotic plaques, which can complicate endovascular intervention.
- Clinicians should be aware of the limitations of CTA and MRA in assessment of vertebral origin stenosis.
- Catheter angiography is often the diagnostic test of choice for the evaluation of severe, symptomatic vertebrobasilar ischemia, and insufficiency.

2.7.6 High-Yield Facts

- Lesions affecting the vertebral artery origin are usually atherosclerotic in etiology.
- Cervical vertebral artery dissections commonly affect the V3 segment of the artery.
- Bowhunter's syndrome can be easily diagnosed using a combination of clinical criteria as well as noninvasive imaging using CTA with provocative maneuvers.
- The subclavian steal syndrome can be diagnosed when a vertebral artery is not apparent on 2D-TOF but is apparent on gadolinium bolus MRA.

Further Reading

[1] Khan S, Rich P, Clifton A, Markus HS. Noninvasive detection of vertebral artery stenosis: a comparison of contrast-enhanced MR angiography, CT angiography, and ultrasound. Stroke. 2009; 40(11):3499–3503

[2] Tahmasebpour HR, Buckley AR, Cooperberg PL, Fix CH. Sonographic examination of the carotid arteries. Radiographics. 2005; 25(6):1561–1575

[3] Taylor WB, III, Vandergriff CL, Opatowsky MJ, Layton KF. Bowhunter's syndrome diagnosed with provocative digital subtraction cerebral angiography. Proc Bayl Univ Med Cent. 2012; 25(1):26–27

Chapter 3

Intracranial Steno-Occlusive Disease

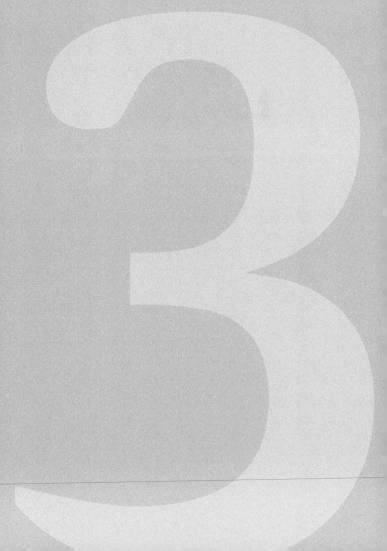

3 Intracranial Steno-Occlusive Disease

3.1 Moyamoya Disease

3.1.1 Clinical Case

A 23-year-old female with mild right arm weakness and headache (▶ Fig. 3.1).

3.1.2 Description of Imaging Findings and Diagnosis

Diagnosis

Watershed infarct in the left cerebral hemisphere. High FLAIR signal in the pial arteries over the left hemisphere with sulcal hyperintensity. Absence of MCA flow void on the left. Angiogram confirms diagnosis of moyamoya.

3.1.3 Background

Moyamoya disease is an idiopathic steno-occlusive disease primarily affecting the terminus of the internal carotid artery and proximal anterior and middle cerebral arteries. The disease is histopathologically characterized by intimal hyperplasia and medial thinning. Intimal hyperplasia is caused by the proliferation of smooth muscle cells. The medial thinning is secondary to the degradation and apoptosis of smooth muscle cells and the degradation of connective tissue matrix from matrix metalloproteinase activity. Vessel occlusion occurs as a result of intimal hyperplasia and luminal thrombosis. Moyamoya collaterals are dilated perforating arteries that represent a combination of preexisting lenticulostriate perforators and newly developed vessels. Owing to increased flow, these arteries have fragmented elastic lamina, thinned media, and are prone to microaneurysm formation, which can result in hemorrhage.

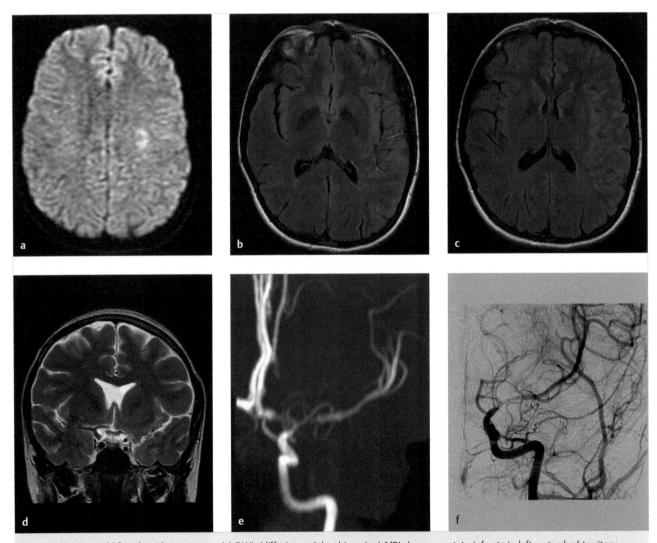

Fig. 3.1 A 23-year-old female with moyamoya. (**a**) DWI (diffusion weighted imaging) MRI shows punctate infarcts in left watershed territory. (**b**) T2/FLAIR (fluid attenuation inversion recovery) MRI shows hyperintensity in the distal left MCA vessels. (**c**) Axial T2/FLAIR MRI shows sulcal hyperintensity as well. (**d**) Coronal T2 MRI shows the loss of normal left MCA and ICA flow voids. (**e**) TOF MRA shows typical ICA terminus occlusion of moyamoya. (**f**) Left common carotid artery (CCA) angiogram shows narrowing of left ICA terminus and proximal M1 and A1 segments.

Moyamoya has a bimodal age distribution with an early childhood peak and a middle age peak. Approximately, 70% of moyamoya patients present during childhood. The disease is more common in, but not exclusive to, the East Asian populations. In children, ischemic stroke is the primary presentation while in adults the primary presentation is that of intracranial hemorrhage. Moyamoya disease is idiopathic and sometimes familial. Moyamoya syndrome is secondary to conditions such as radiation induced vasculopathy, NF1, Down's syndrome, tuberous sclerosis, and sickle-cell disease.

3.1.4 Imaging Findings

Moyamoya disease is often first identified using standard MRI protocols without the aid of vascular imaging (▶ Fig. 3.2). On T2-weighted imaging there is often loss of the normal M1 segment flow voids, greater than the normal degree of flow voids in the basal ganglia and sulcal FLAIR hyperintensity consistent with the "ivy sign." The areas of sulcal FLAIR hyperintensity are usually accompanied by enhancement on post-contrast imaging and are reflective of slow filling leptomeningeal collaterals that can also be seen in other condition of slow flow in the distal vasculature. Younger moyamoya patients often present with signs of cerebral ischemia including watershed infarcts and/or chronic cortical infarctions affecting the external watershed zones.

Both MRA and CTA are useful imaging modalities in evaluating the angioarchitecture of moyamoya disease. In 80% of cases, moyamoya disease is bilateral and affects the ICA termini. In 20% of cases, moyamoya disease is unilateral. In cases in which moyamoya disease is bilateral, it is possible that the disease state could be at different stages of progression on each side (▶ Fig. 3.3). One of the key distinguishing features of moyamoya disease is the presence of robust lenticulostriate collaterals, which create a "puff of smoke" appearance. There are sometimes robust choroidal collaterals as well. It is important to point out that lenticulostriate collaterals are not always present in moyamoya, particularly in early and advanced cases. In advanced cases, there will be occlusion of the supraclinoid ICA with much of the intracranial blood supply provided by the vertebrobasilar system and external carotid arteries.

Collateral vessels should be closely inspected to evaluate the presence of microaneurysms, which can rupture and result in hemorrhage. Intraparenchymal hemorrhage in moyamoya is often the result of a ruptured lenticulostriate collateral aneurysm, whereas intraventricular hemorrhage is usually the result of a ruptured distal choroidal artery aneurysms. Hemorrhage is the most common presentation for elderly patients with moyamoya (▶ Fig. 3.4).

There is overlap in the appearance of moyamoya with other steno-occlusive diseases such as atherosclerosis and vasculitis. High-resolution vessel wall imaging (VWI) with MRI has emerged as a useful tool to differentiate these entities. Several studies comparing the HR-VWI characteristics of moyamoya disease and intracranial atherosclerosis have demonstrated that these two diseases can in most cases be readily distinguished. Unlike atherosclerosis, moyamoya disease is often characterized by mild concentric vessel wall enhancement in the acute phase or no enhancement at all in the subacute phase. Moyamoya disease seems to lack the thicker enhancement patterns seen with vasculitis as well. Concentric wall enhancement in the distal ICA and proximal MCA is present in 90% of moyamoya disease patients, involving both symptomatic and asymptomatic segments with the degree of enhancement is generally lower than that seen with atherosclerosis. It has been suggested that the concentric enhancement may result from the intimal hyperplasia, although it is possibly also due to the associated inflammation. Moyamoya disease is typically characterized by negative remodeling (i.e., vessel wall thinning/shrinking), whereas atherosclerosis more commonly demonstrates positive remodeling (vessel wall thickening). Areas of negative remodeling and vessel obliteration demonstrate variable degrees of enhancement (▶ Fig. 3.5).

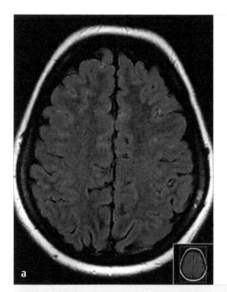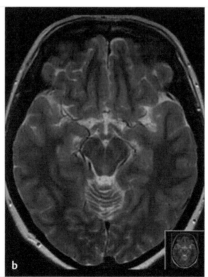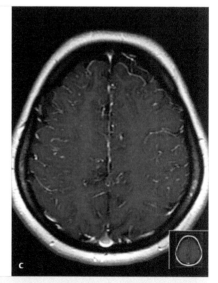

Fig. 3.2 Bilateral Moyamoya on MRI. (**a**) Axial T2/FLAIR MRI shows sulcal hyperintensity from slow flow of leptomeningeal vessels. (**b**) Axial T2 weighted MRI shows absent bilateral MCA flow voids. (**c**) Axial post-contrast MRI shows sulcal enhancement, also related to slow flow from leptomeningeal collaterals.

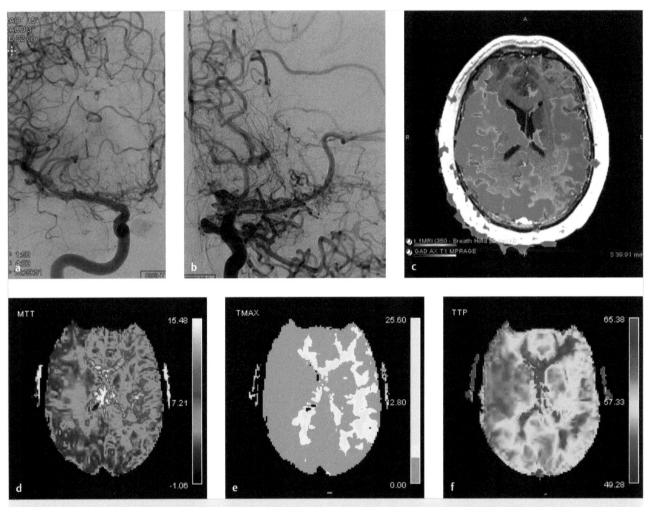

Fig. 3.3 Moyamoya at different stages. (**a–b**) Right ICA angiogram shows occlusion of the right anterior cerebral artery (ACA), which is now supplied by lenticulostriate collaterals, but a patient MCA. Left ICA angiogram shows occlusion of both the ACA and MCA with puff of smoke lenticulostriate collaterals supplying the distal left MCA. (**c**) Cerebrovascular reserve study using breath-hold technique shows decreased cerebral vascular reserve (CVR) in the left MCA territory but normal CVR in the right hemisphere. (**d–f**) Dynamic susceptibility contrast MR perfusion studies show decreased perfusion in the left MCA territory on MTT, $T_{max,}$ and time to peak (TTP) maps.

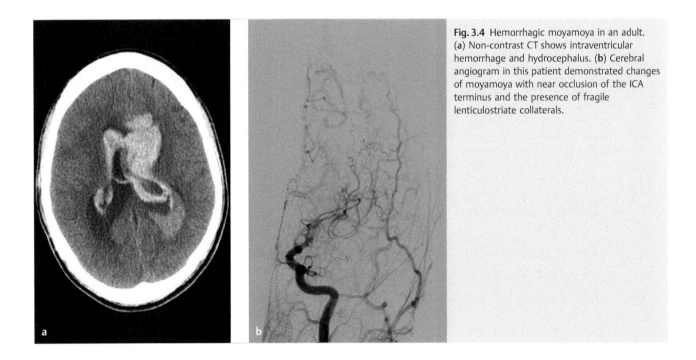

Fig. 3.4 Hemorrhagic moyamoya in an adult. (**a**) Non-contrast CT shows intraventricular hemorrhage and hydrocephalus. (**b**) Cerebral angiogram in this patient demonstrated changes of moyamoya with near occlusion of the ICA terminus and the presence of fragile lenticulostriate collaterals.

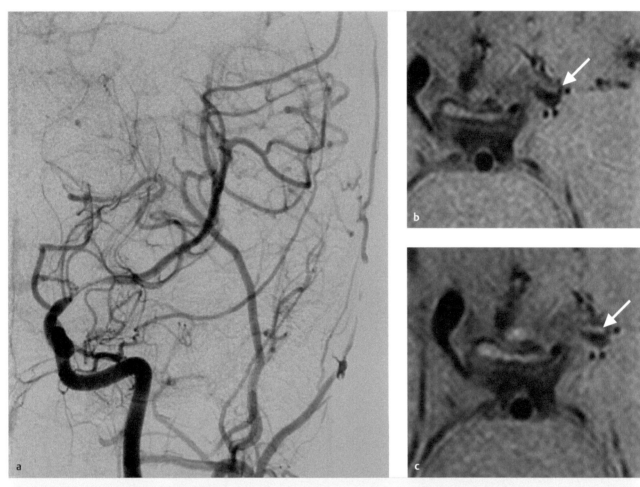

Fig. 3.5 VWI in moyamoya. (a) Left ICA angiogram shows changes of moyamoya with high-grade stenosis of the left ICA terminus. (b) Pre- and (c) post-contrast VWI study shows minimal faint enhancement of the left ICA terminus and negative remodeling (i.e., shrinkage) of the vessel (arrows).

Table 3.1 Suzuki Stages of Moyamoya

Stage	Angiographic Description
I	Stenosis of ICA bifurcation
II	Dilated ACA, MCA, and narrowed ICA bifurcation with moyamoya changes
III	Stenosis of MCA and ACAs with increased moyamoya vessels
IV	Disappearance of MCA and ACA with fine moyamoya vessels
V	Disappearing intracerebral portion of ICA with shrinking moyamoya vessels
VI	Disappearance of moyamoya vessels with collateral formation from ECA only

Abbreviations: ICA, Internal carotid artery; ACA, Anterior cerebral artery; MCA, Middle carotid artery; ECA, External carotid artery.

3.1.5 What the Clinician Needs to Know

- General information regarding Suzuki stages of each affected vessel in moyamoya disease (▶ Table 3.1)
- Presence and location of aneurysms affecting collateral vessels
- Evidence of prior ischemic injury including internal and external watershed territories
- Impaired cerebrovascular reserve

- Size of superficial temporal artery (STA) and occipital artery on affected sides for bypass planning

3.1.6 High-Yield Facts

- Moyamoya disease in the young typically presents with ischemia, whereas moyamoya disease in the elderly presents with hemorrhage.
- Aneurysms affecting the lenticulostriate and choroidal collaterals are a well-known cause of hemorrhage in moyamoya patients.
- Typical MRI findings include the loss of T2 flow voids in the MCAs, robust flow voids in the basal ganglia.

Further Reading

[1] Suzuki J, Takaku A. Cerebrovascular "moyamoya" disease. Disease showing abnormal net-like vessels in base of brain. Arch Neurol. 1969; 20(3): 288–299

[2] Horie N, Morikawa M, Nozaki A, Hayashi K, Suyama K, Nagata I. "Brush Sign" on susceptibility-weighted MR imaging indicates the severity of moyamoya disease. AJNR Am J Neuroradiol. 2011; 32(9):1697–1702

[3] Brinjikji W, Mossa-Basha M, Huston J, Rabinstein AA, Lanzino G, Lehman VT. Intracranial vessel wall imaging for evaluation of steno-occlusive diseases and intracranial aneurysms. J Neuroradiol. 2017; 44(2):123–134

3.2 Intracranial Atherosclerosis

3.2.1 Clinical Case

A 73-year-old male with recurrent posterior circulation ischemic stroke (▶ Fig. 3.6).

3.2.2 Description of Imaging Findings and Diagnosis

Diagnosis

Stenosis of the mid basilar artery with a vulnerable enhancing plaque. Strokes are likely secondary to embolic phenomenon related to the vulnerable plaque.

3.2.3 Background

Intracranial atherosclerosis is the most common cause of intracranial vessel narrowing in the adult population. Atherosclerosis is most commonly seen in adult patients with cardiovascular risk factors. It is more common in East Asian and African populations than in Caucasian populations and is thought to be one of the most common causes of stroke worldwide. Intracranial atherosclerosis can affect a single large vessel segment (supraclinoid ICA, M1 segment, basilar artery, etc.), be bilateral and appear similar to moyamoya or have multifocal involvement of large- and medium-sized vessels with an imaging appearance similar to CNS vasculitis.

It is important to understand the histological characteristics of intracranial atherosclerosis in order to better understand imaging appearance. Traditionally, intracranial atherosclerosis

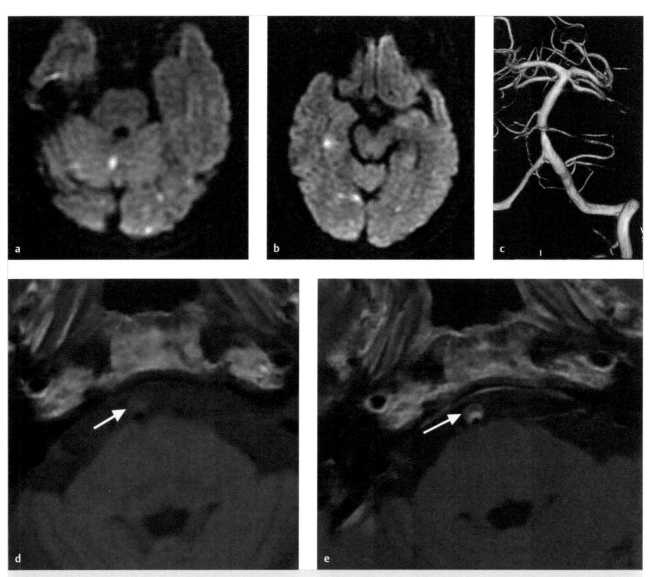

Fig. 3.6 A 73-year-old male with recurrent embolic posterior circulation strokes secondary to vulnerable plaque. (**a**) and (**b**) Axial DWI MRI shows multiple posterior circulation infarcts involving the cerebellum, hippocampus, and bilateral occipital lobe. (**c**) CTA demonstrates a high-grade stenosis of the mid basilar artery. (**d**) Pre-contrast high-resolution VWI shows an eccentric atherosclerotic plaque of the mid basilar artery (*arrow*). (**e**) Post-contrast MRI shows the robust enhancement of the plaque suggesting that this is an active, hot plaque (*arrow*).

was thought to occur as a result of endothelial dysfunction resulting in the infiltration of lipids into the intima, vascular wall inflammation, and remodeling. Recent evidence suggests that the vasa vasorum and adventitia are key players in the development of intracranial atherosclerosis as the vasa vasorum are responsible for transporting inflammatory cells to the adventitia, thus initiating and perpetuating inflammatory cascades. This assertion is supported by histologic and imaging studies, which demonstrate the proliferation of vasa vasorum in patients with intracranial atherosclerotic disease. Histologic studies demonstrate that atherosclerotic plaques with intraplaque hemorrhage, lipid-rich necrotic core, and other unstable features have increased the proliferation of fragile vasa vasorum, suggesting that vasa vasorum are involved in plaque progression. Vasa vasorum proliferation plays a key role in the positive remodeling (i.e., wall thickening) seen on HR-VWI of intracranial atherosclerotic diseases.

3.2.4 Imaging Findings

Conventional luminal imaging techniques (i.e., CTA, Digital Subtraction Angiography [DSA], and MRA) are nonspecific in the evaluation of intracranial atherosclerotic disease. The typical imaging manifestation is a focal area of narrowing involving an intracranial vessel. The most common locations include the cavernous/supraclinoid ICA, vertebral artery, and basilar artery. However, atherosclerosis can affect any intracranial vessel. When evaluating any imaging modality for intracranial atherosclerosis the three most important factors the neuroradiologist should consider are (1) the mechanism of stroke, (2) the degree of stenosis, and (3) the vulnerability and location of the plaque. Intracranial atherosclerosis can result in stroke due to (1) occlusion of perforator vessels (i.e., brainstem perforator or lenticulostriates) (▶ Fig. 3.7), (2) emboli from a vulnerable plaque (▶ Fig. 3.6), or (3) hemodynamic "watershed-type" infarcts due to flow limitation from high degree of stenosis (▶ Fig. 3.8).

CTA and MRA are the two most commonly used imaging techniques for evaluating intracranial atherosclerosis. These techniques allow for the assessment of degree of stenosis and location/length of the plaque. When reviewing CTA/MRA images, careful attention should be paid to determine the relationship of the plaque/narrowing to the perforating vessels. Stenosis degree should be measured. The technique for measuring the degree of stenosis in intracranial atherosclerosis is the WASID criteria.

CTA allows for the excellent delineation of intracranial artery anatomy and is more accurate than MRA in assessing luminal stenosis. However, CTA has limitations related to bony artifacts when evaluating the cavernous ICAs. CTA, particularly multiphase CTA, is a potentially useful tool in the assessment of collateral blood flow in patients with intracranial atherosclerosis. TOF-MRA and contrast-enhanced MRA are commonly used in the evaluation of intracranial atherosclerosis. TOF-MRA generally overestimates the degree of stenosis as low-flow distal to the lesion can result in signal loss. However, there is value in seeing the loss of flow signal distal to a lesion as it highly suggests that the lesion is flow limiting. Contrast MRA is less susceptible to flow-related artifacts.

Perfusion imaging is essential to imaging intracranial atherosclerosis as hypoperfusion is a common cause of stroke in these patients. CTP and MR perfusion studies can be used to identify hypoperfused areas that could be potentially salvageable with revascularization therapies (▶ Fig. 3.9).

High-resolution VWI has been shown to be a valuable tool in the evaluation of intracranial atherosclerosis (▶ Fig. 3.6, ▶ Fig. 3.7, ▶ Fig. 3.8, ▶ Fig. 3.9). Typically, atherosclerotic plaque appears as eccentric wall thickening and enhancement. Intrinsic high T1 signal on fat saturated T1-sequences (50% higher than temporalis muscle) represents intraplaque hemorrhage. T2-weighted HR-VWI can also be used to characterize these lesions as most lesions have a thin juxtaluminal band of T2 hyperintensity with an underlying T2 hypointense component. This thin juxtaluminal band presumably represents a fibrous cap. T2 hypointense internal areas have been shown to correlate with areas of foamy macrophages on pathologic specimens imaged at 7 Tesla with a dedicated surface coil. Positive remodeling, which occurs in a majority of cases of atherosclerosis, is essentially wall thickening due to adventitial proliferation and intraplaque hemorrhage, whereas negative remodeling is reflective of shrinkage of the vessel wall. Positive remodeling has been associated with vulnerable plaques and can be present in the absence of stenotic disease. It is important to realize that non-stenotic intracranial atherosclerosis can result in symptoms from obstruction of lenticulostriate ostia along the superior aspect of the MCA and rupture of non-stenotic plaque resulting in distal emboli.

In addition to its value in the diagnosis of intracranial atherosclerosis, HR-VWI is also a valuable tool in the identification of vulnerable and culprit plaques. Studies strongly suggest that enhancement characteristics and extent of remodeling of intracranial atheromatous plaques can serve as biomarkers of plaque activity. Current evidence indicates that all symptomatic atherosclerotic plaques enhance, whereas asymptomatic plaques variably enhance. In fact, plaque enhancement is associated with a 35-times higher odds of symptomatic status. Degree of enhancement of symptomatic plaque seems to decrease over a period of weeks following an acute ischemic stroke. Enhancement characteristics can help identify culprit plaques in patients with acute ischemic stroke.

3.2.5 What the Clinician Needs to Know

- Degree of stenosis and downstream perfusion status determined with either perfusion imaging or multiphase CTA
- Plaque characteristics including enhancement and intrinsic T1 signal
- Plaque location in relation to smaller perforator vessels (i.e., lenticulostriates, brainstem perforators, etc.)
- Do the location and characteristic of the plaque correlate with the type of stroke the patient has?

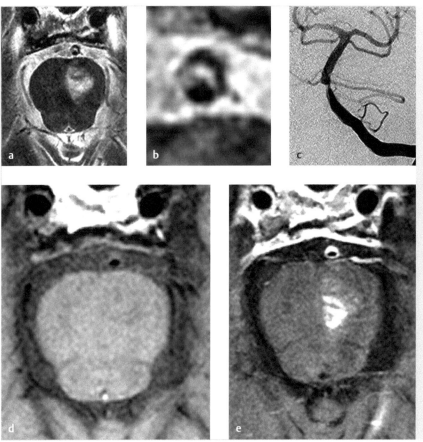

Fig. 3.7 Basilar artery atherosclerotic plaque resulting in brainstem perforator infarct. (a) High-resolution T2 weighted VWI MRI shows a brainstem perforator infarct. Note the hyperintense fibrous cap. (b) Magnified view of the basilar artery shows a small perforator arising from the vessel at the location of the plaque. Essentially, the plaque began to involve the origin of the perforator vessel thus resulting in the perforator infarct. (c) Conventional angiogram shows the focal severe narrowing and the proximity of multiple perforator vessels to the plaque. (d) Pre-contrast T1 VWI shows the plaque with positive vessel wall remodeling. (e) Post-contrast T1-W VWI shows the robust enhancement of the plaque suggesting it is a vulnerable and active plaque.

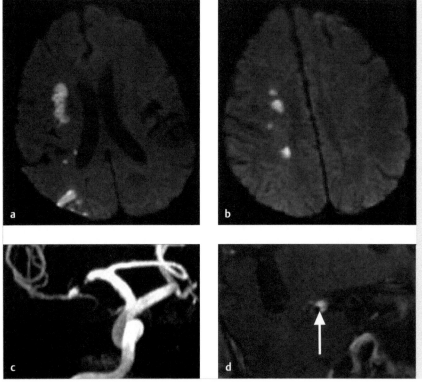

Fig. 3.8 Watershed infarcts from right MCA stenosis. (a) and (b). DWI MRI shows watershed infarcts in the right MCA territory. (c) MRA shows a focal stenosis of the distal M1. (d) Post-contrast VWI MRI shows positive vessel wall remodeling and robust plaque enhancement consistent with a vulnerable and active plaque (arrow).

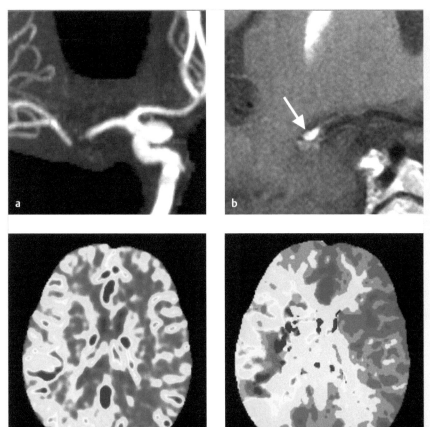

Fig. 3.9 Right MCA perfusion defect in setting of active atheromatous plaque. (a) MRA shows a high-grade stenosis of the distal right MCA. (b) VWI MRI shows enhancement of a nodular plaque at the distal right MCA. (c) CBV map shows increased CBV in the sulci of the right MCA territory related to vessel engorgement of leptomeningeal collaterals. (d) T_{max} map shows increased T_{max} in the whole right MCA territory consistent with hypoperfusion.

3.2.6 High-Yield Facts

- Intracranial atherosclerosis can be present in the absent of any degree of stenosis and vulnerable plaques can have substantial positive remodeling.
- Plaque morphology and stability, collateral status, and downstream perfusion status are as important as the degree of stenosis in risk stratification of intracranial atherosclerosis.
- Enhancing plaques on VWI-MRI are associated with higher rates of future embolic events.

Further Reading

[1] Brinjikji W, Mossa-Basha M, Huston J, Rabinstein AA, Lanzino G, Lehman VT. Intracranial vessel wall imaging for evaluation of steno-occlusive diseases and intracranial aneurysms. J Neuroradiol. 2017; 44(2):123–134

[2] Yu JH, Kwak HS, Chung GH, Hwang SB, Park MS, Park SH. Association of Intraplaque Hemorrhage and Acute Infarction in Patients With Basilar Artery Plaque. Stroke. 2015; 46(10):2768–2772

[3] Majidi S, Sein J, Watanabe M, et al. Intracranial-derived atherosclerosis assessment: an in vitro comparison between virtual histology by intravascular ultrasonography, 7 T MRI, and histopathologic findings. AJNR Am J Neuroradiol. 2013; 34(12):2259–2264

3.3 Intracranial Dissection

3.3.1 Clinical Case

A 45-year-old female with sudden onset neck pain and severe headache (▶ Fig. 3.10).

3.3.2 Description of Imaging Findings and Diagnosis

Diagnosis

Focal narrowing of the intradural right vertebral artery. Intrinsic high T1 signal in the vessel wall without any enhancement. Findings consistent with intracranial dissection.

3.3.3 Background

Spontaneous intracranial arterial dissections (IADs) are thought to represent an uncommon but underdiagnosed cause of stroke. The prevalence of IAD is highly variable depending on the population as it only represents a small minority of all cervicocephalic dissections in European populations but a majority of dissections in Asian populations. Intracranial dissections can affect both pediatric and adult populations and the mean age at presentation is about 50 years. A vast majority of intracranial

dissections affect the posterior circulation with the V4 segment of the vertebral artery being the most common site. Bilateral V4 segment IAD affects up to 10% of patients.

IADs can present with headache (80%), cerebral ischemia (30–50%), or subarachnoid hemorrhage (SAH) (30–50%). A combination of SAH and ischemia at time of presentation is exceedingly rare. IADs resulting in stenotic disease are histopathologically characterized by disruption of the endothelium, intima, and internal elastic lamina with the penetration of blood in between the vessel wall planes with longitudinal extension. Stenosis and occlusion of the parent vessel in the setting of dissection is the result of a subintimal or subadventitial hematoma causing mass effect on the lumen. Mural hematoma can also involve and occlude perforating vessels. Reopening of the lumen distal to the entry site can result in distal embolism, resulting in acute ischemic stroke. Dissections resulting in SAH are due to penetration of blood into the subadventitial space or through the adventitia.

3.3.4 Imaging Findings

Examples of ways in which intracranial dissections can present are provided in figures ▶ Fig. 3.11, ▶ Fig. 3.12, ▶ Fig. 3.13, ▶ Fig. 3.14. Specific diagnostic criteria for intracranial dissections have been put forth and are summarized in ▶ Table 3.2. Factors that can differentiate intracranial dissection from other

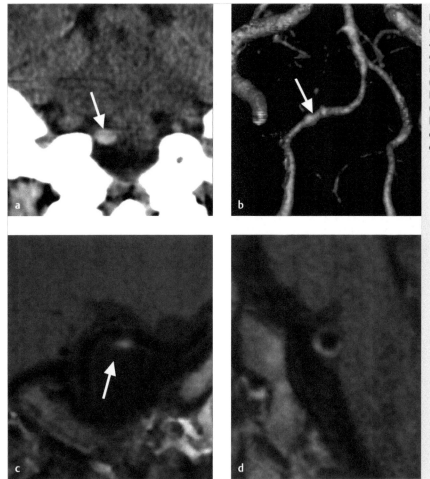

Fig. 3.10 Intradural vertebral artery dissection. (a) Non-contrast CT shows a focal hyperdensity adjacent to the right medulla (*arrow*). (b) CTA demonstrates a string of beads pattern of the intradural right vertebral artery (*arrow*). (c) Oblique sagittal T1 pre-contrast VWI shows high T1 signal in the vessel wall (*arrow*). (d) Sagittal T1 pre-contrast VWI MRI shows high T1 signal in the vessel wall confirming the diagnosis of an intradural vertebral artery dissection with intramural hematoma.

occlusive or dilated arteriopathies are present in ▸ Table 3.3. On luminal imaging, intracranial dissections have a wide range of manifestations including the appearance of a double lumen, fusiform aneurysmal dilatation, pseudoaneurysm formation, luminal narrowing, and occlusion. Ultimately, some of these imaging appearances may be nonspecific on conventional imaging as there is a broad differential diagnosis for focal aneurysmal dilatations, stenosis, and occlusions, including poststenotic dilatation in the setting of atheromatous disease. While subintimal dissections are readily recognizable on luminal imaging from the appearance of the true and false lumen, subadventitial dissections may be more difficult to detect and diagnose.

T1 weighted HR-VWI has been shown to be helpful in the detection of high signal intramural hematoma associated with subadventitial dissections. HR-VWI has also been shown to be sensitive in detecting characteristics such as intimal flap and double lumen, findings which are specific to dissection. Vessel wall contrast enhancement is sometimes seen in intracranial dissection and is thought to be secondary to a combination of slow blood flow in the false lumen, inflammation, and enhancement of the vasa vasorum. Whereas both dissections and atherosclerotic plaque with intraplaque hemorrhage can demonstrate luminal narrowing with T1 hyperintensity, and eccentric vessel wall enhancement, other findings including an intimal flap, double lumen, or clear crescentic false lumen should indicate dissection. T2 W VWI has also been shown to be useful in characterizing intracranial dissections as the intramural hematoma can demonstrate hyperintensity or hypointensity depending on the age of the dissection. High-resolution susceptibility weighted imaging has a high sensitivity for detecting intramural hematoma.

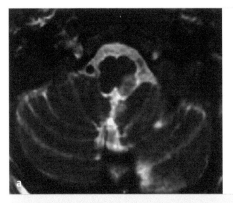 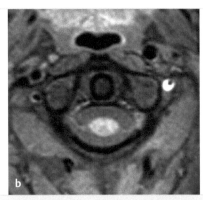 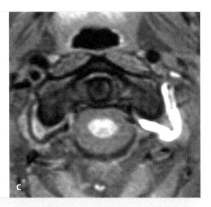

Fig. 3.11 Lateral medullary infarct secondary to dissection involving the medullary perforators. (**a**) T2 weighted MRI shows a lateral medullary infarct. (**b-c**). T1 pre-contrast MRI with fat saturation shows a dissection involving the distal vertebral artery with intramural hematoma.

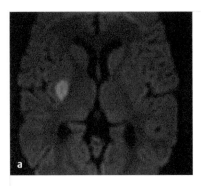 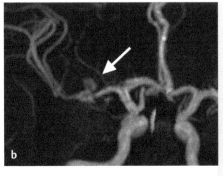

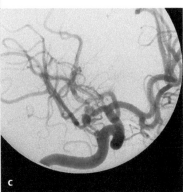 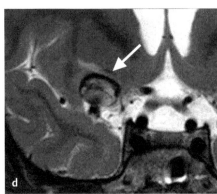

Fig. 3.12 Rapid remodeling of a dissection into a partially thrombosed aneurysm. (**a**) A 12-year-old child presented with sudden onset left-sided hemiparesis secondary to basal ganglia infarct. (**b**) TOF MRA shows a focal narrowing of the distal right MCA with a post-stenotic aneurysmal dilatation and another narrowing extending to the M2 s (*arrow*). (**c**) Conventional angiogram confirms the presence of the MCA dissection and associated aneurysm. (**d**) Two years later, the aneurysm continued to grow. At this point, it is a partially thrombosed aneurysm (*arrow*).

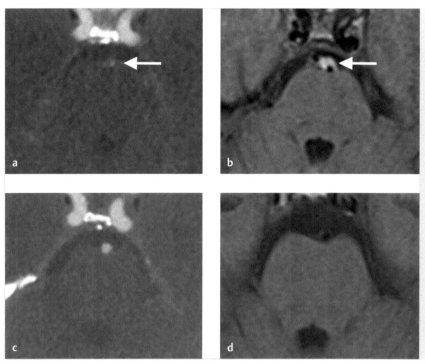

Fig. 3.13 Basilar artery dissection which spontaneously healed on aspirin. (**a**) CTA demonstrates a high-grade stenosis of the basilar artery (*arrow*). (**b**) T1 pre-contrast MRI demonstrates high intramural T1 signal consistent with dissection (*arrow*). (**c**) Four months later, the vessel spontaneously recanalized and (**d**) the intramural hematoma resolved.

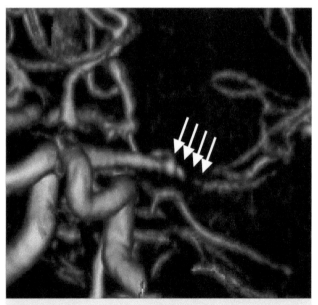

Fig. 3.14 Intracranial M1 dissection with string of beads appearance in a patient with Marfan's syndrome (*arrows*).

Table 3.2 Diagnostic Criteria for Intracranial Dissection

One of the following three features should be present

1. Fusiform or irregular dilatation at a non-branching site of an intracranil artery with at least one of the following criteria

    Intramural hematoma

    Intimal flap

    Double lumen

    Rapid change in morphology

    Focal stenosis or string of pearls sign

2. Long filiform or irregular stenosis of an intracranial artery with at least one of the following criteria

    Intramural hematoma

    Intimal flap

    Double lumen

    Rapid change in morphology

    Focal stenosis or string of pearls sign

3. Occlusion of an intracranial artery that recanalizes in either a fusiform or irregular aneurysmal dilatation at a non-branching site or a long filiform irregular stenosis

3.3.5 What the Clinician Needs to Know

- Imaging sequelae of intracranial dissection including infarction or SAH.
- Proximity of the dissected vessels to smaller perforator vessels (i.e., lateral medullary perforators, brainstem perforators, and lenticulostriates).
- Degree of luminal compromise and presence of intraluminal thrombus, which can result in further ischemic stroke.

Studies on the serial imaging of untreated IADs have shown that these lesions heal in multiple ways including focal aneurysmal dilatation, persistent stenosis or occlusion, or recanalization and normalization of vessel caliber. Serial imaging with HR-VWI and MRA may prove useful to follow the remodeling process.

Table 3.3 Factors Differentiating Intracranial Dissection from Other Arteriopathies

Differential Diagnosis	Factor Favoring Intracranial Dissection
Atherosclerotic stenosis	Isolated stenosis, rapid change in degree of stenosis, or development of aneurysmal dilatation, young age
Vasospasm due to subarachnoid haemorrhage	Intracranial arterial narrowing on the day of ictus
Reversible cerebral vasoconstriction syndrome	Narrowing of one, rather than multiple arteries, stenosis persisting > 3 months, dynamic change in lesion, mural hematoma
Vasculitis	Narrowing of one rather than multiple arteries, no vessel wall enhancement, mural hematoma
Fusiform aneurysm without dissection	Acute symptoms, mural hematoma, dynamic change in lesion, double lumen, or intimal flap
Dolichoectasia	Acute symptoms, mural hematoma, dynamic change in lesion, double lumen, or intimal flap
Thromboembolic occlusion	Mural hematoma or recanalization with long segment stenosis, fusiform aneurysm, string of pearls sign, or intimal flap/double lumen
Transient cerebral arteriopathy	Mural hematoma. TCA typically presents with enhancement

Abbreviation: TCA, Transverse cervical artery.

- Key differentiators of intracranial dissection from other possible etiologies of focal stenosis or dilatation of an intracranial vessel.
- Intracranial dissection has a substantially higher prevalence and incidence in Asian populations when compared to Caucasian populations.

3.3.6 High-Yield Facts

- Unruptured intracranial dissections at presentation (i.e., those with headache or ischemic stroke only) rarely rupture. Meanwhile, ruptured intracranial dissections have a high rate of re-hemorrhage.
- Intramural hematoma is the primary differentiator of IAD from other forms of steno-occlusive disease.
- Dissecting aneurysms presenting with hemorrhage rarely have associated intramural hematoma.

Further Reading

[1] Debette S, Compter A, Labeyrie MA, et al. Epidemiology, pathophysiology, diagnosis, and management of intracranial artery dissection. Lancet Neurol. 2015; 14(6):640–654

[2] Krings T, Choi IS. The many faces of intracranial arterial dissections. Interv Neuroradiol. 2010; 16(2):151–160

[3] Brinjikji W, Mossa-Basha M, Huston J, Rabinstein AA, Lanzino G, Lehman VT. Intracranial vessel wall imaging for evaluation of steno-occlusive diseases and intracranial aneurysms. J Neuroradiol. 2017; 44(2):123–134

3.4 Reversible Cerebral Vasoconstriction Syndrome (RCVS)

3.4.1 Clinical Case

A 44-year-old female severe thunderclap headache (▶ Fig. 3.15).

3.4.2 Description of Imaging Findings and Diagnosis

Diagnosis

Multifocal intracranial stenoses involving the distal cerebral vasculature. Given age, clinical presentation, and imaging findings, differential diagnoses included RCVS and vasculitis.

3.4.3 Background

Reversible cerebral vasoconstriction syndrome, also known as Call-Fleming syndrome, is an increasingly recognized cause of thunderclap headache and delayed ischemia, particularly in younger adults. Thunderclap headache is occasionally accompanied by seizures and focal neurological symptoms. In a vast majority of patients, the symptoms resolve spontaneously over 2–3 weeks and demonstrate significant improvement, when patients receive calcium channel blockers. Permanent neurological deficits or death are very rare. While many cases remain idiopathic, known predisposing factors or overlapping disease entities for RCVS include pre-eclampsia/eclampsia, recreational drug abuse, decongestants, migraine medications, and sexual activity. RCVS is a diagnosis of exclusion and other causes of vascular narrowing and SAH should be ruled out. Work-up should include CT and CTA, lumbar puncture, and MRI. A detailed clinical history should be obtained and f/u imaging may be of importance.

RCVS is thought to result from alterations in cerebrovascular tone secondary to various exogenous and endogenous factors. Experimental studies demonstrate that the vasospasm is the result of shortening and overlapping smooth muscle cells resulting in wall thickening and luminal stenosis. Arterial inflammation is absent in RCVS. The disease typically affects small- and medium-sized arteries in the first stages of the disease and then subsequently affects more proximal and larger vessels.

3.4.4 Imaging Findings

On conventional luminal imaging, RCVS is often characterized by vasoconstriction affecting multiple vascular territories with a beaded appearance of medium- and large-sized arteries. However, within the first 5 days of presentation, angiographic evaluation can be unremarkable. In up to one-third of patients, there is no vasoconstriction for up to 1 week. Over time (weeks), the vasospastic changes of RCVS can progress in a centripetal direction (i.e., from distal vessels to proximal/circle of Willis vessels). The key differentiator between RCVS and other causes of vascular narrowing is the fact that RCVS resolves over the course of a few weeks and demonstrates resolution when being treated with calcium antagonists (▶ Fig. 3.15). On non-contrast CT, a small amount of distal/sulcal SAH can

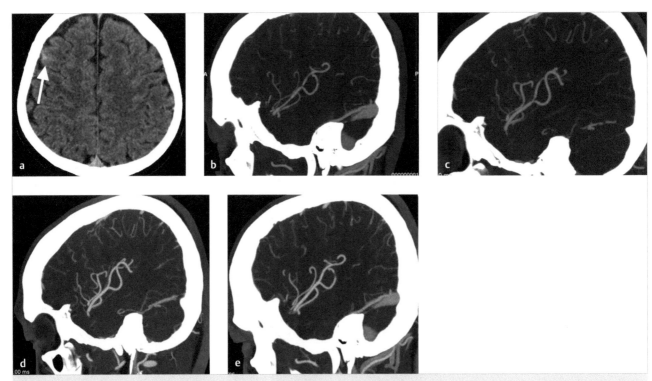

Fig. 3.15 Sulcal SAH in a patient with RCVS. (**a**) Non-contrast CT shows a sulcal SAH overlying the right frontal lobe (*arrow*). (**b**) Sagittal CTA of the right MCA shows multifocal vessel constriction. (**c**) Sagittal CTA of the left MCA also shows multifocal vessel constriction. (**d**) Repeat CTA showing the right MCA territory 2 months later shows reversal of the vascular narrowing. (**e**) Same for the left MCA territory. Findings are consistent and classic for RCVS.

be present. MRI can also demonstrate sulcal SAH on FLAIR as well as other complications such as watershed infarcts or posterior reversible encephalopathy syndrome. It is important to point out that not all sulcal FLAIR hyperintensities are related to SAH and that it can be due to slow flow in constricted arteries. Patients can occasionally present with intraparenchymal hemorrhage as well.

Because RCVS has a similar angiographic appearance to CNS vasculitis and other causes of intracranial vascular narrowing, research has been performed using high-resolution VWI in differentiating these two entities. A number of studies have now demonstrated that unlike vasculitis, RCVS typically demonstrates no or minimal enhancement of the affected vascular segments, likely reflecting the absence of active inflammation (▶ Fig. 3.16). Mild wall thickening, a reflection of the shortening and overlapped smooth muscle cells, can be present in some cases (▶ Fig. 3.17). One study demonstrated that vessel wall thickening resolves during follow-up imaging of most patients which correlates with improved imaging findings on transcranial doppler (TCD) and luminal imaging.

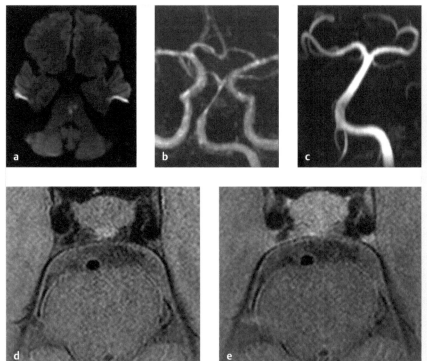

Fig. 3.16 A 45-year-old female presenting with right-sided weakness and severe headache. (a) Axial DWI MRI shows a left paramedian pontine infarct in a perforator distribution. (b) MRA demonstrates long-segment narrowing of the basilar artery. Findings were thought to be due to dissection. (c) Two months later, repeat MRA demonstrates reversal of basilar artery narrowing. (d) Pre- and (e) post-contrast VWI demonstrate no vessel wall enhancement, no intramural hematoma, and no atheromatous disease.

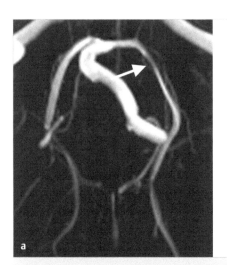
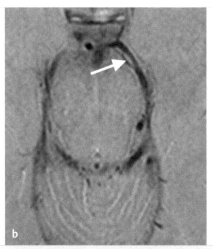
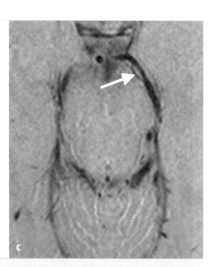

Fig. 3.17 RCVS with vessel wall thickening on VWI. (a) MIP MRA shows areas of focal narrowing in the left posterior cerebral artery (PCA) in this patient with severe thunderclap headache who was on decongestants (arrow). (b) Pre-contrast VWI MRI shows vessel wall thickening in the P2 segment (arrow). (c) Post-contrast VWI MRI shows no enhancement in the area of vessel wall thickening (arrow).

3.4.5 What the Clinician Needs to Know

- Distribution of vascular narrowing and compromised blood vessels
- Presence of RCVS complications including SAH, ischemic stroke, or posterior reversible encephalopathy syndrome (PRES)
- Ideal timing of repeat imaging (4–6 weeks post-presentation), if diagnosis of RCVS is considered
- A lack of vasoconstriction at the time of thunderclap headache does not exclude a diagnosis of RCVS

3.4.6 High-Yield Facts

- A feature common to all RCVS triggers is that they increase sympathetic tone.

- RCVS is not a benign disease and is sometimes complicated by ischemic stroke, sulcal SAH, PRES, and intraparenchymal hemorrhage.
- RCVS progresses in a centripetal direction-going from the periphery to the central intracranial vessels.

Further Reading

[1] Ducros A. Reversible cerebral vasoconstriction syndrome. Lancet Neurol. 2012; 11(10):906–917

[2] Miller TR, Shivashankar R, Mossa-Basha M, Gandhi D. Reversible Cerebral Vasoconstriction Syndrome, Part 1: Epidemiology, Pathogenesis, and Clinical Course. AJNR Am J Neuroradiol. 2015; 36(8):1392–1399

[3] Miller TR, Shivashankar R, Mossa-Basha M, Gandhi D. Reversible Cerebral Vasoconstriction Syndrome, Part 2: Diagnostic Work-Up, Imaging Evaluation, and Differential Diagnosis. AJNR Am J Neuroradiol. 2015; 36(9):1580–1588

3.5 Primary CNS Vasculitis

3.5.1 Clinical Case

A 56-year-old female with recurrent ischemic strokes, headaches, and encephalopathy.

3.5.2 Description of Imaging Findings and Diagnosis

Diagnosis

Multiple enhancing areas of T2 hyperintensity involving multiple vascular territories in the setting of multifocal intracranial stenoses involving the distal cerebral vasculature. Findings consistent with vasculitis.

3.5.3 Background

Primary angiitis of the central nervous system (PACNS) is a rare, idiopathic, form of vasculitis. The estimated incidence is 2–4 cases per 1,000,000 person-years. The male:female ratio of PACNS is 2:1 and the mean age of presentation is 50 years. The most common presenting symptoms include headache, cognitive impairment, and encephalopathy. Stroke and neurological deficits occur in roughly 40% of patients. Headache in PACNS is usually insidious and progressive and not a "thunderclap headache" that is common in RCVS. Given the nonspecific nature of PACNS symptoms there is often a 6–12 month delay in diagnosis. Secondary causes of vasculitis including infection, malignancy, and CNS manifestations of systemic vasculitides are substantially more common than PACNS but can have a similar neurological presentation.

The most common histopathologic pattern in PACNS is granulomatous vasculitis in which giant cells with associated lymphocytes, plasma cells, and histiocytes infiltrate the vessel wall. Unlike extracranial vasculitis, PACNS is typically not characterized by vasa vasorum involvement as the vasa vasorum are characteristically absent in affected branch vessels. Historically, CNS vasculitis has been very difficult to diagnose using both clinical and imaging criteria. The diagnosis of vasculitis is typically made through cortical and leptomeningeal biopsies, which are known to have sensitivities ranging from 50–75%. Furthermore, affected vessels are often below the resolution of conventional angiography, which has a sensitivity 30–90% depending on the study.

In order to make a diagnosis of PACNS, all three of the following criteria need to be met:
- History or clinical findings of an acquired neurological deficit of unknown origin after a thorough initial basic assessment.
- Cerebral angiogram with classic features of vasculitis or a CNS biopsy sample showing vasculitis.
- No evidence of systemic vasculitis or any other disorder to which the angiographic or pathological features could be secondary.

3.5.4 Imaging Findings

MRI is the imaging modality of choice for evaluation of PACNS as 90–100% of patients will have abnormal findings. On T2/FLAIR weighted imaging, white matter hyperintensities can be seen in the subcortical white matter, deep gray matter, deep white matter, and cerebral cortex. Often, infarcts are seen in "atypical" locations such as the corpus callosum. Infarcts are present in 50% of cases and are usually bilateral, involve multiple vascular territories and affect cortical and subcortical regions. Various ages of the infarcts may be present. Enhancing mass-like areas with surrounding vasogenic edema and mass effect are present in 15% of cases. Another common pattern is diffuse small-vessel ischemic disease. Overall, gadolinium enhancement of T2 hyperintense lesions is present in 30% of cases. Leptomeningeal enhancement is seen in up to 15% of cases and may be an ideal site for biopsy. Intraparenchymal and SAH is present in roughly 10% of cases, but unlike RCVS, the SAH is generally not sulcal (▶ Fig. 3.18).

MRA and CTA are useful in identifying the multifocal areas of vascular narrowing associated with PACNS and other forms of vasculitis. There is usually involvement of distal vessels (i.e., M3, M4, P3, P4, A3, A4, etc.); however, involvement of larger vessels can be present. DSA is often performed for these patients as many distal cortical vessels are well below the spatial resolution of CTA and MRA. If vasculitis is suspected, we pre-medicate patients with steroids prior to diagnostic angiography as contrast agents can aggravate distal vascular narrowing and thus may lead to distal infarcts.

HR-VWI has emerged as a key tool in the diagnosis of CNS vasculitis. Affected vessels are typically characterized by mild smooth vessel wall thickening of medium- and small-sized arteries and **concentric** enhancement (▶ Fig. 3.19). In some cases, vasculitis can demonstrate a circumferential, but considerably eccentric enhancement pattern. The smooth, intense, homogeneous, and concentric enhancement pattern is one key to differentiating vasculitis from atheromatous disease (eccentric heterogeneous variable enhancement) and RCVS (minimal to no enhancement). Distribution of disease is another key difference between vasculitis and atheromatous disease as vasculitis more often affects vessels distal to the MCA bifurcation and the ACA and posterior communicating arteries. It is important to note that PACNS can also manifest as smooth eccentric wall enhancement and thickening. In these cases, other features such as lack of positive remodeling and clinical findings may be important clues to differentiate it from atherosclerosis. One major advantage of VWI is its ability to identify inflammation of small vessels such as lenticulostriate arteries due to enhancement of the perivascular tissues. In an early MRI study of patients with primary CNS vasculitis, one author noted that 66% of patients had prominent perivascular enhancement in the Virchow Robbin spaces, which resolved with immunosuppressant treatment.

HR-VWI may play a role in monitoring response to therapy as well. Vessel wall enhancement can diminish significantly with medical treatment on the order of weeks or months. The utility of vessel wall enhancement as a biomarker for true response to clinical treatment seems promising, but needs further investigation (▶ Fig. 3.20).

It is important to point out that there is a subset of PACNS, which is angiography negative but biopsy positive. In this subset, small arteries or arterioles, which are below the resolution of cerebral angiography are affected. These patients often present with cognitive dysfunction and have leptomeningeal or parenchymal enhancing lesions on MRI.

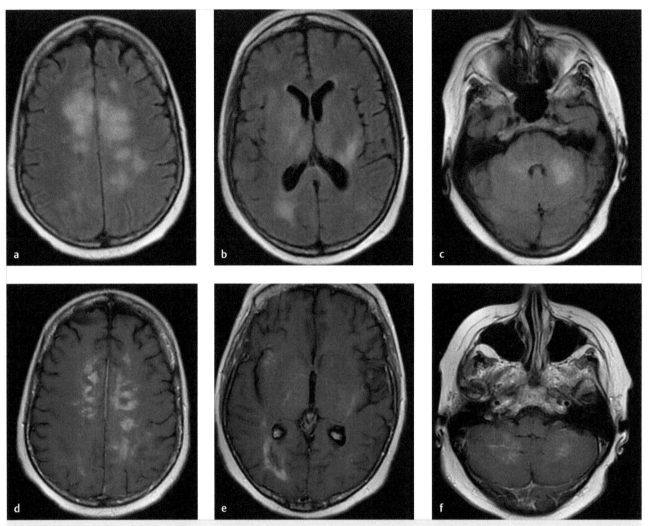

Fig. 3.18 Conventional imaging findings in vasculitis. (**a–c**). T2/FLAIR images demonstrate multifocal T2/FLAIR hyperintensities involving deep white matter and gray matter structures. (**d–f**). Many of these areas are associated with enhancement on T1 post-gad imaging.

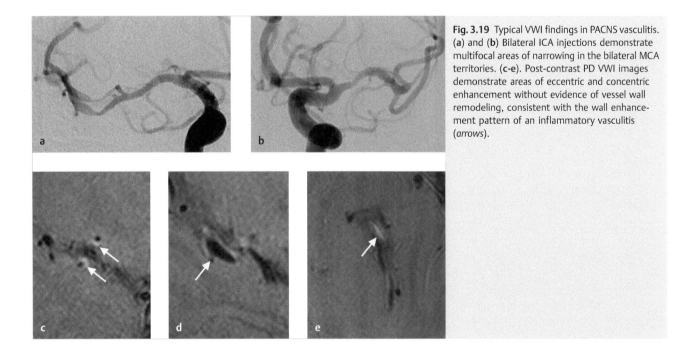

Fig. 3.19 Typical VWI findings in PACNS vasculitis. (**a**) and (**b**) Bilateral ICA injections demonstrate multifocal areas of narrowing in the bilateral MCA territories. (**c-e**). Post-contrast PD VWI images demonstrate areas of eccentric and concentric enhancement without evidence of vessel wall remodeling, consistent with the wall enhancement pattern of an inflammatory vasculitis (*arrows*).

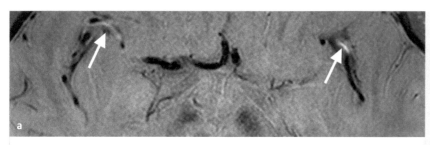

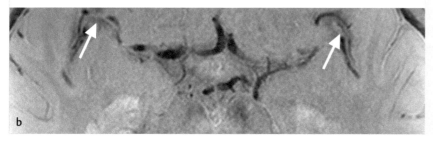

Fig. 3.20 Response to steroid therapy on VWI in a patient with PACNS. (**a**) Pre-treatment PD post-contrast VWI exam demonstrates multifocal areas of concentric vessel wall enhancement typical of an inflammatory vasculitis (*arrows*). (**b**) Following a 12 week course of corticosteroid, there is near complete resolution of vessel wall enhancement (*arrows*).

3.5.5 What the Clinician Needs to Know

- Distribution of vascular narrowing and compromised blood vessels.
- Presence of PACNS complications including ischemic stroke, SAH, mass-like lesions, and intraparenchymal enhancement.
- The location of leptomeningeal enhancement is a good target for a biopsy.
- The diagnostic yield of leptomeningeal biopsy and cerebral angiography is not 100%. Often times, multiple biopsies or vascular imaging studies will need to be performed to make the correct diagnosis.

3.5.6 High-Yield Facts

- PACNS affecting larger intracranial vessels tends to have a more fulminant course.

- A small proportion of PACNS cases are angio-negative and biopsy positive. These patients often present with cognitive dysfunction.
- VWI can be useful in distinguishing PACNS from other causes of vascular narrowing. VWI in PACNS shows multifocal areas of concentric vessel wall enhancement.

Further Reading

[1] Birnbaum J, Hellmann DB. Primary angiitis of the central nervous system. Arch Neurol. 2009; 66(6):704–709
[2] Salvarani C, Brown RD, Jr, Hunder GG. Adult primary central nervous system vasculitis. Lancet. 2012; 380(9843):767–777
[3] Brinjikji W, Mossa-Basha M, Huston J, Rabinstein AA, Lanzino G, Lehman VT. Intracranial vessel wall imaging for evaluation of steno-occlusive diseases and intracranial aneurysms. J Neuroradiol. 2017; 44(2): 123–134

Chapter 4

Intracranial Aneurysms

4

4 Intracranial Aneurysms

4.1 Imaging of Unruptured Saccular Aneurysms

4.1.1 Clinical Case

A 73-year-old female with severe frontal headache and cognitive decline (▶ Fig. 4.1).

4.1.2 Description of Imaging Findings and Diagnosis

Diagnosis

Giant partially thrombosed aneurysm with associated perianeurysmal edema. Digital subtraction angiography (DSA) demonstrates a large luminal component but there is an obvious mismatch between the size of the aneurysm on DSA and the size on MRI.

4.1.3 Background

Saccular cerebral aneurysms comprise roughly 90% of all cerebral aneurysms and are the most common cause of nontraumatic subarachnoid hemorrhage (SAH). The prevalence of saccular aneurysms in the general population ranges from 2 to 8% depending on the region (higher prevalence in Japan and Finland). Two-thirds of aneurysm patients are women. Among patients with intracranial aneurysms, 10–20% have multiple lesions. Saccular aneurysms are associated with a variety of abnormal connective tissue diseases; however, most aneurysms are sporadic. Patients with connective tissue disease or a family history of intracranial aneurysms will often undergo screening for intracranial aneurysms even when asymptomatic.

Saccular aneurysms are histologically characterized by disruption of the internal elastic lamina at the entrance site/neck of the aneurysm. The histopathologic features of the intima, media, and adventitia are the prime determinants of aneurysm natural history. Unruptured aneurysms are characterized by an intact endothelium and smooth muscle layer with the absence of inflammatory cells in the vessel wall. In contradistinction, ruptured and unstable aneurysms are characterized by endothelial disruption, absence of smooth muscle cells, and inflammatory cell infiltration into the media and adventitia. Adventitial inflammation results in media thinning, promoting aneurysm formation. Histopathologic studies have demonstrated that unstable aneurysms are also characterized by wall thinning, organizing thrombus, and the increased expression of inflammatory markers.

Management of unruptured aneurysms (i.e., to treat or not to treat) is one of the major dilemmas in cerebrovascular medicine. In the United States, for example, roughly 30,000 patients/year suffer from an aneurysmal SAH whereas somewhere between 5 and 10 million people have an unruptured aneurysm. A number of decision aids have been published to guide in the management of these lesions (▶ Table 4.1). However, the primacy of imaging findings in guiding treatment decisions remains undisputed.

4.1.4 Imaging Findings

The role of the diagnostic neuroradiologist in evaluation of a suspected aneurysm patient is to (1) detect the aneurysm, (2) characterize the aneurysm, and (3) determine the effect the aneurysm is having on the surrounding nonvascular structures.

Both CT angiography and MR angiography are excellent imaging modalities for the detection of cerebral aneurysms.

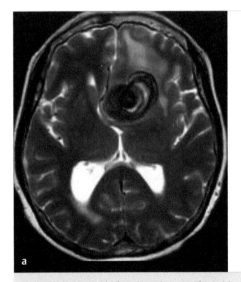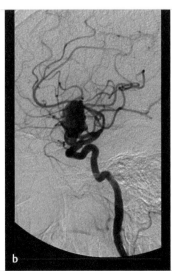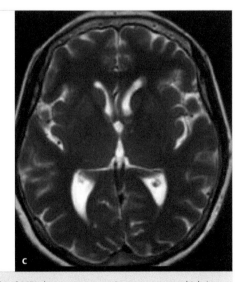

Fig. 4.1 A 73-year-old female with severe frontal headache and cognitive decline. (a) T2-weighted MRI demonstrates a giant aneurysm which is projecting into the inferior left frontal lobe. There is a laminated appearance to the aneurysm wall consistent with thrombus. There is also a substantial amount of vasogenic edema. (b) Left ICA cerebral angiogram shows a large paraophthalmic aneurysm; however, the aneurysm size on luminal imaging is substantially smaller than that on cross-sectional imaging. (c) Following flow diversion treatment, MRI performed 30 months later demonstrates resolution of the edema and mass effect. The patient's symptoms improved.

Table 4.1 PHASES and ELAPSS Score

	ELAPSS SCORE Points	PHASES SCORE Points
Earlier SAH		
Yes	0	1
No	1	0
Location of Aneurysm		
ICA	0	0
ACA/Acom	0	4
MCA	3	2
Pcom/Posterior	5	4
Age		
<= 60y	0	NA
>60y (per 5y)	1	NA
<70y	NA	0
>= 70y	NA	1
Population		
North America, China, Europe	0	0
Japan	1	3
Finland	7	5
Aneurysm Size, mm		
1–2.9	0	0
3–4.9	4	0
5–6.9	10	0
7–9.9	13	3
10–19.9	22	6
>= 20 mm	22	10
Aneurysm Shape		
Regular	0	NA
Irregular	4	NA
Hypertension		
Yes	NA	1
No	NA	0

Abbreviations: PHASES, Population, Hypertension, Age, Size, Earlier SAH, Site; ELAPSS, Earlier SAH, Location, Age, Population, Size, and Shape.

A number of modern series have found that multi-detector row CTA and the time of flight MRA have sensitivities and specificities of greater than 90% in the detection of cerebral aneurysms measuring 3 mm or larger. When evaluating these angiographic images, there are a few key principles to keep in mind to increase one's ability to detect a cerebral aneurysm. First, one must evaluate both the thin-cut source images as well as the thick-cut maximum intensity projection images. MIP images allow most aneurysms to "pop-out," but occasionally one can be tricked into thinking that a prominent vascular loop is an aneurysm if thin-cut images are not used to verify the finding on the MIPs. Thin-cut images also allow for the detection of smaller aneurysms, which are concealed on the maximum intensity projections (MIPs). Thin slices are also useful in evaluating aneurysms of the cavernous sinus/carotid siphon, especially on CTA. Second, it is important to review all multiplanar reformatted images as some aneurysms are more obvious when viewed

in the coronal and sagittal planes. Third, a 3D representation of the circle of Willis is invaluable for aneurysm detection. Each bifurcation point should be closely inspected and each potential finding should be verified on source images. Whenever a patient has one aneurysm, always look for more. The most common site to find a second aneurysm is in the same location as the first aneurysm, but on the contralateral side (i.e., mirror image aneurysms) (▶ Fig. 4.2).

Characterization of the aneurysm is essential to determining treatment options. Measurements should be obtained of the aneurysm neck, aneurysm height, and aneurysm width. The maximum neck width of the aneurysm is important in treatment planning as wide necked aneurysms often require stent-assisted coiling, flow diversion, or surgical clipping, whereas narrow-necked aneurysms can be treated with simple endovascular coiling. The shape of the aneurysm should be described as smooth (i.e., no surface irregularity, well rounded), lobulated (i.e., two more or less equally sized lobules), or having a daughter sac (i.e., a small outpouching arising from the aneurysm sac). Saccular and lobulated aneurysms have been shown to have more favorable natural histories than those which have daughter sacs (▶ Fig. 4.3).

The orientation of the aneurysm is also important (inferior, superior, posterior, anterior, etc.). For example, an Acom aneurysm that points superiorly or posteriorly is favorable for endovascular management due to the presence of perforators draped over the aneurysm sac, whereas one directed inferiorly is favorable for surgical clipping as it is difficult to get a good working projection for endovascular treatment. The relationship of the aneurysm with branch vessels (i.e., is the vessel coming from the aneurysm neck) and smaller perforators in the vicinity of the aneurysm (i.e., thalamoperforators, heubner, anterior temporal artery, lenticulostriates, etc.) is essential. Anatomic variants (i.e., hypoplastic or absence Pcom or A1, fenestration, MCA trifurcation vs. bifurcation, etc.) can also affect treatment decisions.

The relationship between the aneurysm and adjacent non-vascular structures is something that is often overlooked when evaluating an intracranial aneurysm patient. For aneurysms located along the cavernous ICA, careful attention should be paid to the relationship between the aneurysm and the sphenoid sinus as large or giant cavernous carotid aneurysms can erode in the sinus and result in life-threatening epistaxis (▶ Fig. 4.4). For ICA aneurysms, the relationship between the aneurysm and the clinoid process is helpful in determining if a lesion is intradural or extradural as those below the anterior clinoid process are considered extradural (and not at risk of SAH), whereas those above are intradural (and at risk of SAH). For those at are paraclinoid, some are intradural and some are extradural. The relationship between aneurysms and the cranial nerves needs to be commented on and can best be evaluated on high resolution fast imaging employing steady-state acquisition fast imaging employing steady-state acquisition (FIESTA) imaging (▶ Fig. 4.5). Paraophthalmic and Acom/ACA aneurysms can exert substantial mass effect on the optic nerve. Pcom, basilar tip, and PCA aneurysms can cause mass effect on the oculomotor nerve. The relationship between the aneurysm and the adjacent cerebral parenchyma is also important. Large and giant aneurysms can sometimes exert substantial mass effect on the adjacent brain parenchyma and result in edema and neurological deficit even in the absence of rupture (▶ Fig. 4.1, ▶ Fig. 4.2). This is

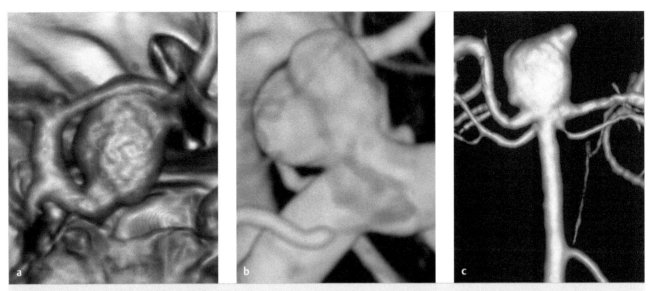

Fig. 4.2 Different aneurysm morphologies. (a) 3D reconstructed CTA demonstrates a large paraclinoid aneurysm with a smooth morphology. (b) 3DRA demonstrates a lobulated paraophthalmic aneurysm with two equal sized lobules. (c) 3DRA demonstrates a large basilar tip aneurysm with a small daughter sac.

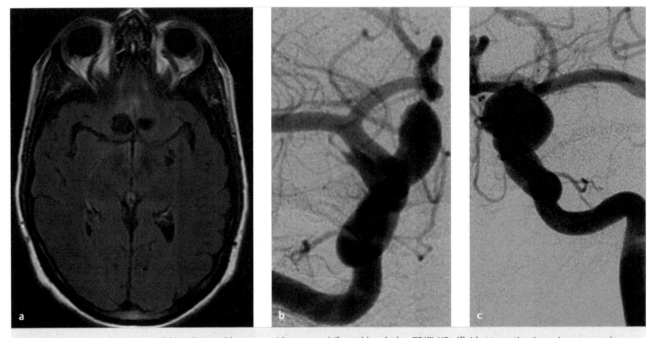

Fig. 4.3 Mirror image aneurysms. (a) A 43-year-old woman with a severe bifrontal headache. T2/FLAIR (fluid attenuation inversion recovery) demonstrates bilateral aneurysms, which project into the bilateral gyrus rectus with associated edema. (b) Right ICA cerebral angiogram demonstrates an 8-mm right paraclinoid aneurysm and (c) Left ICA cerebral angiogram demonstrates a 10-mm paraclinoid aneurysm. Given the presence of edema and headaches, these aneurysms were thought to be symptomatic and were both treated.

especially true for giant thrombosed aneurysms, which are sometimes mistaken for large extra-axial tumors.

4.1.5 What the Clinician Needs to Know

- Anatomic characteristics of the aneurysm including size, neck width, location, orientation, and relationship to branch vessels.
- Morphology of the aneurysm including presence of lobulations or daughter sac.
- Aneurysm multiplicity.
- Relationship between the aneurysm and adjacent nonvascular tissues including osseous structures, cranial nerves, and brain parenchyma.

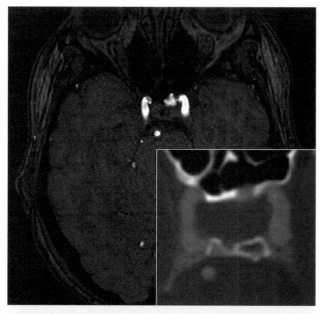

Fig. 4.4 Cavernous ICA aneurysm projecting into sphenoid sinus. TOF MRA shows an 8-mm cavernous ICA aneurysm with a daughter sac, which is projecting into the sphenoid sinus. Inset image shows an osseous defect in the posterior wall of the sphenoid sinus.

4.1.6 High-Yield Facts

- Saccular aneurysm rupture risk is dictated primarily by size (large size → more rupture) and location (i.e., Acom/ACA and posterior circulation aneurysms at higher risk of rupture).
- The term giant aneurysm is typically reserved for aneurysms which are 25 mm or larger. These lesions often have intraluminal thrombus and can exert mass effect on surrounding structures.
- Mirror image aneurysms are the most common location for patients with multiple aneurysms.

Further Reading

[1] HaiFeng L, YongSheng X, YangQin X, et al. Diagnostic value of 3D time-of-flight magnetic resonance angiography for detecting intracranial aneurysm: a meta-analysis. Neuroradiology. 2017; 59(11):1083–1092

[2] Turan N, Heider RA, Roy AK, et al. Current Perspectives in Imaging Modalities for the Assessment of Unruptured Intracranial Aneurysms: A Comparative Analysis and Review. World Neurosurg. 2018; 113:280–292

[3] Krings T, Piske RL, Lasjaunias PL. Intracranial arterial aneurysm vasculopathies: targeting the outer vessel wall. Neuroradiology. 2005; 47 (12):931–937

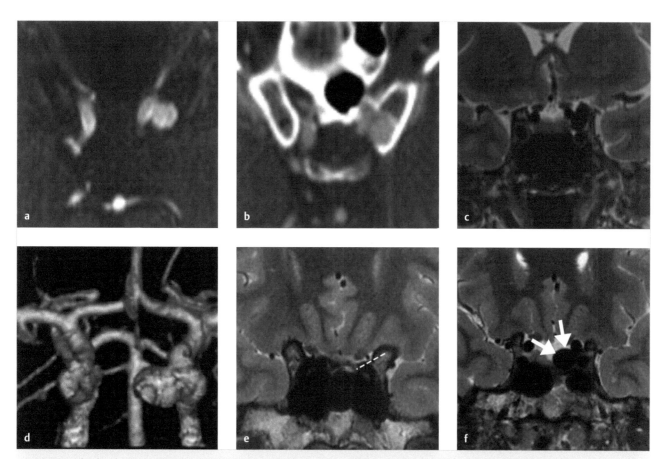

Fig. 4.5 Intradural and extradural cavernous ICA aneurysms. (**a**) Laterally projecting 4-mm aneurysm of the cavernous ICA. (**b**) On CTA, the aneurysm is below the left clinoid process. (**c**) On the coronal T2 MRI, the aneurysm is entirely below the left clinoid process and is thus extradural. (**d**) 3D reconstruction of a CTA shows a medially projecting aneurysm arising from the cavernous ICA. (**e**) Coronal T2 MRI shows the distal dural ring (dashed line). (**f**) Coronal T2 weighted MRI shows the aneurysm which is clearly projecting into the subarachnoid space, and above the distal dural ring.

4.2 Imaging of Ruptured Aneurysms

4.2.1 Clinical Case

A 73-year-old female with sudden onset severe headache followed by decreased level of consciousness. Current GCS is 11 (▸ Fig. 4.6).

4.2.2 Description of Imaging Findings and Diagnosis

Diagnosis

Intraparenchymal hemorrhage in the bilateral frontal lobes, greater on the right, with associated diffuse SAH. CTA demonstrates a small pericallosal aneurysm pointing toward the right.

4.2.3 Background

Saccular cerebral aneurysms are the most common cause of nontraumatic SAH. Rupture of a cerebral aneurysm results in the extravasation of blood into the subarachnoid space, which triggers a cascade of events that can result in severe disability or death. Failure to diagnose and treat an aneurysmal SAH can

result in further impairment due to aneurysm rebleeding and delayed cerebral ischemia from cerebral vasospasm. Although lumbar puncture is the gold standard for the diagnosis of SAH, CT has emerged as the diagnostic modality of choice with sensitivity and specificity of over 99% in the first days after the SAH.

The diagnostic neuroradiologist's job does not stop at the identification of the SAH and the culprit aneurysm. Rather, the neuroradiologists is responsible for obtaining and relaying all the information that is required to make a determination regarding the ideal management strategy for the aneurysm; namely, factors that will determine whether the aneurysm will be clipped or coiled.

4.2.4 Imaging Findings

An imaging checklist in the evaluation of ruptured aneurysms is provided in ▸ Table 4.2. The first task of the neuroradiologist is to properly localize the aneurysm. At most institutions, CT angiography is the imaging modality of choice and is performed prior to conventional angiography. The use of thin-slice multidetector row CTA with MIP and 3D reconstructions allows for a 90% sensitivity and specificity for detection of intracranial aneurysms. One clue regarding the location of the aneurysm is identifying the region of the densest hematoma. For example, dense subarachnoid blood in the left sylvian fissure should prompt one to closely inspect the left MCA bifurcation while

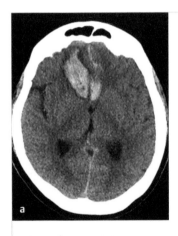
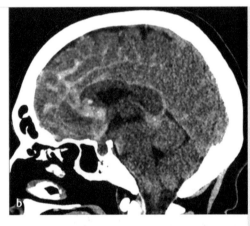
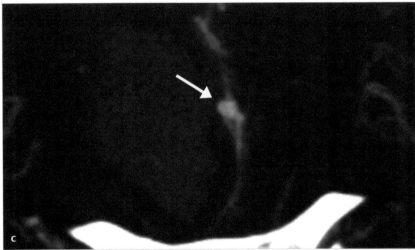

Fig. 4.6 Subarachnoid and intraparenchymal hemorrhage secondary to ruptured pericallosal artery aneurysm. (**a**) Non-contrast CT demonstrates a dense intraparenchymal hematoma in the bilateral inferior frontal lobes, greater on the right. (**b**) Sagittal reconstructed CT shows diffuse subarachnoid blood as well. (**c**) CTA shows a 4-mm pericallosal artery aneurysm which is pointing to the right, in the region of the dense hematoma (*arrow*).

dense blood in the interhemispheric fissure should prompt one to closely examine that ACA/Acom complex. Whenever a patient has one aneurysm, always look for more. The most common site to find a second aneurysm is in the same location as the first aneurysm, but on the contralateral side (i.e., mirror image aneurysms). A good rule of thumb is that posterior circulation aneurysms and aneurysms along the ICA typically go to coiling while those of the MCA go to clipping.

Neuroradiologists need to determine and characterize in the aneurysm configuration and geometry. Measurements of the height, width, and neck width are needed for treatment planning. Aneurysms which are narrow-necked are more amenable to simple coiling while wider neck aneurysms will require coiling with adjuvant techniques or clipping (▶ Fig. 4.7).

Two factors that are commonly underreported in diagnostic neuroradiology reports include the projection of the aneurysm and the proximity of large vessels or perforators to the aneurysm neck and dome. For example, at the Acom complex, aneurysms which project inferiorly are typically reserved for clipping as it is difficult to get a working projection on

biplane; while, aneurysms which project superiorly are reserved for coiling due to the presence of perforators draping over the aneurysm itself (▶ Fig. 4.8). Regarding the presence of nearby vessels, any time perforators are surrounding the aneurysm neck or dome, coiling is preferred. Meanwhile, whenever there is a vessel coming from the aneurysm neck, clipping is preferred. Any calcifications at the aneurysm neck need to be identified as these can complicate clipping procedures and may sway the treatment decision toward coiling (▶ Fig. 4.9).

In addition to aneurysm characterization, assessment of the cerebrovascular tree for other aneurysms, anatomical variations (i.e., hypoplastic vessels, fenestrations, fetal PCA, etc.), atherosclerosis, and elongative arteriopathies is important for treatment planning.

Lastly, roughly 10–20% of ruptured aneurysm patients have multiple intracranial aneurysms. Unless these aneurysms are in a single operative field or operative bed, most practitioners hesitate to treat multiple aneurysms in a single operation, even in the setting of a SAH (▶ Fig. 4.10). Thus, it is important to be able to determine, with a reasonable level of confidence, which aneurysm is the culprit aneurysm. Blood distribution is the first important hint (▶ Table 4.3). Regarding aneurysm characteristics, factors such as irregular morphology, larger size, presence of a bleb or daughter sac, local vasospasm, and a high aspect ratio (i.e., height to neck width) are imaging findings which suggest that an aneurysm may be the culprit in setting of SAH and multiple aneurysms.

Table 4.2 Imaging Checklist

Non-Contrast CT Findings	Aneurysm Characteristics
SAH Extent	Location
SAH Distribution	Size
Large Clot/Parenchymal Hemorrhage	Multiplicity
Intraventricular Hemorrhage	Neck Size and Dome-to-Neck Ratio
Hydrocephalus	Irregular Morphology
	Calcified Neck or Dome
Anatomic Characteristics	
Proximity to perforator vessels	**Aneurysm Etiology**
Vessels coming from neck	Saccular
Elongative arteriopathy	Dissecting
Anatomic Variants	Partially thrombosed
Atheroscleroisis	Traumatic
Local Vasospasm	Mycotic

4.2.5 What the Clinician Needs to Know

- Is there a "life-threatening situation" such as herniation, large clot, intraventricular hemorrhage, or hydrocephalus?
- Location and number of aneurysms, and, if there are multiple aneurysms, location of the culprit lesion.
- Aneurysm morphology including size, lobulations, daughter sacs, proximity to perforators, or other large vessels.
- Any issues which would result in challenging endovascular access.

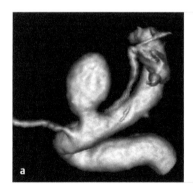
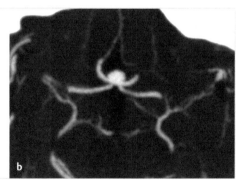

Fig. 4.7 Examples of narrow and wide necked aneurysms. (**a**) The 9-mm paraophthalmic aneurysm with a narrow neck and wide dome. (**b**) Broadnecked anterior communicating artery aneurysm.

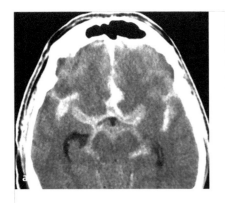
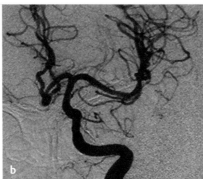
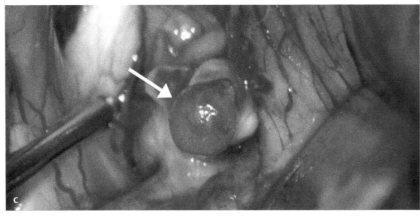

Fig. 4.8 Inferiorly projecting Acom aneurysm. (a) Non-contrast CT shows dense SAH in the interhemispheric fissure. (b) Cerebral angiogram shows an inferiorly projecting Acom aneruysm. (c) Surgical photograph shows the inferiorly pointing anterior communicating artery aneurysm (arrow).

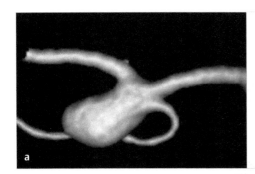
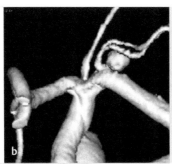

Fig. 4.9 Consideration of surrounding vessels. (a) Anterior communicating artery aneurysm with a vessel arising from the aneurysm neck. This may be better treated surgically. (b) Left M1 aneurysm with a large perforator trunk arising close to the aneurysm neck and perforators draping over the aneurysm. This would be better treated endovascularly.

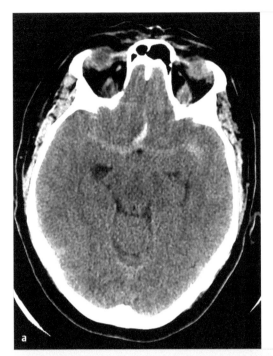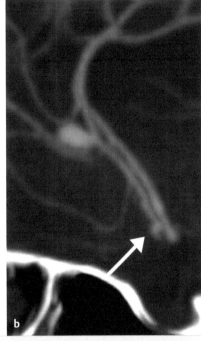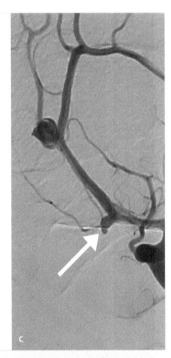

Fig. 4.10 Multiple aneurysms, which one ruptured? (**a**) Non-contrast CT shows SAH with dense blood around the region of the anterior communicating artery. There was no blood in the distality of the interhemispheric fissure. (**b**) CTA shows two aneurysms, a small anterior communicating artery aneurysm with a tiny inferiorly projecting daughter sac (*arrow*) and a larger, 5-mm pericallosal artery aneurysm. (**c**) DSA confirms the presence of both aneurysms and better delineates the tiny daughter sac (*arrow*). In this case, both aneurysms were coiled as they were in the same vascular territory and there was some uncertainty as to which one bleed. However, we think it was probably the Acom.

Table 4.3 Hemorrhage Distribution and Aneurysm Location

Hemorrhage Distribution	Most Likely Aneurysm Location
Interhemispheric Fissure at Suprasellar Cistern	Acom/ACA
Distal Interhemispheric Fissure	Pericallosal
Distal Sylvian Fissure	MCA
Proximal Sylvian Fissure	Pcom
Perimedullary, Unilateral	PICA
Infratentorial, Symmetric	Basilar Tip

Abbreviations: Acom, Anterior communicating artery; ACA, Anterior cerebral artery; MCA; Middle cerebral artery; Pcom, Posterior communicating artery; PICA, posterior inferior cerebellar artery.

4.2.6 High-Yield Facts

- In the setting of multiple aneurysms, size, morphology, hemorrhage distribution, and local vasospasm can help identify the target lesion.
- Aneurysms in close proximity to small perforators are better managed endovascularly, while those with vessels coming from the neck are better treated with surgery.
- Thin-slice CTA with MIPS and 3D reconstructions are essential for detection of smaller aneurysms.

Further Reading

[1] HaiFeng L, YongSheng X, YangQin X, et al. Diagnostic value of 3D time-of-flight magnetic resonance angiography for detecting intracranial aneurysm: a meta-analysis. Neuroradiology. 2017; 59(11):1083–1092

[2] Turan N, Heider RA, Roy AK, et al. Current Perspectives in Imaging Modalities for the Assessment of Unruptured Intracranial Aneurysms: A Comparative Analysis and Review. World Neurosurg. 2018; 113:280–292

[3] Krings T, Piske RL, Lasjaunias PL. Intracranial arterial aneurysm vasculopathies: targeting the outer vessel wall. Neuroradiology. 2005; 47(12):931–937

[4] Karttunen AI, Jartti PH, Ukkola VA, Sajanti J, Haapea M. Value of the quantity and distribution of subarachnoid haemorrhage on CT in the localization of a ruptured cerebral aneurysm. Acta Neurochir (Wien). 2003; 145(8):655–661, discussion 661

4.3 Imaging of Non-Saccular Aneurysms

4.3.1 Clinical Case

An 83-year-old male with multiple cranial neuropathies and headache (▶ Fig. 4.11).

4.3.2 Description of Imaging Findings and Diagnosis

Diagnosis

Fusiform and dolichoectatic partially thrombosed basilar trunk aneurysm exerting mass effect on multiple lower cranial nerves.

4.3.3 Background

Non-saccular aneurysms comprise 10% or less of all intracranial aneurysms. These lesions are due to multiple different causes, which each may necessitate a different type of treatment. The role of the diagnostic neuroradiologist in these instances is to raise awareness of the underlying cause of the aneurysm which will impact treatment. The aim of this section is to raise the awareness that aneurysms may be a *symptom* of an underlying disease rather than a disease entity by themselves. The most commonly reported pathomechanical types of non-saccular intracranial aneurysms include atherosclerotic, dissecting, blister, mycotic, oncotic, traumatic, and immunodeficient aneurysms.

Variables including clinical history, patient demographics, and aneurysm morphological characteristics are key to distinguishing between these entities. Furthermore, by obtaining an accurate classification of the aneurysm, appropriate systemic work-up and treatment can be pursued. A summary of typical demographic characteristics and clinical history characteristics for non-saccular aneurysms is provided in ▶ Table 4.4.

4.3.4 Imaging Findings

Imaging findings of non-saccular aneurysms are summarized in ▶ Table 4.5. Below, we will describe the salient features of the most common types of non-saccular intracranial aneurysms.

Dolichoectatic and fusiform aneurysms most commonly affect the vertebrobasilar circulation. These aneurysms are sometimes referred to as atherosclerotic aneurysms as well. These aneurysms result from the diffuse degradation of the internal elastic lamina of an entire vessel segment (i.e., V4 segment, vertebral artery, M1 segment, etc.). These types of aneurysms are characterized by non-saccular dilatations involving the entire vessel wall for a segment. This results in the formation of an aneurysm without a neck. These lesions typically have a very poor natural history and are prone to high rates of growth, mass effect, and rupture. They are often fusiforme in shape and are associated with a high rate of acute ischemic stroke due to their propensity to form intraluminal thrombus which goes on to occlude the ostia of perforator vessels. In fact, perforator infarction in the setting of a vertebrobasilar fusiform aneurysm is thought to be a harbinger for acute growth or rupture of the lesion. Distal emboli can also result from intraluminal thrombus. Large

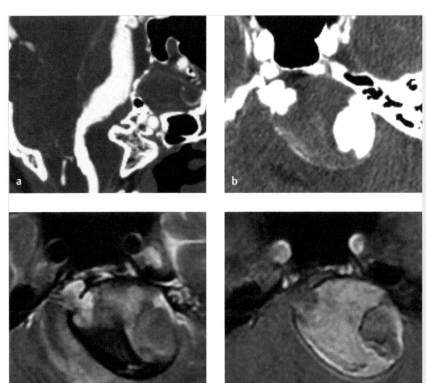

Fig. 4.11 Partially thrombosed dolichoectatic and fusiform basilar aneurysm with mass effect. **(a)** MPR CTA demonstrates a holobasilar aneurysm with a large amount of luminal thrombus. **(b)** Axial CTA shows the aneurysm with a large amount of luminal thrombus. The aneurysm is compressing the brainstem. **(c)** Axial T2 weighted MRI shows marked mass effect of the aneurysm on the pons with a large amount of vasogenic edema. Note the aneurysm consuming the whole pre-pontine cistern, thus compressing multiple cranial nerves. **(d)** Post-contrast MRI shows enhancement of the luminal thrombus suggesting that it has been present for a long duration and neovascularized.

Table 4.4 Summary of Typical Clinical Findings in Patients with Non-saccular Aneurysms

Aneurysm Type	Patient Demographics	Comorbidities	Presentation
Fusiform	Older patients, more common in males	Hypertension, smoking, peripheral artery disease, abdominal aortic aneurysms	Ischemic stroke, SAH, headache, cranial neuropathy
Dissecting	Younger patients, more common in males	Connective tissue diseases	Acute headache, ischemic stroke very rare, SAH
Blood Blister	Younger patients, more common in females	None	SAH
Oncotic	Younger patients, equal M:F	Atrial myxoma	Ischemic stroke, SAH, intraparenchymal hemorrhage
Mycotic	Younger patients, equal M:F	Endocarditis, valvular infection	Ischemic stroke, SAH, intraparenchymal hemorrhage, cerebritis, fever
Immunodeficient	Children and adolescents, equal M:F	Severe combined immunodeficiency, HIV	Ischemic stroke

Abbreviation: SAH, Subarachnoid hemorrhage.

Table 4.5 Typical Conventional Imaging Findings in Patients with Non-saccular Aneurysms

Aneurysm Type	Luminal Imaging Characteristics	Most Common Location
Fusiform	Fusiform dilatation of a long segment of an intracranial vessel. No identifiable neck. May see intraluminal thrombus. May be associated with dolichoectasia as well	Vertebral and basilar arteries, cavernous/supraclinoid ICAs, M1 segment
Dissecting	Focal fusiform dilatation of an intracranial blood vessel usually with a proximal stenosis/string of pearl sign. Dynamic change in lesion shape on follow-up	Non-branching segments including vertebral artery, basilar artery, M1 segment and distal PCA/MCA vessels
Blood Blister	Tiny bump on the vessel wall associated with an area of dense SAH. Sensitivity with CTA/MRA very low	Always located on dorsal wall of supraclinoid ICA opposite the origin of the Pcom and anterior choroidal artery. No branch point identified.
Oncotic	Usually small, irregularly shaped aneurysm in a distal vessel. Often associated with an area of sulcal SAH	Typically involve distal MCA territory as they form due to vessel wall infiltration of tumor emboli
Mycotic	Usually small, irregularly shaped aneurysm in a distal vessel. Often associated with an area of sulcal SAH	Typically involve distal MCA territory as they form due to vessel wall infiltration of septic emboli
Immunodeficient	Fusiform morphology	Basilar artery

Abbreviations: ICA, Internal carotid artery; PCA, Posterior cerebral artery; MCA, middle cerebral artery; CTA, CT angiography; MRA, MR angiography.

dolichoectatic and fusiform aneurysms are also known to be associated with substantial cranial nerve and brainstem mass effect, especially since they are also associated with some degree of vessel tortuosity. Hydrocephalus is also a common presentation from brainstem mass effect and compression of the fourth ventricle (▶ Fig. 4.12). 10% of dolichoectatic and fusiform aneurysm patients have additional abdominal aortic aneurysms.

Dissecting aneurysms were at least partially discussed in the section on intracranial dissections. As mentioned previously, intracranial dissections can present with headache, ischemia or SAH. Unruptured dissecting aneurysms (i.e., those presenting with headache or stroke) rarely rupture as the aneurysm has found a "release" of its intraluminal pressure. On the other hand, ruptured dissecting aneurysms have a high rate of re-rupture (exceeding the re-rupture rate of saccular aneurysms, especially in poor grade patients). The key factor distinguishing a dissecting aneurysm from other types of non-saccular aneurysms is the focal proximal stenosis prior to the aneurysmal dilatation. Intramural T1 signal or hemorrhage is rare in dissecting aneurysms but is a highly specific imaging finding (▶ Fig. 4.13). These lesions occur along straight segments of vessels, and not at bifurcation site.

Blood blister aneurysms are defined as aneurysms along the dorsal (anterior) wall of the supraclinoid ICA opposite the origin of the posterior communicating artery and anterior choroidal artery. They form due to an acute tear in the entire vessel wall. These lesions are very small, have a shallow broad neck and about one-third are occult on CTA. If a CTA is negative but there is dense SAH on one side of the suprasellar cistern, one should suspect a blood blister aneurysm and go to angiography (▶ Fig. 4.14). Unruptured blood blister aneurysms are by definition nonexistent and their treatment is as such biased by numismatic strabism of the operator.

Oncotic and mycotic aneurysms have very similar appearances. Oncotic aneurysms are typically due to cerebral emboli from cardiac myxoma. One recently published study found that patients with cardiac myxoma who present with ischemic stroke are at high risk of developing oncotic aneurysms, sometimes over a decade following the initial ischemic stroke. Oncotic tissue grows into the vessel wall to form the aneurysm. Mycotic aneurysms result from septic emboli in the setting of endocarditis or valvular infection. Infectious particles stimulate neutrophil infiltration and elastase secretion resulting in focal vessel wall weakening. Mycotic and oncotic aneurysms have very similar characteristics angiographically as they are gener-

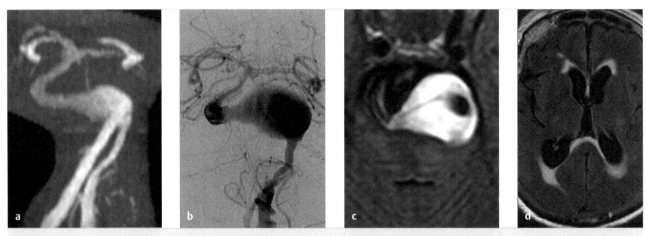

Fig. 4.12 Dolichoectatic basilar trunk aneurysm presenting with hydrocephalus. (**a**) MIP TOF MRA shows the large basilar trunk fusiform aneurysm in the setting of a dolichoectatic basilar artery. (**b**) Cerebral angiogram shows the giant basilar trunk aneurysm and marked dolichoectasia of the basilar artery. (**c**) Axial T2/FLAIR MRI shows mass effect of the aneurysm and compression of the fourth ventricle. (**d**) Axial FLAIR MRI shows hydrocephalus with periventricular T2/FLAIR hyperintensity consistent with transependymal flow of CSF.

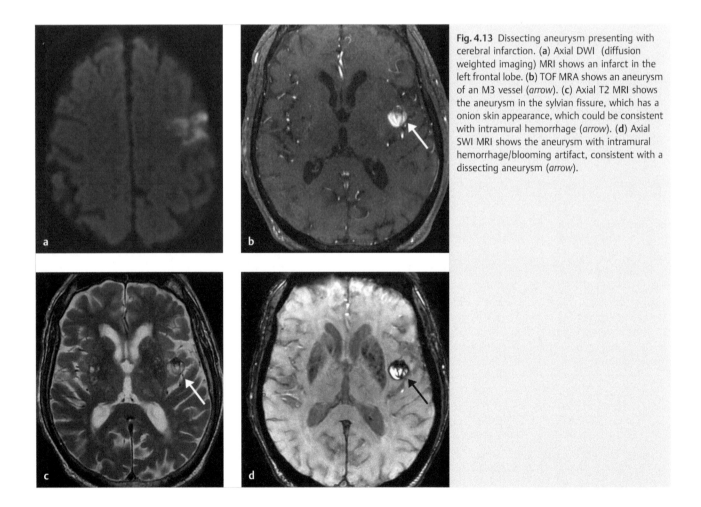

Fig. 4.13 Dissecting aneurysm presenting with cerebral infarction. (**a**) Axial DWI (diffusion weighted imaging) MRI shows an infarct in the left frontal lobe. (**b**) TOF MRA shows an aneurysm of an M3 vessel (*arrow*). (**c**) Axial T2 MRI shows the aneurysm in the sylvian fissure, which has a onion skin appearance, which could be consistent with intramural hemorrhage (*arrow*). (**d**) Axial SWI MRI shows the aneurysm with intramural hemorrhage/blooming artifact, consistent with a dissecting aneurysm (*arrow*).

ally small (2–3 mm), multiple, and can have irregular shapes appearing saccular, fusiform, or even resembling mushrooms. They are often associated with adjacent sulcal SAH, parenchymal hemorrhage or infarction (► Fig. 4.15). Infectious aneurysms can resolve spontaneously with antibiotic therapy. However, both oncotic and mycotic aneurysms can rapidly enlarge. CTA is the preferred imaging modality for screening and follow-up due to its higher spatial resolution and ability to image the entire distality of the cerebral vasculature (MRA often requires a black saturation band at the skull vertex).

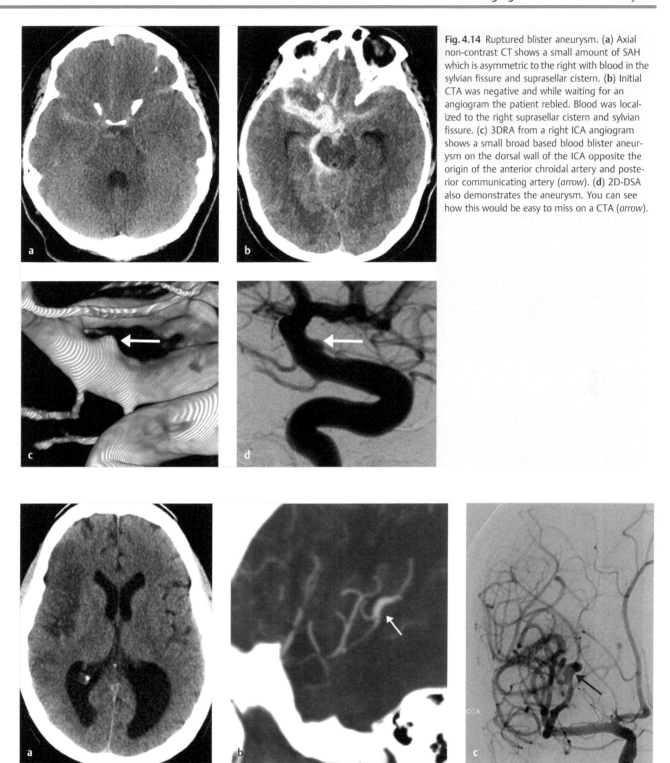

Fig. 4.14 Ruptured blister aneurysm. (**a**) Axial non-contrast CT shows a small amount of SAH which is asymmetric to the right with blood in the sylvian fissure and suprasellar cistern. (**b**) Initial CTA was negative and while waiting for an angiogram the patient rebled. Blood was localized to the right suprasellar cistern and sylvian fissure. (**c**) 3DRA from a right ICA angiogram shows a small broad based blood blister aneurysm on the dorsal wall of the ICA opposite the origin of the anterior chroidal artery and posterior communicating artery (*arrow*). (**d**) 2D-DSA also demonstrates the aneurysm. You can see how this would be easy to miss on a CTA (*arrow*).

Fig. 4.15 Mycotic aneurysm presenting with cerebral infarction. (**a**) Axial non-contrast CT in this patient with endocarditis shows a right MCA distribution infarct. (**b**) CTA demonstrates a fusiform aneurysm of an M3 branch (*arrow*). (**c**) AP right ICA cerebral angiogram shows a dilated and fusiform mycotic aneurysm (*arrow*). This appearance is typical for these aneurysms.

Immunodeficient aneurysms are the rarest form of aneurysm. They are most commonly seen in young children with congenital immunodeficiencies or patients with HIV/AIDS. The pathogenesis of these lesions is unclear. Typical imaging appearance is multifocal fusiform enlargement of intracranial arteries. Because immunodeficient aneurysms are often accompanied by a vasculitis, these lesions are commonly associated with ischemic stroke as well.

4.3.5 What the Clinician Needs to Know

- Type of aneurysm as well as the potential etiology of the aneurysm. For example, if a mycotic aneurysm is suspected, the radiologist should prompt the clinician to perform a work-up for endocarditis or other central infection.
- Effect of aneurysm on adjacent nonvascular structures (i.e., acute ischemic stroke from distal emboli, SAH from aneurysm rupture, cranial nerve mass effect).
- Aneurysm multiplicity (especially important in fusiform, infectious, or oncotic aneurysms).
- Aneurysm size, location, morphology, and anatomy.

4.3.6 High-Yield Facts

- Fusiform aneurysms predominantly affect the posterior circulation and have a poor natural history with high rates of growth, rupture, and ischemic stroke. Close follow-up of these lesions is warranted. Furthermore, AAA screening should be recommended in these patients.
- Blood blister aneurysms are often occult on CTA and can be difficult to identify angiographically as well. These lesions have high rates of rehemorrhage. If the CTA is negative and blood is primarily on one side of the suprasellar cistern, a blood blister aneurysm should be suspected.
- Oncotic and mycotic aneurysms have similar morphologies and imaging characteristics. They prefer the MCA territory because that is where most of the blood flow (and septic emboli and tumor emboli) goes. Multiplicity is the rule with these lesions.

Further Reading

[1] Brinjikji W, Morris JM, Brown RD, et al. Neuroimaging Findings in Cardiac Myxoma Patients: A Single-Center Case Series of 47 Patients. Cerebrovasc Dis. 2015; 40(1–2):35–44

[2] Nasr DM, Brinjikji W, Rouchaud A, Kadirvel R, Flemming KD, Kallmes DF. Imaging Characteristics of Growing and Ruptured Vertebrobasilar Non-Saccular and Dolichoectatic Aneurysms. Stroke. 2016; 47(1):106–112

[3] Sacho RH, Saliou G, Kostynskyy A, et al. Natural history and outcome after treatment of unruptured intradural fusiform aneurysms. Stroke. 2014; 45 (11):3251–3256

[4] Krings T, Lasjaunias PL, Geibprasert S, Pereira V, Hans FJ. The aneurysmal wall. The key to a subclassification of intracranial arterial aneurysm vasculopathies? Interv Neuroradiol. 2008; 14(September) Suppl 1:39–47

[5] Krings T, Mandell DM, Kiehl TR, et al. Intracranial aneurysms: from vessel wall pathology to therapeutic approach. Nat Rev Neurol. 2011; 7(10):547–559

4.4 Vessel Wall Imaging for Intracranial Aneurysms

4.4.1 Clinical Case

A 63-year-old female with severe headache lasting five days. Head CT was negative, however, lumbar puncture showed xanthochromia (▶ Fig. 4.16).

4.4.2 Description of Imaging Findings and Diagnosis

Diagnosis

Large basilar tip and posterior communicating artery aneurysms. There is concentric enhancement of the posterior communicating aneurysm suggesting this may be the ruptured aneurysm.

4.4.3 Background

Intracranial aneurysms are biologically complex lesions that are related to different underlying etiologies. While the morphologic characteristics of different intracranial aneurysms have been well classified, many histopathologic and imaging studies have demonstrated that much of the pathophysiology of these lesions involves the vessel wall. Vessel wall pathology can include thrombus, dissection, inflammation, and increased vasa vasorum. A summary of the histopathologic, VWI characteristics, and luminal imaging characteristics of the below-described lesions is provided in ▶ Table 4.6.

4.4.4 Imaging Findings

HR-VWI is potentially useful for the evaluation of the natural history of intracranial saccular aneurysms. Vessel wall enhancement in unruptured aneurysms lesions is thought to be secondary to vessel wall inflammation and increased density of vasa vasorum; variables associated with morphological modification and higher risk of rupture of intracranial aneurysms. Concentric wall enhancement is seen in nearly 90% of growing and ruptured aneurysms and only 30% of stable aneurysms (▶ Fig. 4.17). Overall, aneurysm wall enhancement is a sensitive, but not specific marker for aneurysm instability. It is conceivable to view aneurysm wall enhancement as a biomarker for aneurysm vulnerability and rupture, possibly necessitating more urgent treatment as opposed to conservative management, particularly in saccular aneurysms. Aneurysm wall enhancement has been shown in several cases to be useful in the setting of SAH in patients with multiple intracranial aneurysms. A number of series of patients with multiple intracranial aneurysms and SAH have found that ruptured aneurysms demonstrated significant vessel wall enhancement while the unruptured aneurysms lacked enhancement. The significance of non-circumferential wall enhancement in saccular aneurysms is still up in the air (▶ Fig. 4.18).

The primary VWI characteristic of dissecting aneurysms is the presence of acute intramural hemorrhage resulting in a crescent-shaped region of high T1 signal. There is often an area of luminal narrowing immediately proximal to the aneurysmal dilatation. Dissecting aneurysms also tend to form at locations other than branching points and are characterized by irregular shapes. A number of studies have used high resolution VWI to

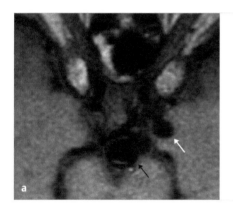
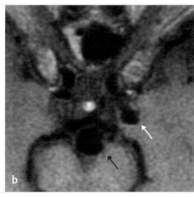

Fig. 4.16 Basilar tip and posterior communicating artery aneurysm with vessel wall imaging (VWI). (**a**) Non-contrast T1 VWI study demonstrates a posterior communicating artery (*white arrow*) and basilar tip (*black arrow*) aneurysm. (**b**) Post-contrast imaging shows enhancement of the wall of the posterior communicating artery aneurysm (*white arrow*) and no enhancement of the basilar tip aneurysm (*black arrow*). The posterior communicating artery aneurysm was treated acutely.

Table 4.6 Summary of VWI Findings in Various Types of Intracranial Aneurysms

Aneurysm Type	VWI Characteristics
Saccular	Unruptured: Typically lack vessel wall enhancement on T1CE imaging. Ruptured/Growing: Concentric vessel wall enhancement on T1CE imaging in ~90% of cases
Fusiform	Intrinsic T1 hyperintensity and gadolinium enhancement possibly associated with growth
Dissecting	Crescentic T1 Hyperintensity, Enhancement of Wall/Pseudolumen, Intimal Flap
Partially Thrombosed	Onion skin pattern with peripheral T1 hyperintensity in thrombosed portion. Lack of enhancement→ decreased growth rates
Mycotic/Oncotic	Circumferential enhancement usually present, significance is uncertain
Partially Thrombosed	Onion skin pattern with peripheral T1 hyperintensity in thrombosed portion. Lack of enhancement→ dereased growth rates

Abbreviation: T1CE, T1 contrast enhanced.

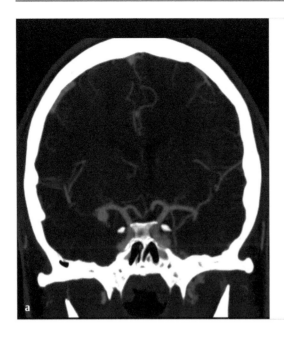
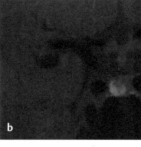
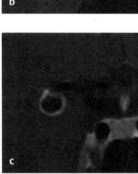

Fig. 4.17 Example of robust and circumferential wall enhancement. (a) Coronal MIP of a CTA shows an inferiorly projecting right MCA aneurysm. (b) Pre-contrast T1 VWI sequence and (c) Post-contrast T1 VWI sequence show robust circumferential enhancement of the aneurysm.

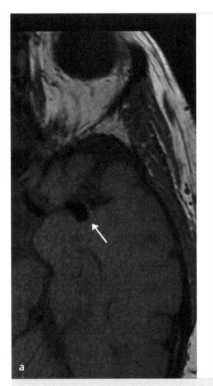
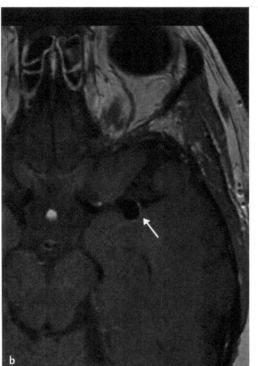
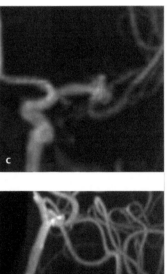
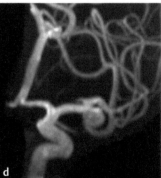

Fig. 4.18 Mild wall enhancement in a growing MCA bifurcation aneurysm. (a) Pre-contrast T1 VWI and (b) Post-contrast T1 VWI show mild wall enhancement of a left MCA bifurcation aneurysm (*arrows*). (c) MRA from the time of initial evaluation shows a 4-mm MCA bifurcation aneurysm. (d) The aneurysm grew to 7 mm in a 1-year period.

characterize dissecting aneurysms. High-resolution VWI has been shown to be more sensitive than conventional multise-quence MRI/MRA in detecting intramural high signal, which is a specific but not sensitive feature of these lesions (▶ Fig. 4.19). Two studies of intracranial dissecting aneurysms have demon-strated that 3 T T1-weighted black-blood VWI is also effective in detecting intimal flaps and the double-lumen sign, which are often difficult to detect with noninvasive luminal imaging

techniques such as MRA and CTA. Abnormal vessel wall en-hancement on black-blood imaging secondary to slow blood flow in the false lumen and/or proliferation of the vasa vaso-rum have also been described. Being able to differentiate dis-secting aneurysms with acute intramural hemorrhage from fusiform and saccular aneurysms is important as dissecting aneurysms may be associated with a more malignant natural history and often require treatment with techniques such as

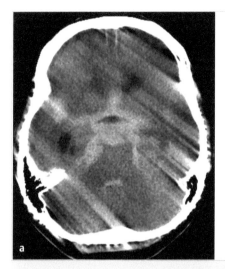 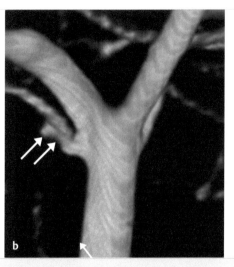 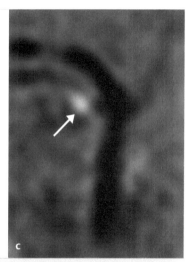

Fig. 4.19 Example of a dissecting SCA aneurysm. (**a**) Non-contrast CT shows diffuse SAH. (**b**) 3DRA shows an irregular aneurysm with a tiny intimal flap at the SCA origin (*arrows*). (**c**) Pre-contrast VWI shows mural T1 hyperintensity, findings consistent with a dissecting aneurysm (*arrow*).

parent vessel occlusion, intracranial stenting or flow diversion. It is important to point out that not all dissecting aneurysms have intramural hemorrhage as this resolves in the chronic stage of the dissection.

Fusiform aneurysms with or without thrombus are complex lesions, which have many potential etiologies. Some authors suggest that many of these lesions, especially those with intramural hematoma, are the result of healed dissections. Many of these aneurysms result from fragmentation of the internal elastic lamina with intimal neovascularization and intramural hemorrhage. Vessel wall inflammation has also been suggested to play a role in the growth and formation of these lesions. The presence of intramural hemorrhage within these lesions generally portends a poor prognosis. Several studies with conventional resolution MRI suggest that mural T1 hyperintensity consistent with intramural hemorrhage and enhancement of the aneurysm wall with gadolinium predict aneurysm growth.

4.4.5 What the Clinician Needs to Know

- Pre-gadolinium enhancement characteristics of the aneurysm including intrinsic T1 hyperintensity, intramural thrombus, and areas of wall thickening.
- Degree of enhancement of the aneurysm sac as well as the location of aneurysm sac enhancement.

- In setting of multiple aneurysms and SAH, the enhancing aneurysm is often the culprit lesion.

4.4.6 High-Yield Facts

- Concentric wall enhancement of a cerebral aneurysm is a sensitive but not specific sign of wall instability and future growth and rupture. Aneurysms without wall enhancement have low growth rates.
- Mural T1 signal in fusiform aneurysms is associated with increased risk of growth and rupture.
- Intramural hemorrhage is present in some, but not all, dissecting aneurysms. Chronic dissecting aneurysms are sometimes indistinguishable from fusiform aneurysms.

Further Reading

[1] Krings T, Mandell DM, Kiehl TR, et al. Intracranial aneurysms: from vessel wall pathology to therapeutic approach. Nat Rev Neurol. 2011; 7(10):547–559

[2] Brinjikji W, Mossa-Basha M, Huston J, Rabinstein AA, Lanzino G, Lehman VT. Intracranial vessel wall imaging for evaluation of steno-occlusive diseases and intracranial aneurysms. J Neuroradiol. 2017; 44(2):123–134

[3] Lehman VT, Brinjikji W, Mossa-Basha M, et al. Conventional and high-resolution vessel wall MRI of intracranial aneurysms: current concepts and new horizons. J Neurosurg. 2018; 128(4):969–981

4.5 Post-Aneurysm Treatment Imaging

4.5.1 Clinical Case

A 63-year-old female with history of previously coiled distal PICA aneurysm. Routine follow-up MRA (▶ Fig. 4.20).

4.5.2 Description of Imaging Findings and Diagnosis

Diagnosis

TOF MRA demonstrates blooming artifact from coils and laminated thrombus in the aneurysm dome. No evidence of recurrence. However, gadolinium bolus MRA demonstrates a large recurrence, which was confirmed on angiography.

4.5.3 Background

Follow-up imaging is mandatory for all intracranial aneurysm patients who have undergone treatment. Aneurysm recurrence is – depending on the initial presentation (ruptured vs unruptried – type of underlying vascular pathology) a fairly common phenomenon following endovascular coiling as roughly 20% of aneurysms recur and require retreatment. Aneurysms treated with flow diverters can have a poor response to therapy and require the placement of additional flow diverters. Even surgically clipped aneurysms can recur and many surgeons closely surveille their clipped patients. Identifying aneurysm recurrences is important because aneurysm recurrences and remnants continue to be at risk of rupture.

Given the costs and risks associated with cerebral angiography, many centers have moved toward noninvasive imaging to follow-up surgically or endovascularly treated patients. As expected, CTA and MRA are the two most commonly used imaging techniques for aneurysm follow-up. More recently, there has been interest in cone-beam CT for aneurysm follow-up as well.

Timing of post-treatment aneurysm imaging varies from center to center. In cases of an occluded aneurysm or one with a small neck remnant which is stable and unchanged, follow-up imaging is usually obtained at 3–6 months, 12–24 months, 3–5 years, and then every 3–5 years thereafter. If there is increase in size of the neck remnant then follow-up imaging is performed on a yearly basis. In cases where the remnant is large enough to warrant treatment, DSA is recommended.

4.5.4 Imaging Findings

Coil embolization is the most common form of intracranial aneurysm treatment. Endosaccular coils are composed of platinum, which can result in substantial streak artifact on CTA and blooming artifact on MRA. Over the past several years, it has become clear that gadolinium bolus MR angiography is the ideal conventional imaging technique for the evaluation of intracranial aneurysm recurrence following coil embolization therapy. When compared to TOF imaging, gadolinium bolus MR angiography is associated with higher rates of major and minor recurrence detection. In cases where there is a contraindication

to gadolinium-based contrast agents 3D-TOF MRA is sufficient with sensitivity and specificity values of > 85% (▶ Fig. 4.21, ▶ Fig. 4.22). In evaluating a coiled aneurysm, a simple three-point scale can be reported: (1) complete occlusion (i.e., no neck filling or contrast in the coil interstices), (2) neck remnant (contrast opacification of the neck but no filling of coil interstices), and (3) aneurysm remnant (contrast opacification of the aneurysm sac itself or filling of the coil interstices). Due to substantial metallic streak artifact, CTA is not suitable for the follow-up of coiled aneurysms.

Flow diversion and stent-assisted coiling are becoming more commonplace in the treatment of intracranial aneurysms. Again, the most commonly used follow-up imaging modality for stent-treated aneurysms is MR angiography. On MR, stents appear as a tiny endoluminal signal void. MR imaging of stents is difficult due to a combination of magnetic susceptibility and the faraday cage effect. Contrast enhanced MRA is preferable for the follow-up of stent- and flow-diverter treated aneurysms due to the fact that there is less signal loss in the parent vessel and more signal at the neck of the aneurysm. It is important to point out that even CE-MRA results in overdiagnosis of in-stent stenosis. In-stent stenosis is a very rare (< 5%) and generally benign complication of stent or flow diverter treatment. However, in some cases it can be severely flow limiting. In cases where there is a high concern for in-stent stenosis, CTA or DSA should be considered. CE-MRA has a sensitivity and specificity of 83 and 100%, for detecting aneurysm recurrence, compared to values of 50 and 100%, for TOF MRA, respectively. In addition to assessing aneurysm filling and parent vessel patency, the patency of any branch vessels covered by the aneurysm should be noted as up to 20% of branch vessels covered with flow diverter stent become occluded over time. CTA can be useful in flow-diverter treated aneurysms, especially for the evaluation of parent vessel patency. However, any time there is a coil mass in the aneurysm the utility of CTA is limited.

An important fact to point out for flow diversion is that because flow diversion does not involve placing anything in the aneurysm sac itself, over time, aneurysms will shrink in size and completely resolve. ▶ Fig. 4.23 demonstrates a case of a giant cavernous ICA aneurysm with mass effect which completely resolved following flow diversion.

One technique which is gaining interest in the field of post-treatment aneurysm imaging is flat-panel detector CTA using intravenous contrast (▶ Fig. 4.24). With improvements in modern-day flat panel detectors, we are now able to achieve high-quality imaging of stent and flow diverter treated aneurysms. This type of imaging has to be performed in the angiography suite and optimal work flows for routine implementation of this type of imaging have yet to be established. Flat panel CTA does allow for an excellent evaluation of stent wall apposition, stent kinking, and intrasaccular flow due to its high spatial resolution.

For clipped aneurysms, the most practical imaging technique is CTA. There is just too much blooming artifact from metallic clips to allow for accurate assessment of the aneurysm neck and parent vessel on MRA, even with metallic artifact corrections. MDCTA is not perfect either, but gives one the best shot at evaluating the parent artery and presence of neck remnant. Flat panel detector CTA and CTA with digital subtraction techniques are currently being evaluated for follow-up of clipped aneurysms and show promise. However, these techniques are not widely available.

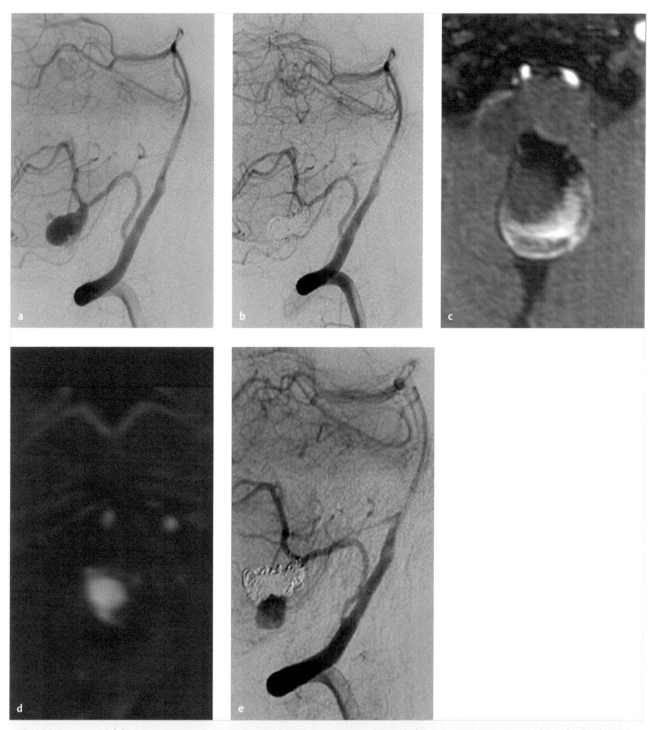

Fig. 4.20 Recurrence of dissecting PICA aneurysm seen only on post-contrast MRA. (**a**) Large dissecting PICA aneurysm involving the distal PICA. (**b**) Immediate post-coiling angiogram shows complete obliteration. (**c**) TOF MRA shows blooming artifact from the coils and laminated thrombus in the aneurysm. (**d**) However, contrast enhanced MR angiography (CE-MRA) shows a large aneurysm recurrence with contrast in the pouch. (**e**) Follow-up angiogram shows a large recurrence of the aneurysm.

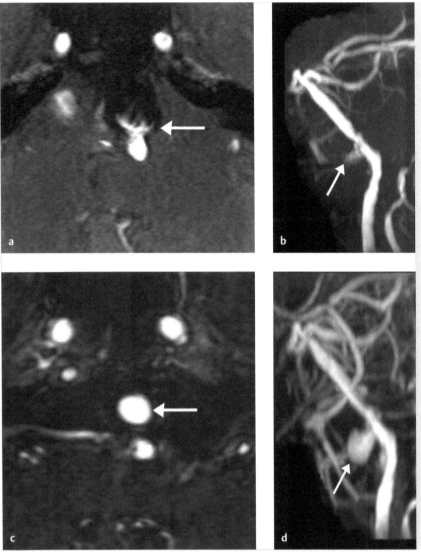

Fig. 4.21 Recurrent basilar trunk aneurysm seen best on CE-MRA. (a–b) TOF MRA shows blooming artifact from the coil and a small recurrence (*arrow*). (c–d) CE MRA shows a much larger recurrence which is even more prominent on the 3D MIP (*arrow*).

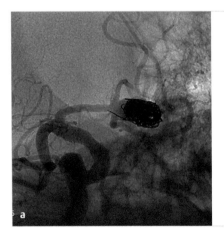
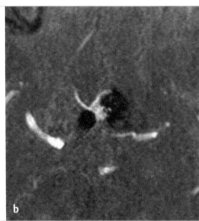

Fig. 4.22 Blooming artifact from a coil detachment zone. (a) Coiled Acom aneurysm with a small tail projecting into the A1 segment. This coil has a ferromagnetic component at the detachment zone. (b) On the CE MRA, there is a large recurrence and there is blooming artifact in the A1 segment from the ferromagnetic component. Make sure not to mistake this for a migrated coil!

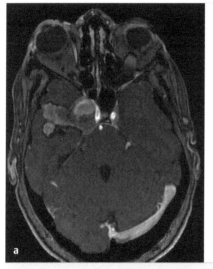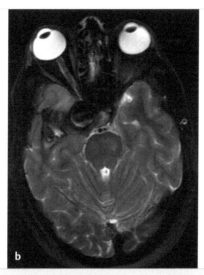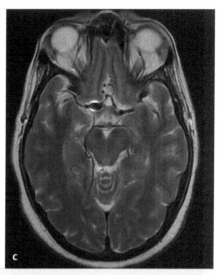

Fig. 4.23 Giant ICA aneurysm which completely remodels with flow diversion. (**a**) Bolus MRA shows a giant cavernous ICA aneurysm which is largely thrombosed and has a large secondary lobule or daughter sac. (**b**) T2 MRI also confirms the presence of the aneurysm with some associated mass effect on the temporal lobe. (**c**) 18 months following flow diverter treatment the aneurysm has completely resolved as has the mass effect. This is typical of flow diverter treated aneurysms.

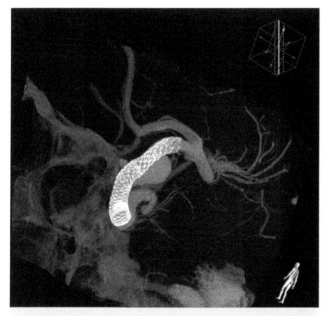

Fig. 4.24 IV CTA of a paraclinoid aneurysm treated with a single-flow diverter.

4.5.5 What the Clinician Needs to Know

- For coiled aneurysms: the presence of neck remnant or aneurysm remnant

- For stent-treated aneurysms: residual aneurysm filling, in-stent stenosis, branch vessel patency, and wall apposition
- For clipped aneurysms: how well one can see the parent vessel and how reliable the imaging modality will be for recurrence evaluation, presence of neck remnant or aneurysm remnant, and patency of branch vessels

4.5.6 High-Yield Facts

- Gadolinium bolus MRA is the preferred imaging modality for the assessment of aneurysm filling for aneurysms treated using endovascular techniques.
- Gadolinium bolus MRA will over-estimate degree of in-stent stenosis for flow diverter and stent-treated aneurysms. In cases where there is a high clinical concern for in-stent stenosis, a CTA or DSA should be considered.
- MDCTA and flat panel IV-CTA are the best imaging modalities for evaluation of clipped aneurysms.

Further Reading

[1] Soize S, Gawlitza M, Raoult H, Pierot L. Imaging Follow-Up of Intracranial Aneurysms Treated by Endovascular Means: Why, When, and How? Stroke. 2016; 47(5):1407–1412

[2] Hänsel NH, Schubert GA, Scholz B, et al. Implant-specific follow-up imaging of treated intracranial aneurysms: TOF-MRA vs. metal artifact reduced intravenous flat panel computed tomography angiography (FPCTA). Clin Radiol. 2018; 73(2):218.e9–218.e15

[3] Kaufmann TJ, Huston J, III, Cloft HJ, et al. A prospective trial of 3T and 1.5T time-of-flight and contrast-enhanced MR angiography in the follow-up of coiled intracranial aneurysms. AJNR Am J Neuroradiol. 2010; 31(5):912–918

Chapter 5

Cerebral Arteriovenous Malformations (AVMs) and Dural Arteriovenous Fistulas (dAVFs)

5 Cerebral Arteriovenous Malformations (AVMs) and Dural Arteriovenous Fistulas (dAVFs)

5.1 Evaluating AVM Angioarchitecture

5.1.1 Clinical Case

A 47-year-old female with new seizures (▶ Fig. 5.1).

5.1.2 Description of Imaging Findings and Diagnosis

Diagnosis

Fistulous type arteriovenous malformation (AVM) in the left parietal lobe with multiple feeding arterial aneurysms, a markedly hypertrophied MCA branch suggesting a fistulous component, multiple intranidal aneurysms, large venous pouches, and a long draining vein.

5.1.3 Background

Brain AVMs are substantially rarer than intracranial aneurysms with an estimated prevalence of 20 per 100,000 people. These lesions are thought to form either in utero or early in life; however, there are a few reported cases of de novo AVMs developing in adult patients. AVMs can have a wide range of presentations including rupture, seizures, headache, cognitive decline, weakness, sensory changes, or bruit. The risk of rupture of a brain AVM is estimated to be 2–3% per year. A simple formula proposed for determining a patient's lifetime risk of an AVM bleed is 105-(patient age in years).

There are a variety of characteristics that need to be considered when evaluating an AVM. Perhaps, the most well-known AVM grading scheme is the Spetzler-Martin Grade, which grades AVMs on a 1–5 scale based on size, eloquence, and venous drainage to determine the patient's risk of neurological deficit after *surgical* resection (▶ Table 5.1). This scale neither

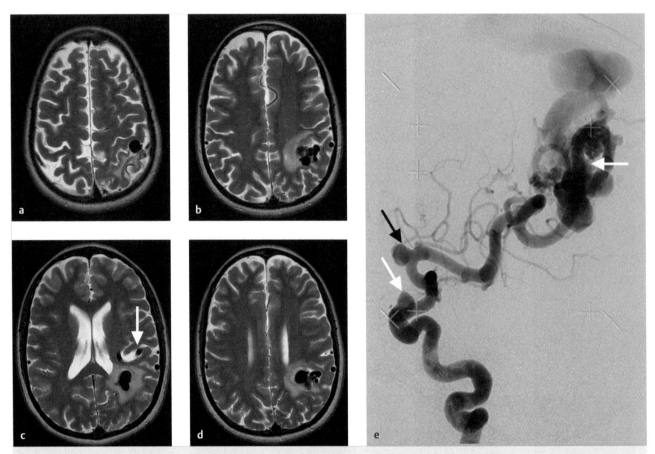

Fig. 5.1 A 47-year-old female with seizure. **(a-d)** Four slices of a T2-weighted MRI demonstrate an AVM with a relatively compact nidus in the left parietal lobe. There is a markedly hypertrophied left MCA branch, which feeds the AVM (*white arrow*). The AVM has a large venous pouch with associated surrounding edema and thrombus. **(e)** Left ICA cerebral angiogram shows a tortuous course of the left cervical ICA. There are proximal flow-related aneurysms of the paraophthalmic ICA and MCA bifurcation (*diagonal arrows*). There are feeding arterial aneurysms of the distal left MCA. There is a fistulous component to the AVM (*horizontal white arrow*), which dives into large venous pouches and ectasias. The draining vein is markedly dilated and has a long course. The fistulous component, thrombosed venous pouch with edema, and long course of the draining vein are all risk factors for seizures in this AVM patient.

Table 5.1 AVM Angioarchitectural Characteristics

Segment	Angioarchitectural Feature	Definition
Feeding Artery	Arterial dilation	≥ 50% increase in vessel diameter
Feeding Artery	Proximal flow-related aneurysm	Aneurysm located in CoW, but not on an AVM-feeding vessel
Feeding Artery	Distal flow-related arterial aneurysm	Aneurysm located along direct feeder of AVM
Feeding Artery	Perinidal angiogenesis	Indirect supply to periphery of AVM from branches of artery other than feeder
Feeding Artery	Number of feeding arteries	Number of arteries which either form fistulous components or converge on the nidus
AV Connection	Fistulous component	Direct transition of artery to vein with no nidus
AV Connection	Intranidal aneurysm	Aneurysm located within the AVM nidus
AV Connection	Nidus component	Plexiform connection between artery and vein
AV Connection	En passage nidus	Multiple smaller vessels arising from a single large vessel go on to supply nidus
AV Connection	Terminal nidus	Feeding artery terminates in plexiform nidus
AV Connection	Diffuse nidus	Large nidus with intermingled brain
AV Connection	Compact nidus	Sharp nidus with no intermingled brain
Venous Drainage	Venous ectasia	Markedly dilated vein
Venous Drainage	Long course of draining vein	≥ 3-cm superficial course of draining vein
Venous Drainage	Venous outflow stenosis	Reduction of 50% or more in vessel diameter
Venous Drainage	Pseudophlebitic pattern	Tortuous engorged cerebral veins in the venous phase of the brain circulation
Venous Drainage	Venous reflux	Reflux of draining vein into cortical or deep venous system
Venous Drainage	Number of draining veins	Number of veins which drain the AVM nidus
Venous Drainage	Deep versus superficial venous drainage	Drainage into the Internal Cerebral Vein or galenic venous system versus cortical venous drainage into the superior sagittal sinus or transverse/sigmoid sinuses

Abbreviations: AVM, Arteriovenous Malformations; AV, Arteriovenous.

evaluates natural history nor does it determine risk factors or success rates of radiosurgical or embolization treatment and thus cannot be used to characterize the risk of hemorrhage or potential success and complication rates of treatments other than surgery. Through extensive study of the imaging characteristics of brain AVMs, we now have a better understanding of which angioarchitectural characteristics are important for understanding AVM natural history, pathophysiology, and treatment decisions. In this chapter, we focus on defining various angioarchitectural terms, which will be expounded on in later chapters. These terms are summarized in ▶ Table 5.1.

5.1.4 Imaging Findings

It is helpful to compartmentalize AVM angioarchitecture into three components: (1) arterial, (2) arteriovenous connection, and (3) draining veins. Each of these components have certain features which can either change natural history, affect clinical management, or influence the clinical presentation.

AVMs can have one or multiple feeding artery. Usually, the dominant feeding artery is large, whereas additional arterial feeders are smaller in caliber. Characterizing the feeding arterial branch locations, sizes, and tortuosity is important for surgical or endovascular planning purposes. Very high-flow AVMs can be associated with tortuosity of the cervical arteries as well. Occasionally, very superficial AVMs, which are large and have bled, can develop dural arterial feeders from the external carotid artery (ECA). These are difficult to identify without the help of conventional angiography. Arterial feeders should also be characterized as en-passage (i.e., multiple branch arteries supplying the nidus from a dominant arterial branch), or direct (i.e., single artery going directly into the nidus). Lastly, feeding arterial aneurysms should

be identified and characterized as they are at risk of rupture due to the high-flow conditions associated with brain AVMs. Up to 20% of brain AVMs have a feeding arterial aneurysm either along the arterial pedicle just proximal to the nidus or flow-related aneurysms along branch vessels in the circle of Willis, even contralateral to the AVM. A substantial proportion of cases have multiple feeding arterial aneurysms (▶ Fig. 5.1).

Another arterial phenomenon that provides some insight into AVM pathophysiology and symptomatic presentation is pernidal angiogenesis. In some cases, AVMs demand so much blood flow that they begin to recruit secondary feeding arteries, which go on to provide more blood flow for the dominant arterial feeder(s). This results in hypertrophy of leptomeningeal collaterals in the periphery of the AVM. On MRI, they are often dilated and tortuous vessels coursing along the sulci but lack the compact appearance of a nidus. Identifying these vessels is important because errant embolization, radiotherapy, or surgical resection of neoangiogenesis can result in infarction of normal brain (▶ Fig. 5.2).

The arteriovenous connection is the weakest angioarchitectural point of the brain AVM. The location of the nidus in relationship to eloquent brain tissue is important. A list of eloquent regions in supplied in ▶ Table 5.2. Nidus size is important for planning surgical, endovascular, and radiosurgical interventions. It is best to measure the nidus in three dimensions to calculate a volume as certain volume thresholds indicate a poor response to radiosurgical treatment (i.e., more than 12cc). Niduses should be characterized as diffuse or compact. Most niduses are compact and do not have any intervening brain tissue. A diffuse nidus is defined as a nidus in which there is normal brain tissue interspersed between the vessels. AVMs should also be evaluated to determine if there are multiple intervening niduses (so-called multi-compartment AVMs). Some brain AVMs can stimulate

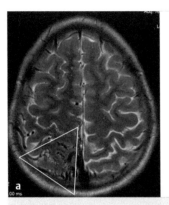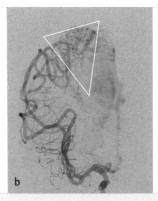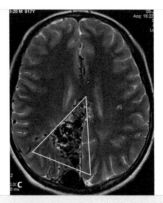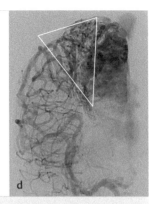

Fig. 5.2 Neoangiogenesis versus nidus. (**a**) Axial T2-weighted MRI shows a wedge-shaped region of increased vascularity (*white triangle*). These vessels are all within the sulci and do not have an organized appearance like a nidus. This is a typical appearance of neoangiogenesis. (**b**) AP Right ICA angiogram shows these vessels as they course to the right paramedial AVM. They are hypertrophied leptomeningeal collaterals and there is no arteriovenous shunting arising from these branches (*white triangle*). (**c**) Axial T2-weighted MRI shows the actual nidus in this patient, a wedge-shaped nidus with no normal intervening brain tissue. The vessels are much more compact (*white triangle*). (**d**) AP right ICA cerebral angiogram shows the compact nidus with arteriovenous shunting (not marked). The perinidal angiogenesis is just lateral to it and you can see the more disorganized, non-compact appearance of the perinidal angiogenesis (*white triangle*).

Table 5.2 Spetzler-Martin Grading Score

AVM size	Adjacent eloquent cortex	Draining veins
Under 3 cm = 1	Non-eloquent = 0	Superficial only = 0
3–6 cm = 2	Eloquent* = 1	Deep veins = 1
Over 6 cm = 3		

*Eloquent location was defined as the sensorimotor, language or visual cortex, hypothalamus, thalamus, brainstem, cerebellar nuclei, or regions directly adjacent to these structures.

the formation of direct arteriovenous fistulas without an intervening nidus-identification of such lesions requires careful following of the course of all feeding arteries and draining veins. These fistulous components shunts can result in arterial steal phenomenon and nonhemorrhagic neurological deficits. Intranidal aneurysms should be identified and any change in size or shape of these lesions should be closely monitored. Intranidal aneurysms have been shown to portend a higher risk of rupture and are often the rupture point of hemorrhagic brain AVMs and are often located in the center of the hematoma.

The draining vein is often neglected when evaluating AVM angioarchitecture, but it often holds the key to understanding the AVM presentation and natural history. Radiologists are often inclined to describe the location and direction of the draining veins (i.e., deep and superficial), but this only helps in understanding operative risk and not clinical presentation or natural history. Venous ectasia, colloquially referred to as venous aneurysms, are associated with a higher rupture risk. These ectasias can become partially thrombosed as well resulting in mass effect. Stenosis of the draining vein is also associated with higher rupture risk as it leads to increased pressure in the nidus. Stenosis is most common at the junction between the draining vein and the dural venous sinus but can happen anywhere. Evidence of venous congestion surrounding the AVM

should also be evaluated. This is best demonstrated by the presence of dilated transmedullary veins on CTA or SWI MRI. Venous congestion is often related to outflow obstruction secondary to venous stenosis or thrombosis and can result in hemorrhage or nonhemorrhagic neurological symptoms. Last, the course of the draining pial vein is important to comment on. A long pial course of the draining vein portends a higher rate of seizure and other nonhemorrhagic neurological presentations. The reason for this being the fact that a long draining vein under high pressure will not be able to drain normal parenchyma as well. In such cases, it is not uncommon to see venous congestion in the affected territory (▶ Fig. 5.1, ▶ Fig. 5.3).

5.1.5 What the Clinician Needs to Know

- Basic AVM characteristics including size, location, eloquence of surrounding brain, and venous drainage patterns
- Angioarchitectural weak points of the brain AVM including intranidal aneurysms, flow-related aneurysms, venous ectasias, venous stenosis, deep venous drainage, single venous drainage and posterior fossa location
- Presence of dilated cortical and transmedullary veins, which can influence the presentation of an unruptured AVM

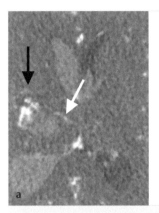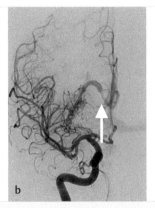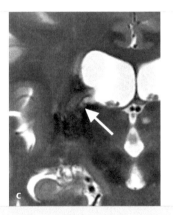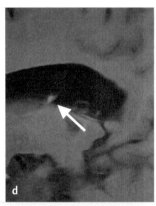

Fig. 5.3 Draining vein stenosis resulting in thrombosis. (**a**) Ruptured AVM in the right thalamocapsular region. The nidus is easily identified (*black arrow*). However, the medially coursing draining vein appears to be narrowed or poorly opacified (*white arrow*). (**b**) Right ICA cerebral angiogram demonstrates the AVM and the focal draining vein stenosis (*white arrow*). (**c**) 6 months later, repeat MRI demonstrates a curvilinear T2-hyperintense structure in the location of the draining vein (*white arrow*). (**d**) The vein was T1 hyperintense as well (*white arrow*). In the interim, the stenotic draining vein thrombosed resulting in resolution of the brain AVM. In this case, the draining vein stenosis was a risk factor for hemorrhage, and contributed to spontaneous resolution of the AVM.

5.1.6 High-yield Facts

- AVM characteristics associated with the higher risk of future hemorrhage include prior hemorrhage, intranidal aneurysm, venous stenosis or ectasia, deep venous drainage, single venous drainage, and deep or posterior fossa location.
- AVM characteristics associated with a higher risk of nonhemorrhagic neurologic deficits include a high-flow shunt, venous congestion or outflow obstruction, long pial course of the draining vein, and arterial steal.
- Spetzler-Martin score is associated with surgical risk and not natural history.

Further Reading

[1] Geibprasert S, Pongpech S, Jiarakongmun P, Shroff MM, Armstrong DC, Krings T. Radiologic assessment of brain arteriovenous malformations: what clinicians need to know. Radiographics. 2010; 30(2):483–501

[2] Mokin M, Dumont TM, Levy EI. Novel multimodality imaging techniques for diagnosis and evaluation of arteriovenous malformations. Neurol Clin. 2014; 32(1):225–236

[3] Leclerc X, Gauvrit JY, Trystram D, Reyns N, Pruvo JP, Meder JF. [Cerebral arteriovenous malformations: value of the non invasive vascular imaging techniques]. J Neuroradiol. 2004; 31(5):349–358

5.2 Evaluating the Ruptured Brain AVM

5.2.1 Clinical Case

A 47-year-old female with sudden onset severe headache and the loss of consciousness.

5.2.2 Description of Imaging Findings and Diagnosis

Diagnosis

Ruptured vermian AVM with intraparenchymal and intraventricular hemorrhage with an intranidal aneurysm, which is projecting directly into the large hematoma (▶ Fig. 5.4).

5.2.3 Background

Ruptured brain AVMs present a major clinical challenge for surgical and endovascular neurovascular specialists. One of the key challenges in managing these lesions is deciding when and how to treat the lesion. Unlike ruptured intracranial aneurysms, current recommendations state that it is preferable to wait at least a month before attempting to cure a patient of a ruptured AVM. The reasons for this are two-fold. First, many studies suggest that patients who are rehabilitated and then undergo AVM resection may experience better outcomes than those who are treated in the acute phase. Second, in some cases, the hematoma from the AVM rupture can compress part of the nidus or one of the draining veins making part of the AVM invisible on imaging. Tackling the lesion while there is a hematoma could lead to incomplete treatment. There is no ambiguity when it comes to emergency decompressive surgery or hematoma evacuation for patients who have large hematomas causing mass effect. However, even in these cases, resection of the AVM is not recommended.

There is a growing body of literature suggesting that targeted treatment of intranidal and feeding arterial aneurysms in ruptured brain AVMs in the acute phase may be of benefit. In patients with an AVM-associated aneurysm and a ruptured brain AVM, the rate of rehemorrhage is 11% per patient-month, whereas it is just 1% per patient-month without an aneurysm. Because of this, it is imperative for neuroradiologists to identify any and all angiographic weak points within a ruptured AVM. The neuroradiologists should ask herself "what part of the AVM ruptured?" whenever encountered with a ruptured AVM. Among ruptured AVMs, associated aneurysms are the cause of hemorrhage in roughly 50% of cases.

5.2.4 Imaging Findings

Again, when assessing angiographic weak points in an already ruptured brain AVM, it helps to compartmentalize AVM angioarchitecture into three components: (1) feeding arteries, (2) arteriovenous connection/nidus, and (3) draining veins. Each of these components have certain features, which can affect the clinical management of patients with ruptured AVMs.

Feeding arterial aneurysms are present in roughly 20% of ruptured brain AVMs. The pathophysiological basis for these lesions is thought to be an underlying vascular defect or a result of the dynamic interaction between hemodynamic stress, vasoactive substances, and functional alterations from vascular remodeling. There are three types of flow-related aneurysms, each with different levels of severity. First, unrelated aneurysms are aneurysms which form in the intracranial circulation but are remote from the AVM itself. These lesions can rupture just like any other intracranial aneurysm but the site of the rupture is remote from the AVM itself. An example of an unrelated aneurysm would be a left MCA aneurysms in a patient with an AVM in the right frontal lobe. Regarding flow-related aneurysms, we have proximal and distal flow-related aneurysms. Proximal flow-related aneurysms are located on a vessel that is proximal to the artery, which is directly feeding the AVM. These aneurysms are located on the ICA, circle of Willis, MCA (M1 segment or bifurcation) or vertebrobasilar trunk. An example of a proximal flow-related aneurysm would be a left M1 segment aneurysm in a patient with a left sylvian fissure AVM supplied by M2/M3 branches.

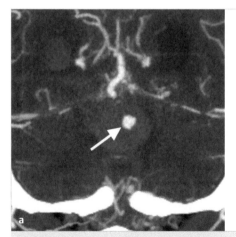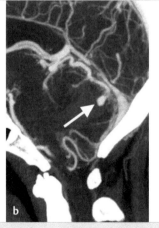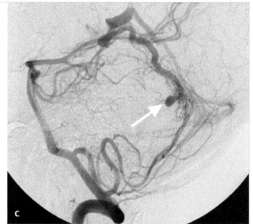

Fig. 5.4 Ruptured vermian AVM with intranidal aneurysm projecting into the hematoma. (a) Coronal CTA demonstrates a large vermian hematoma with a 4-mm aneurysm (*arrow*) projecting directly into the hemorrhage cavity. (b) Sagittal CTA confirms the aneurysm, projecting anteriorly into the hemorrhagic cavity (*arrow*). (c) Left vertebral artery cerebral angiogram shows the AVM on the posterior surface of the vermis with a draining vein along the vermian surface. The intranidal aneurysm is projecting anteriorly, as on the CTA (*arrow*).

Distal flow-related aneurysms are located along the artery, which is directly supplying the AVM (▶ Fig. 5.5). There is a direct relationship between the proximity of the aneurysm to the AVM and the risk of rupture.

Intranidal aneurysms are present in up to 50% of ruptured AVMs. These lesions form as weak points within an already weak nidus and, when present, are often the culprit for the hemorrhage. Oftentimes, the intranidal aneurysm will project directly into the hematoma cavity, and when that happens, one can be certain that the aneurysm itself was the culprit for the hemorrhage. Conveying this information is important because targeted endovascular or surgical treatment can be performed to exclude the intranidal aneurysm while leaving the rest of the AVM intact.

Bleeding can result from draining vein pathology as well. Venous ectasias and varices, colloquially referred to as venous aneurysms can rupture. These hemorrhages can vary from large intraparenchymal hematomas or local hemorrhage solely surrounding the venous varix (▶ Fig. 5.6). Ruptured venous varices are often associated with local thrombosis as well. Targetting treatment to these lesions is difficult without targeting the AVM in its entirety, but the presence of a ruptured venous varix spells a poorer natural history for the already ruptured

AVM and may prompt earlier treatment. AVM rupture can also result from draining vein stenosis or occlusion/thrombosis. Draining vein stenosis or thrombosis can cause rupture due to the associated increased in intranidal blood pressure. Stenosis of the draining vein is also associated with higher rates of re-rupture as well and may prompt earlier treatment (▶ Fig. 5.7). Occasionally, draining vein thrombosis/stenosis can result in rupture and subsequent obliteration of the AVM. Stenosis is most common at the junction between the draining vein and the dural venous sinus but can happen anywhere.

A point should be made about negative CTA/MRA/DSA in a patient with a suspected AVM. A small proportion of brain AVMs are micro-AVMs, defined as lesions which measure 1 cm or less in size. When these lesions rupture they are often completely compressed by the surrounding hematoma and may be occult on conventional angiography and cross-sectional imaging. In cases where there is no clear etiology for the hemorrhage or when an AVM is suspected (i.e., younger patient with occipital hematoma), repeat imaging should be performed around 3 months post-hemorrhage. Such imaging should include DSA and CTA/MRA. If these imaging tests are negative then a repeat CTA/MRA at around 6–12 months is reasonable.

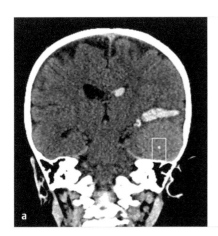
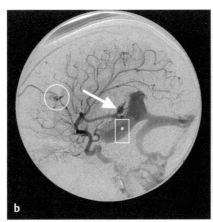

Fig. 5.5 Distal feeding arterial aneurysm in a patient with a direct pial AV fistula. (**a**) Coronal NCCT shows a hemorrhage in the left temporal lobe as well as intraventricular hemorrhage in the temporal horn and left lateral ventricle. There is a giant venous varix displacing the left temporal lobe superiorly (*). (**b**) Left ICA cerebral angiogram shows a direct pial AV fistula along the undersurface of the left temporal lobe. There is a distal feeding arterial aneurysm, which is likely the culprit of the rupture (*arrow*). Note the presence of a second AVM supplied by a frontal branch of the left MCA (*circle*).

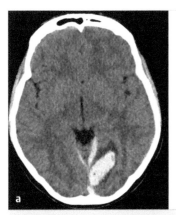
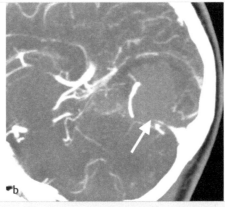
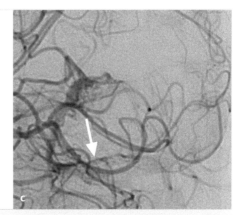

Fig. 5.6 Left occipital hematoma from AVM with draining vein stenosis. (**a**) Non-contrast CT shows a left occipital hematoma with vasogenic edema surrounding it. (**b**) Sagittal reconstructed CTA shows a large vessel along the periphery of the hematoma, which is likely the draining vein. However, we lose track of the vessel as it courses toward the sinus (*arrow*). This is suggestive of a draining vein stenosis or occlusion, which was likely the culprit of the hematoma. (**c**) Left vertebral artery digital subtraction angiography (DSA) shows the nidus and draining vein. There is definitely a draining vein stenosis (*arrow*). This AVM was treated acutely due to the risk of hemorrhage.

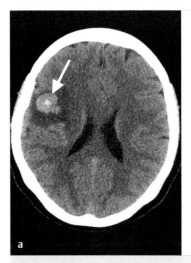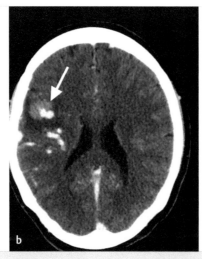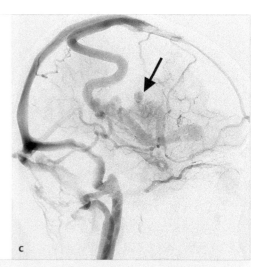

Fig. 5.7 Ruptured venous varix. (**a**) Non-contrast CT demonstrates a focal area of hemorrhage with surrounding vasogenic edema (*arrow*). (**b**) CTA shows a right frontal AVM. There is a large venous varix associated with the AVM, which is filling with contrast (*arrow*). There is surrounding hemorrhage about the venous varix as well as vasogenic edema. (**c**) Left ICA angiogram shows the superiorly pointing venous varix (*arrow*).

5.2.5 What the Clinician Needs to Know

- Presence of lesions which can be targeted for partial embolization or surgical treatment such as feeding arterial or intranidal aneurysms.
- Venous pathologies which may have resulted in the AVM hemorrhage including venous aneurysms, venous stenosis, or venous occlusion.
- CTA and MRA are not sensitive for detection of smaller AVMs in the setting of a rupture and repeat imaging around three months post-hemorrhage should be considered.

5.2.6 High-yield Facts

- Aneurysms associated with AVMs can be (1) unrelated to the AVM itself (i.e., contralateral), (2) proximal feeding arterial

(i.e., ICA, basilar artery, vertebral artery, M1, CoW), (3) distal (i.e., on the direct arterial feeder), or (4) intranidal.
- Venous aneurysms can rupture and often produce a small hematoma surrounding the venous aneurysm itself.
- Draining vein stenosis/occlusion can result in higher rates of re-rupture of the AVM.

Further Reading

[1] Geibprasert S, Pongpech S, Jiarakongmun P, Shroff MM, Armstrong DC, Krings T. Radiologic assessment of brain arteriovenous malformations: what clinicians need to know. Radiographics. 2010; 30(2):483–501
[2] Mokin M, Dumont TM, Levy EI. Novel multimodality imaging techniques for diagnosis and evaluation of arteriovenous malformations. Neurol Clin. 2014; 32(1):225–236
[3] Leclerc X, Gauvrit JY, Trystram D, Reyns N, Pruvo JP, Meder JF. [Cerebral arteriovenous malformations: value of the non invasive vascular imaging techniques]. J Neuroradiol. 2004; 31(5):349–358

5.3 Evaluating Unruptured AVMs and the Peri-AVM Environment

5.3.1 Clinical Case

A 47-year-old female with sudden onset severe headache and visual aura (▶ Fig. 5.8).

5.3.2 Description of Imaging Findings and Diagnosis

Diagnosis

Unruptured brain AVM in the right occipital lobe. The AVM has a large inferiorly projecting venous pouch. On T2 MRI, the pouch is partially thrombosed and there is severe associated surrounding vasogenic edema.

5.3.3 Background

Unruptured brain AVMs currently present a major management conundrum for neurovascular specialists. Following publication of the ARUBA trial that showed superior outcomes for conservative management over curative therapy for unruptured brain AVMs, there has been some pushback against treatment of these lesions. However, unruptured brain AVMs can result in substantial morbidity and mortality due to their risk of rupture as well as their proclivity to cause neurological symptoms in the absence of rupture.

When evaluating an unruptured AVM, it is important to characterize the lesion using the angioarchitectural features described in sections 5.1 and 5.2. This is especially important for evaluating risk of rupture. However, it is also important to consider how the lesion is interacting and affecting the adjacent brain parenchyma. Aside from hemorrhage, unruptured high-flow shunting AVMs can impact the adjacent brain parenchyma in a variety of ways including hypoxemia, mass effect, venous congestion, and vasogenic edema. These mechanisms can result in focal neurological deficits, seizures, developmental

delay, cognitive decline, headaches, and hydrocephalus. Here, we will describe how one should characterize both the unruptured AVM and peri-AVM environment to better understand the clinical presentation and natural history of an unruptured brain AVM.

5.3.4 Imaging Findings

When determining the rupture risk of a brain AVM, angioarchitecture is key. There are a few salient angioarchitectural findings, which are associated with increased risk of rupture of a previously unruptured brain AVM and they include feeding arterial aneurysms, intranidal aneurysms, venous ectasias, and venous outflow stenoses. The prior two chapters provide representative images for these features.

MRI is the preferred modality for evaluation of the peri-AVM environment. Salient findings in the peri-AVM environment that should be evaluated on MRI include medullary venous congestion, prior AVM bleeding, signs of perilesional arterial steal, presence of a long draining vein (i.e., 3 cm or longer), and AVM-related edema (▶ Table 5.3).

As described in sections 5.1 and 5.2, venous drainage patterns have a substantial effect on the natural history and clinical presentation of brain AVMs. When evaluating the draining vein of a brain AVM, it is important to try to think about how arterialization of the draining vein will affect the normal brain, which was originally draining through this vein (▶ Fig. 5.9). This is especially true in deep brain AVMs that drain into internal cerebral veins or the galenic system as the venous drainage of the deep structures is also dependent on these veins to drain. Venous arterialization can impair the normal physiological gradients of medullary venous drainage and result in medullary venous congestion. On imaging, this will manifest as deep white matter edema with or without dilated transmedullary veins. In extreme cases, medullary venous congestion can result in hydrocephalus from impaired CSF clearance and cognitive dysfunction (▶ Fig. 5.10). Perfusion imaging in these patients will show increased CBV (from venous congestion) and MTT (from delayed transit through the medullary venous system). High flow in the

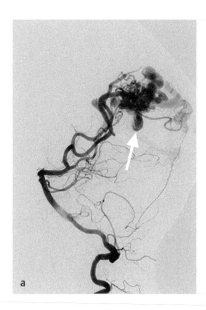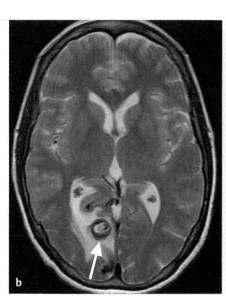

Fig. 5.8 Thrombosed venous varix resulting in edema. **(a)** Left vertebral artery cerebral angiogram shows a 3-cm AVM in the left occipital lobe. The AVM has a large inferiorly projecting venous varix (*arrow*), which, even on angiogram, has a laminated appearance which can be seen in the setting of slow flow or thrombosis. **(b)** Axial T2-weighted MRI shows the partially thrombosed varix with marked surrounding vasogenic edema (*arrow*).

Table 5.3 Summary of Important Parenchymal Imaging Findings for Brain AVM Patients

Vascular Pathology	Parenchymal Finding	Clinical Consequence
Medullary Venous Congestion	Deep white matter edema, dilated medulllary veins	Hydrocephalus from impaired CSF clearance, cognitive dysfunction
Prior AVM Bleeding	T2* artifact surrounding AVM or lining cerebral sulci	Higher risk of future hemorrhage
High flow arteriovenous shunt/arterial steal	Gliosis surrounding the AVM, altered perfusion or autoregulation	Neurological deficit or seizure
Long draining vein	Edema in brain supplied by the draining vein from impaired venous drainage	Seizure, cognitive dysfunction
Large venous pouch	Mass effect and vasogenic edema	Seizure, neurological deficit, hydrocephalus

Abbreviation: CSF, Cerebrospinal fluid.

draining vein can also result in a venopathy and eventual stenosis or thrombosis of the draining vein. If this involves a vein which is also draining normal vein, the patient can suffer a venous infarct in the venous drainage territory (▶ Fig. 5.11).

The presence of a large venous pouch does not only portend a higher risk of rupture, but also can result in mass effect and associated vasogenic edema (▶ Fig. 5.8). Mass effect and edema from a venous pouch can be exacerbated in the setting of acute thrombosis of the pouch itself. Attention should be paid on conventional T1 and T2-weighted imaging for the presence of thrombus or enhancing thrombus in a venous pouch and its associated mass effect. Mass effect can result in focal neurological deficit, seizure activity, or hydrocephalus, if it is in the region of the cerebral aqueduct or other CSF drainage pathways.

Perfusion imaging can provide valuable insights into how an AVM is affecting blood flow in the extranidal brain parenchyma (▶ Table 5.4). One phenomenon that is commonly discussed in the context of brain AVMs is that of "arterial steal." Arterial steal is a process in which increased blood flow through a low-resistance system (i.e., brain AVM) diverts blood flow from a region of normal brain. This results in relative hypotension in these

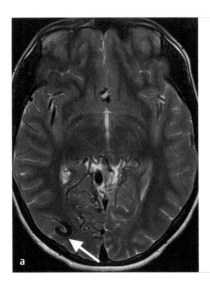
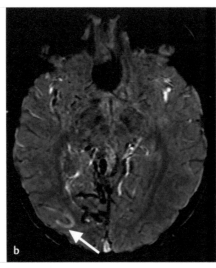

Fig. 5.9 Long, arterialized draining vein in a patient with an occipital AVM. (a) Abnormal vascularity in the medial right occipital lobe secondary to the presence of an occipital AVM. There is a markedly dilated draining vein, which is remote from the AVM itself (*arrow*). (b) SWI imaging shows the vein is hyperintense suggesting it is arterialized. The vein is bright on SWI due to the presence of oxyhemoglobin and it is long because we are several slices below the nidus (*arrow*).

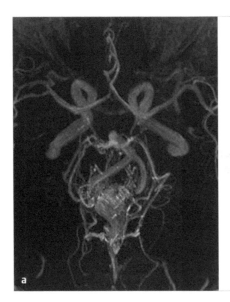
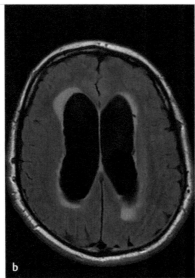

Fig. 5.10 Unruptured brain AVM resulting in hydrocephalus and cognitive dysfunction. (a) TOF MRA shows a large AVM, which was in the pineal region. The AVM did not result in any mass effect but was extremely high flow and had exclusive deep venous drainage. (b) T2/FLAIR (fluid attenuation inversion recovery) MRI shows marked ventricular dilatation and transependymal flow of CSF. This patient's hydrocephalus was the result of impaired CSF resorbition due to severe venous hypertension.

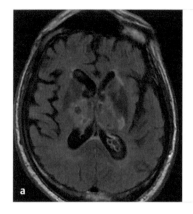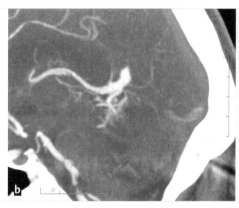

Fig. 5.11 Deep venous infarct secondary to straight sinus thrombosis in patient with vermian AVM. (a) This patient presented with subacute onset of a severe encephalopathy. T2/FLAIR MRI shows bithalamic edema as well as areas of hemosiderin deposition, classic imaging findings of a deep venous infarct. There is also mild hydrocephalus. (b) CTA demonstrates an AVM of the superior vermis, which is draining into the vermian vein. However, the straight sinus is completely thrombosed and absent likely due to a flow-related venopathy.

Table 5.4 Perfusion Imaging Findings in Brain AVM Patients

	CBF	CBV	MTT	Symptoms
Functional Arterial Steal	Dec	Dec	Dec	Seizure
Ischemic Arterial Steam	Dec	Dec	Inc	Focal Neurological Deficit
Venous Congestion	–	Inc	Dec	Focal Neurological Deficit, Seizure, Hemorrhage

Abbreviations: CBF, Cerebral blood flow; CBV, Cerebral blood volume; MTT, Mean transit time; Dec, Decreasing; Inc, Increasing.

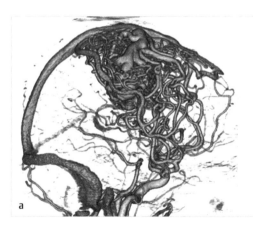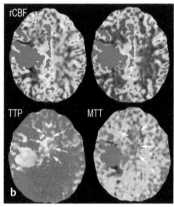

Fig. 5.12 Large right frontal AVM presenting with SMA syndrome with arterial steal phenomenon on perfusion imaging affecting the superior frontal gyrus. (a) 3D reconstructed CTA image shows a large right frontal AVM with superficial venous drainage. (b) CTP with rCBF, time to peak (TTP), and MTT shows increased CBF and decreased TTP and MTT in the AVM region, which is expected given the high flow. However, there is also decreased TTP and MTT in the supplemental motor area as well as normal CBF suggesting a functional arterial steal in this region.

regions and hypoxemia. Studies of CT perfusion in brain AVMs have shown three types of extranidal brain parenchymal perfusion patterns: (1) functional arterial steal, (2) ischemic arterial steal, and (3) venous congestion. In the functional arterial steal pattern, there is decreased CBF, CBV, and MTT (▶ Fig. 5.12). The decreased MTT in these patients reflects a sumping effect from the AVM. In an ischemic arterial steal setting, there is increased MTT and decreased CBF and CBV, which reflects arterial steal from an indirect collateral connection or in an area remote from the nidus in which blood flow is rerouting from normal brain toward the AVM. These perfusion patterns are important as they are associated with AVM-related symptoms. Patients with functional arterial steal most commonly present with seizure while those with ischemic arterial steal most commonly present with focal neurological deficit. Chronic arterial steal of any type can result in local encephalomalacia and gliosis on MRI as well as perinidal angiogenesis and an increased prominence of arterial flow voids surrounding the nidus.

T2* imaging is an essential component to brain AVM imaging. Many patients with "unruptured" brain AVMs have had silent bleeding from a brain AVM, which is best demonstrated on GRE or SWI imaging and hemosiderin staining surrounding the brain AVM itself (▶ Fig. 5.13). This is thought to be associated with a higher rate of future rupture.

5.3.5 What the Clinician Needs to Know

- The presence of angioarchitectural features, which portend a higher risk of rupture including feeding arterial aneurysm, intranidal aneurysm, venous ectasia, and venous outflow stenosis.
- The evidence of medullary venous congestion manifested by deep white matter edema, dilated transmedullary veins, and hydrocephalus.
- The evidence of prior AVM bleeding manifested by T2* artifact surrounding the brain AVM.
- Mass effect from a large venous pouch which may or may not be partially thrombosed.
- Perfusion abnormalities in the brain parenchyma surrounding the AVM.

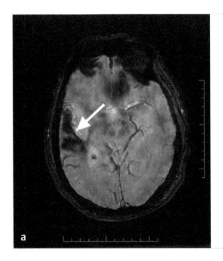 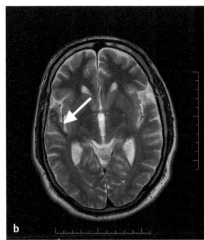

Fig. 5.13 Hemosiderin staining in patient with right temporal AVM and seizure. No known history of rupture. (**a**) SWI image shows hemosiderin staining of the right temporal lobe (*arrow*). (**b**) This is also seen on the T2 MRI as there is subtle hypointensity of the anterior right temporal lobe (*arrow*). This patient was found to have a right temporal AVM, which was later resected.

5.3.6 High-yield Facts

- Perfusion imaging of brain AVMs has demonstrated three distinct perfusion patterns: functional arterial steal, ischemic arterial steal, and venous congestion.
- Edema/T2 signal changes surrounding a brain AVM can be the result of chronic venous congestion or mass effect from a large venous pouch.
- AVMs with surrounding hemosiderin deposition are at higher risk of future rupture.

Further Reading

[1] Krings T, Hans FJ, Geibprasert S, Terbrugge K. Partial "targeted" embolisation of brain arteriovenous malformations. Eur Radiol. 2010; 20(11):2723–2731

[2] Kim DJ, Krings T. Whole-brain perfusion CT patterns of brain arteriovenous malformations: a pilot study in 18 patients. AJNR Am J Neuroradiol. 2011; 32 (11):2061–2066

[3] Shankar JJS, Menezes RJ, Pohlmann-Eden B, Wallace C, terBrugge K, Krings T. Angioarchitecture of brain AVM determines the presentation with seizures: proposed scoring system. AJNR Am J Neuroradiol. 2013; 34(5):1028–1034

5.4 Proliferative Angiopathy

5.4.1 Clinical Case

A 7-year-old presenting with seizures (▶ Fig. 5.14).

5.4.2 Description of Imaging Findings and Diagnosis

Diagnosis

Diffuse AVM involving the entirety of the left frontal lobe with T2/FLAIR hyperintensity of the entire left frontal lobe. Abnormal blood vessels are interspersed with functioning brain tissue. Slow arteriovenous shunting. No discrete nidus. Findings consistent with proliferative angiopathy.

5.4.3 Background

Cerebral proliferative angiopathy comprises up to 4% of all brain AVMs. This entity was first described by Pierre Lasjaunias and is thought to represent a distinct entity or category from a classical brain AVM. Proliferative angiopathy generally presents at a younger age (mean age ~20) and is more common in females. Common presentations include motor or sensory changes, seizures, headaches, and transient ischemic attacks while hemorrhage is very rare. The etiology of proliferative angiopathy is unclear but is thought to be due to aberrant endothelial cell proliferation and angiogenesis as an oversprouting response to cortical hypoxemia. Distinguishing between proliferative angiopathy and a classical brain AVM is important as proliferative angiopathy has a different natural history and thus requires a differentiated therapeutic response.

5.4.4 Imaging Findings

On cross-sectional imaging proliferative angiopathy is characterized by a diffuse network of densely enhancing blood vessels or vascular flow voids that are embedded within and intermingled with normal brain parenchyma. The vascular malformation can involve an entire lobe, multiple lobes, or an entire hemisphere. Perifocal gliosis, sulcal, and ventricular enlargement may be present as a result of the chronic hypoxemia (▶ Fig. 5.14, ▶ Fig. 5.15). In a majority of patients, two or more lobes are affected. Interestingly, despite the large size of the vascular malformation feeding arteries and draining veins are only mildly or moderately enlarged.

Angiographically there are multiple diffuse arterial feeders which are relatively equal in size and contribution to the AVM. Nearly 40% of cases have an associated arterial stenosis, which is rare in classic brain AVMs. Feeding arterial aneurysms are seen in 10% of cases. Nearly 60% of patients have ECA supply to the brain and/or AVM, which makes sense since these lesions form as a response to chronic cortical hypoxemia. Dynamic images typically demonstrate a lack of clear early venous drainage but rather a puddling of contrast within the dilated capillary bed.

Perfusion imaging in cerebral proliferative angiopathy yields a number of interesting findings. Unlike classical brain AVMs, proliferative angiopathy is characterized by oligemia and chronic ischemia in the intra- and perilesional brain tissue. MR perfusion

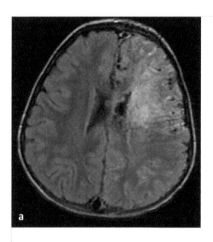
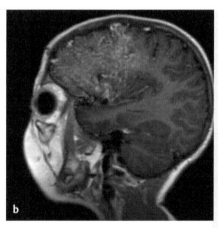
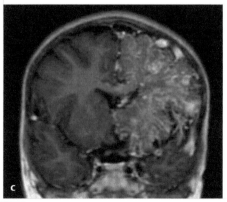
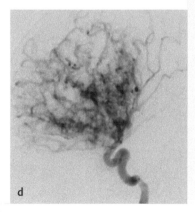

Fig. 5.14 A 7-year-old with seizures secondary to proliferative angiopathy. (**a**) T2/FLAIR MRI shows diffuse T2 hyperintensity of the left frontal lobe as well as multiple enlarged vessels. However, there is no focal nidus. (**b**) Sagittal T1 MRI without contrast shows involvement of the entirety of the left frontal lobe. (**c**) Coronal T1 post-contrast MRI shows diffuse vascular enhancement involving the left frontal lobe and deep structures of the brain. Again, there is no nidus that could be pointed to. (**d**) Left ICA cerebral angiogram shows diffusely increased vascularity of the left frontal lobe. However, there is minimal arteriovenous shunting and the vessels are only mildly hypertrophied. This is a classic case of proliferative angiopathy.

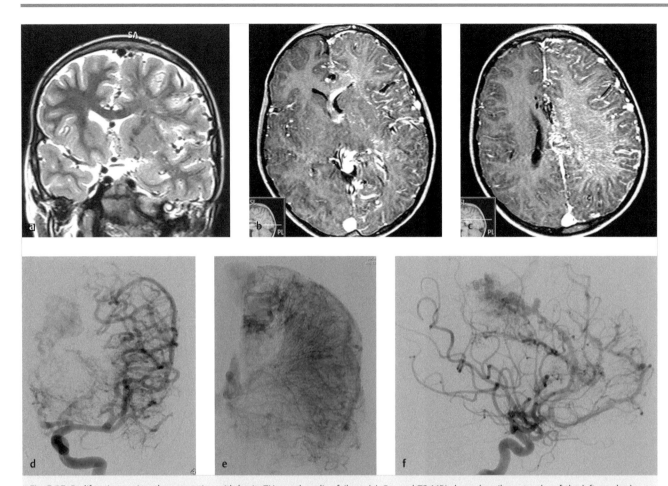

Fig. 5.15 Proliferative angiopathy presenting with bruit, TIAs, and cardiac failure. (a) Coronal T2 MRI shows hemihypertrophy of the left cerebral hemisphere with gyral enlargement. There is also increased vascularity over the entirety of the left cerebral hemisphere. (b) and (c). Axial post-contrast MRI shows diffusely increased vascularity over the left cerebral hemisphere with enhancement of both enlarged cortical veins as well as a dilated and enhancing transmedullary venous system. (d) and (e). Left ICA cerebral angiogram shows moderate enlargement of all MCA branches as well as slow arteriovenous shunting. There is a pseudophlebitic pattern of venous drainage with the dilatation and tortuosity of the medullary venous system. (f) Right ICA cerebral angiogram also shows the arteriovenous shunting. There are feeding arterial aneurysms of the distal anterior cerebral artery (ACA).

and CT perfusion studies on proliferative angiopathy patients show increased CBV and CBF and prolonged MTT and delayed TTP reflecting increased regional vascularity and slow venous drainage. Perfusion abnormalities extend beyond the lesion to unaffected brain parenchyma with low CBF and delayed TTP and MTT indicating abnormal vascular autoregulation with secondary hypoxemia. Studies on cerebrovascular reserve in proliferative angiopathy have demonstrates severe impairment of perilesional cerebrovascular reserve in these patients, substantially more than that seen in brain AVMs presenting with seizures.

5.4.5 What the Clinician Needs to Know

- A holohemispheric brain AVM or a brain AVM, which consumes multiple cerebral lobes is more likely to be proliferative angiopathy than a conventional brain AVM.
- Angiographic findings typical of proliferative angiopathy include normal to moderately sized arterial feeders and draining veins, out of proportion to the large size of the brain AVM, dural arterial supply, proximal arterial stenoses, and lack of clear early venous drainage.

- Perfusion imaging characteristics of proliferative angiopathy include increased CBF and CBV and prolonged MTT and TTP.

5.4.6 High-yield Facts

- Rupture risk in proliferative angiopathy is presumed to be lower than that of a classical brain AVM.
- Perfusion imaging can provide valuable insights regarding chronic brain ischemia and could prompt treatment with pial synangiosis or burr-hole therapy, which has been shown to be effective in these patients.

Further Reading

[1] Lasjaunias PL, Landrieu P, Rodesch G, et al. Cerebral proliferative angiopathy: clinical and angiographic description of an entity different from cerebral AVMs. Stroke. 2008; 39(3):878–885

[2] Vargas MC, Castillo M. Magnetic resonance perfusion imaging in proliferative cerebral angiopathy. J Comput Assist Tomogr. 2011; 35(1):33–38

[3] Geibprasert S, Pongpech S, Jiarakongmun P, Shroff MM, Armstrong DC, Krings T. Radiologic assessment of brain arteriovenous malformations: what clinicians need to know. Radiographics. 2010; 30(2):483–501

5.5 AVMs in CM-AVM, HHT, and Wyburn-Mason Syndrome

5.5.1 Clinical Case

An 8-year-old male with red skin nodules and headache (▶ Fig. 5.16).

5.5.2 Description of Imaging Findings and Diagnosis

Diagnosis

Capillary malformations of the skin and large left cerebellar AVM. Findings consistent with capillary malformation-AVM syndrome secondary to *RASA1* mutation.

5.5.3 Background

An understanding of syndrome-associated AVMs is important for a number of reasons. First, when working with patients who have syndrome-associated AVMs, it is important for clinicians to be aware of the other systemic manifestations of these diseases to allow for appropriate coordination of care, screening, and management. Second, in many cases, secondary CNS manifestations and angioarchitectural features of AVMs can provide a clue regarding whether the AVM is syndrome-associated. Thirdly, the understanding of syndromic AVMs may further our understanding of sporadic brain AVMs. In some cases, the neurologist, neurosurgeon, or neuroradiologist seeing the patient could be the first to suggest the possibility of an underlying syndrome as the culprit for the AVM. A summary of various AVM-associated syndromes is provided in ▶ Table 5.5.

HHT is the most common of the AVM-associated syndromes. HHT is diagnosed clinically using the Curacao criteria including (1) spontaneous and recurrent epistaxis, (2) mucocutaneous telangiectasias, (3) visceral AVMs, and (4), diagnosis of HHT in a first-degree relative using the same criteria. Patients who meet three or more of the four criteria are labeled as "definite HHT" while those with two of the four criteria are labeled as "possible" or "suspected" HHT.

Capillary malformation-arteriovenous malformation (CM-AVM) syndrome is an autosomal dominant inherited disorder. The prevalence of *RASA1* related syndromes is estimated at 1:100000. Patients are affected by multifocal capillary malformations (i.e., Port wine stains) and AVMs and fistulas affecting the multiple tissues including the muscles, bones, gastrointestinal tract, spine, and brain. Approximately, 10–15% of patients with CM-AVM syndrome suffer from various tumors including optic gliomas, superficial basal cell carcinoma, neurofibromas, and vestibular schwannomas. Overall, approximately 10% of patients with *RASA1* mutations have CNS AVMs, 15% have systemic AVMs, and nearly 100% have capillary malformations.

Cerebrofacial arteriovenous metameric syndrome is a segmental neurovascular syndrome, which results from a somatic mutation within the neural crest or cephalic mesoderm prior to migration of these precursor cells to their final location. Wyburn-Mason syndrome (CAMS 2) is one such metameric syndrome, which is characterized by ipsilateral AVMs affecting the face and visual pathway including the eyes, optic nerve, optic tract, and optic radiations. The prevalence of Wyburn-Mason syndrome is far lower than that of HHT and CM-AVM syndrome as only about 50 cases have been reported in the literature. There is no known genetic mutation associated with the disease and most cases are sporadic. Wyburn-Mason syndrome is thought to be the result of a developmental abnormality of the primitive vascular mesoderm of the optic cup and anterior neural tube. These structures give rise to the retinal vessels as well as the vasculature of the midbrain. The developmental insult is thought to occur within the first 7 weeks of gestation and results in persistence of primitive vascular tissue in the retina and midbrain.

5.5.4 Imaging Findings

HHT-associated AVMs are classified as (1) large single-hole pial arteriovenous fistulas (AVF), (2) AVMs with a nidus (typically small, superficial and mono-compartimental), and (3) micro-AVMs or capillary vascular malformation. There are a number of salient features of HHT AVMs that should lead one to consider a diagnosis of HHT if one has not already been established. Micro-AVMs/capillary vascular malformations are considered an HHT-defining feature by some authors. Pial AVFs, especially if multiple are thought to be an exceedingly rare in the sporadic AVM population, but are seen in up to 10% of HHT AVM patients;

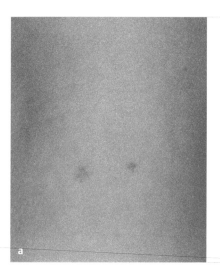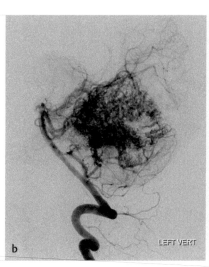

Fig. 5.16 Capillary malformation-AVM syndrome. (a) Photograph of the forearm in this young patient shows two reddish capillary malformations of the skin. (b) Left vertebral artery cerebral angiogram shows a classic nidus-type AVM of the cerebellum. Findings are characteristic of CM-AVM syndrome from a *RASA1* mutation.

Table 5.5 AVM-associated Syndrome Characteristics

Syndrome	Other CNS Manifestations	Systemic Manifestations	Disease Prevalence	AVM Characteristics
Hereditary Hemorrhagic Telangiectasia HHT1 HHT2 Juvenile Polyposis-HHT Overlap	Spinal AVMs, ischemic stroke secondary to pulmonary AVM, cerebral abscess	Pulmonary AVMs, Epistaxis, GI AVMs, Hepatic AVMs, Mucocutaneous telangiectasia, Colon polyps in polyp-associated disease	1:5000 to 1:10000.	Generally smaller than sporadic AVMs. AVM multiplicity an HHT marker. Capillary vascular malformation/micro-AVMs highly prevalent. Pial AVF ~10% of AVMs.
Capillary Malformation-AVM	Spinal AVMs	Face or extremity AVMs. Port wine stains on the face and neck, rarely in the mucosa. Capillary lesions are multifocal. High prevalence of neoplasm.	1:100000	Nidal type AVMs (80%), Pial AVFs (10%) and Vein of Galen Malformation (10%).
Wyburn-Mason Syndrome	Occular/retinal AVMs	Facial AVMs	Rare. ~50 cases reported in literature	Vascular lesions of the orbit, optic tract, optic radiations and occipital lobe.

Abbreviation: CNS, Central nervous system; AVM, Arteriovenous malformation.

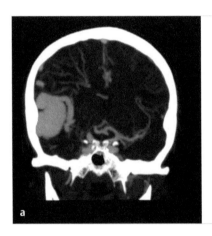 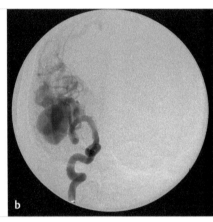

Fig. 5.17 Pial AVF in a patient with HHT. **(a)** Coronal MIP CTA shows a large pial AVF of the right sylvian fissure. The dominant arterial feeder is the enlarge MCA and it drains directly into a dilated venous pouch. **(b)** Right ICA cerebral angiogram better demonstrates the pial AVF with markedly hypertrophied and tortuous ICA and MCA.

thus, the presence of these lesions should trigger an investigation for HHT. Regarding the nidal type AVMs, features which should trigger an investigation for HHT are lesion multiplicity, especially when seen in superficial locations.

Pial AVFs lack a nidus between the feeding artery and draining vein, i.e., are composed of a "single hole" fistula with a dilated venous pouch. These lesions are usually superficially located with only a tiny minority located in the deep portions of the brain. These lesions have many features that portend a poorer natural history including arterial stenoses, feeding artery aneurysms, multiple draining veins, venous ectasia, and a pseudophlebitic pattern (▶ Fig. 5.17).

Nidus-type AVMs are arteriovenous connections with an intervening nidus. About 40% of these lesions are located in eloquent areas and about 15% have deep venous drainage. Over 90% of these lesions have a Spetzler-Martin score of 2 or less. The angioarchitecture of these lesions is typically benign. These lesions tend to measure less than 2 cm and lack features such as arterial stenoses, associated aneurysms, multiple draining veins, venous ectasia, and venous reflux. Associated aneurysms are rare as are signs of long-standing venous hypertension.

Micro-AVMs and capillary vascular malformations lack definite shunting on angiography and have no dilated feeding arteries or veins. These are characterized by a blush of abnormal

vessels in the arterial phase that persists into the late arterial and capillary phase. Angiographically, these lesions are distinct from both capillary telangiectasia and AVMs as these are characterized by the presence of a capillary bed that is abnormally dilated. On conventional MRI, these lesions are characterized as punctuate areas of enhancement within the cerebral or cerebellar sulci and no surrounding susceptibility artifact. These lesions typically measure less than 5 mm in diameter and 80% are superficial (▶ Fig. 5.18).

There is a wide variation in the types of AVMs seen in patients with CM-AVM syndrome (▶ Fig. 5.16). Intracerebral AVMs, AVFs, and vein of galen malformations are more common in this syndrome. In addition, a substantial proportion of patients suffer from facial AVMs and spinal AVMs. Pial AVFs are extremely rare in the general population and are seen at a surprisingly high rate among patients with both HHT and CM-AVM syndrome. The salient feature which distinguishes AVMs associated with CM-AVM syndrome and sporadic AVMs is the presence of vascular malformations on the skin. Because these vascular malformations are difficult to distinguish from the cutaneous lesions seen in HHT patients, having patients be evaluated by an experienced dermatologist is generally strongly recommended.

Patients with Wyburn-Mason Syndrome and other CAMS-type syndromes typically present within the first three decades

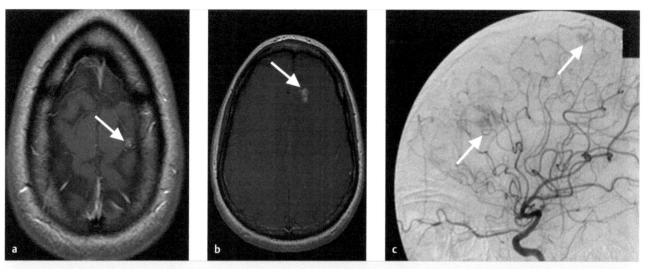

Fig. 5.18 Capillary vascular malformation in HHT. (**a**) and (**b**). Post-contrast MRI shows two foci of enhancement in the left frontal lobe. They are along the cortical surface (*arrows*). (**c**) Left ICA cerebral angiogram shows faint contrast opacification of these lesions (*arrows*). There is no associated arterial hypertrophied and slow, if any, arteriovenous shunting. These lesions are pathognomonic for capillary vascular malformations in the setting of HHT.

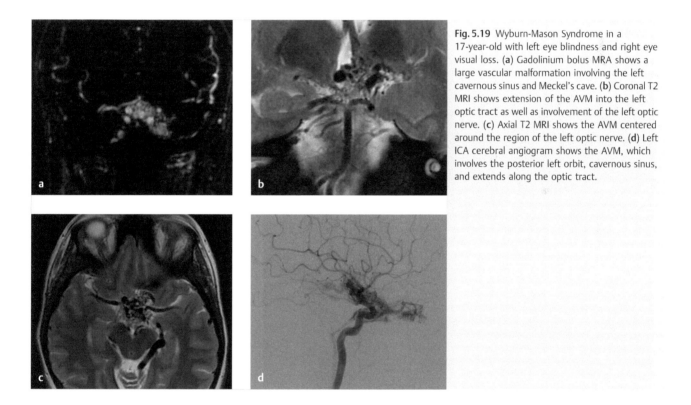

Fig. 5.19 Wyburn-Mason Syndrome in a 17-year-old with left eye blindness and right eye visual loss. (**a**) Gadolinium bolus MRA shows a large vascular malformation involving the left cavernous sinus and Meckel's cave. (**b**) Coronal T2 MRI shows extension of the AVM into the left optic tract as well as involvement of the left optic nerve. (**c**) Axial T2 MRI shows the AVM centered around the region of the left optic nerve. (**d**) Left ICA cerebral angiogram shows the AVM, which involves the posterior left orbit, cavernous sinus, and extends along the optic tract.

of life. The most common manifestation of Wyburn-Mason syndrome is a retinal AVM resulting in the loss of visual acuity and visual field deficits. Retinal AVMs can be variable in size and are often impossible to identify on conventional imaging. Outside of the retina, the most common site of AVMs in Wyburn-Mason is the orbit, followed by the thalamus and hypothalamus, optic chiasm, optic tracts, and optic radiations (▶ Fig. 5.19). Head and neck vascular malformations associated with Wyburn-Mason primarily are located in the distribution of

the trigeminal nerve and can involve the frontal or maxillary sinuses. About ⅓ to ½ of Wyburn-Mason patients present with these malformations.

5.5.5 What the Clinician Needs to Know

• Presence of multiple brain AVMs should prompt a work-up for HHT or CM-AVM syndrome. Dermatological evaluation can be helpful in confirming the diagnosis.

- Multiple brain AVMs along a single metamere (i.e., eye, orbit, optic tract, occipital lobe) is characteristic of CAMS, an AVM syndrome without an associated germ-line mutation.
- Capillary vascular malformations are exclusively found in HHT patients and are considered by many authors an HHT-defining lesion.

5.5.6 High-yield Facts

- Syndrome-associated AVMs often have specific angioarchitectural features that can help distinguish them from sporadic AVMs.
- Hereditary Hemorrhagic Telangiectasia is the most prevalent syndrome that is associated with brain AVMs.

- Pial arteriovenous fistulas are extremely rare in the general population and the presence of one of these lesions should prompt an investigation for an AVM syndrome such as HHT or CM-AVM.

Further Reading

[1] Krings T, Kim H, Power S, et al. Brain Vascular Malformation Consortium HHT Investigator Group. Neurovascular manifestations in hereditary hemorrhagic telangiectasia: imaging features and genotype-phenotype correlations. AJNR Am J Neuroradiol. 2015; 36(5):863–870

[2] Larralde M, Abad ME, Luna PC, Hoffner MV. Capillary malformation-arteriovenous malformation: a clinical review of 45 patients. Int J Dermatol. 2014; 53(4):458–461

[3] Brinjikji W, Iyer VN, Sorenson T, Lanzino G. Cerebrovascular Manifestations of Hereditary Hemorrhagic Telangiectasia. Stroke. 2015; 46(11):3329–3337

5.6 Cranial Dural AVF Angioarchitecture and Classification

5.6.1 Clinical Case

A 64-year-old male with bulbar dysfunction and respiratory distress (▶ Fig. 5.20).

5.6.2 Description of Imaging Findings and Diagnosis

Diagnosis

Hypoglossal canal dural arteriovenous fistula (dAVF) with medullary venous reflux (Cognard Type V).

5.6.3 Background

In contrast to pial AVMs, cranial dAVFs consist of pathological shunts between dura supplying arteries and dural venous sinuses or meningeal/cortical veins in the absence of an intervening nidus. Several pathophysiological mechanisms have been proposed for these lesions with the two most common being (1) various conditions (dural sinus or cortical venous thrombosis, trauma, inflammation, or surgery) inciting abnormal activation of neoangiogenesis promoting anomalous connections between dural arteries and thin-walled venous channels and (2) venous hypertension. Adult dAVFs are generally believed to be acquired

lesions and a substantial proportion result from trauma, craniotomy, venous sinus thrombosis, infection, pregnancy, or tumor. In children, dAVFs are usually congenital and marked by the presence of persistent embryonic vessels.

The clinical manifestations of dAVFs range from "benign" findings such as tinnitus, bruit, and dizziness to more malignant findings such as hemorrhage, focal neurological deficit, cognitive dysfunction, seizure, and dementia/encephalopathy. The natural history and clinical presentation of a dAVF depends in large part on the angioarchitecture and venous drainage patterns. It cannot be emphasized enough that dAVFs are primarily a venous disease and much of the action pathophysiologically and on imaging is on the venous side. Thus, in the classification of dAVFs, the focus is on venous drainage patterns. Lesions which show leptomeningeal/cortical venous drainage/reflux and venous ectasias are associated with significantly higher rates of neurological complications including hemorrhage, seizure, and other focal neurological deficits than those with benign antegrade venous drainage in a large and patent dural venous sinus. Here, we will summarize three commonly used classification systems of dAVF with an emphasis on cross-sectional imaging findings and the implications of these classifications on dAVF natural history.

5.6.4 Imaging Findings

Before delving into the various dAVF classification systems and their clinical significance, a review of the salient angiographic

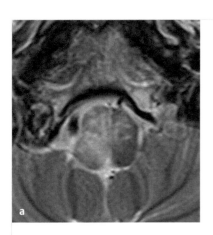
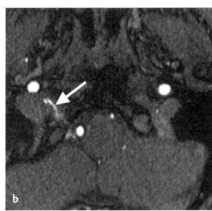
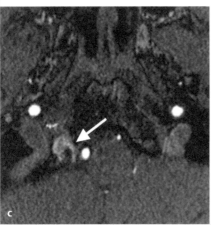
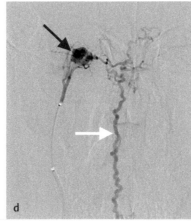

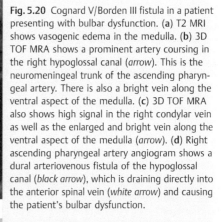

Fig. 5.20 Cognard V/Borden III fistula in a patient presenting with bulbar dysfunction. (**a**) T2 MRI shows vasogenic edema in the medulla. (**b**) 3D TOF MRA shows a prominent artery coursing in the right hypoglossal canal (*arrow*). This is the neuromeningeal trunk of the ascending pharyngeal artery. There is also a bright vein along the ventral aspect of the medulla. (**c**) 3D TOF MRA also shows high signal in the right condylar vein as well as the enlarged and bright vein along the ventral aspect of the medulla (*arrow*). (**d**) Right ascending pharyngeal artery angiogram shows a dural arteriovenous fistula of the hypoglossal canal (*black arrow*), which is draining directly into the anterior spinal vein (*white arrow*) and causing the patient's bulbar dysfunction.

and angioarchitectural (i.e., CTA and MRA) imaging findings in dAVFs is warranted. On the arterial side, the dominant arterial feeders can be easily identified on TOF MRA by the presence of hypertrophied ECA branches with multiple smaller dural or transosseous feeders that converge upon the draining vein (▶ Fig. 5.21). The most common feeders for dAVFs are the posterior division of the middle meningeal artery (MMA), occipital artery, and ascending pharyngeal artery. Hypertrophy of any of these arteries should clue one in to the presence of a dAVF. CTA can also be used but lacks the signal to noise ratio of TOF MRA and streak artifact from adjacent bone can obscure visualization of ECA arterial feeders.

Next is the arteriovenous connection. The site of the arteriovenous connection is identified by the presence of either a collection of smaller arteries converging on a focal site in the dural sinus or a focal dilatation representing the venous pouch with high intravascular signal on TOF MRA and similar density to arterial flow on CTA. dAVFs can have multiple arteriovenous connections so identification of any and all such connections is important for treatment choice.

Characterization of the venous drainage patterns is the most important task when evaluating a dAVF. Drainage directly into a dural venous sinus with antegrade flow is the most benign venous drainage pattern. Reflux of venous flow into a cortical vein or direct venous drainage into a cortical vein is considered a malignant venous drainage pattern (▶ Fig. 5.22). Thus, any abnormally high-flow signal in a cortical vein on TOF should be promptly identified. Venous varices of subarachnoid veins should be identified as they represent a potential rupture point for the dAVF. Lastly, it is important to comment on the patency of the dural venous sinuses as (1) dural venous sinus thrombosis is part of the pathophysiology of dAVFs and (2) drainage of the dAVF into an isolated segment of sinus is associated with a poorer natural history while treatment risks are generally considered to be very low in these types of lesions.

The Borden system is the simplest classification system for dAVFs with three separate grades (▶ Table 5.6).

Borden Type I fistulas drain directly into the dural venous sinus with normal anterograde flow in the draining sinus and the systems which drain the sinus. An example of a Type I fistula would be a transverse-sigmoid fistula in which blood flows the normal expected route of transverse sinus→sigmoid sinus→internal jugular vein. These lesions have an annual hemorrhage rate of 0% and less than 2% of these lesions go on to develop cortical venous drainage.

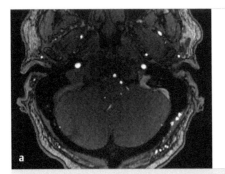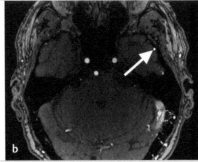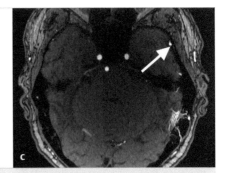

Fig. 5.21 Example of a Cognard I/Borden I fistula on MRA. (a) 3D TOF MRA shows a bright and arterialized left sigmoid sinus and a normal, low-signal right sigmoid sinus. (b) 3D TOF MRA a couple slices higher shows arterialization of the sinus and multiple enlarged transosseous feeders as well as an enlarged MMA (*arrow*). Note how you do not see these arteries on the right. (c) 3D TOF MRA shows the site of the fistula in the wall of the transverse sigmoid junction where all the transosseous feeders converge. Also noted is the enlarged MMA (*arrow*).

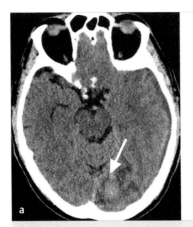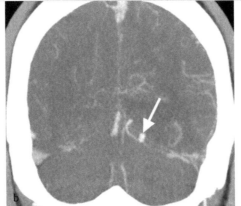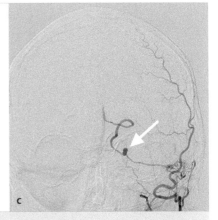

Fig. 5.22 Example of a Cognard IV/Borden III fistula. (a) Non-contrast CT shows a subacute hematoma and associated vasogenic edema in the left occipital lobe (*arrow*). (b) Coronal CTA shows a prominent vein along the inferior aspect of the occipital lobe with a focal venous ectasia/aneurysm (*arrow*). (c) Left ECA angiogram again shows the fistula, which drains directly into a subarachnoid vein/cortical vein and has a venous ectasia/aneurysm (*arrow*).

Table 5.6 Borden and Cognard Classification Schemes

Classifica-tion	Definition	Significance
Borden		
I	Venous drainage directly into dural venous sinus or meningeal vein	Benign natural history
II	Venous drainage into dural sinus with cortical venous reflux	Hemorrhage risk 5%/year
III	Venous drainage directly into cortical veins or in an isolated sinus segment	Hemorrhage risk 10%/year
Cognard		
I	Venous drainage into dural sinus with antegrade flow	Benign natural history
IIa	Venous drainage into dural sinus with retrograde flow	Benign natural history
IIb	Venous drainage into dural sinus with antegrade flow and cortical venous reflux	Hemorrhage risk 5%/year
IIa + b	Venous drainage into dural venous sinus with retrograde flow and cortical venous reflux	Hemorrhage risk 5%/year
III	Venous drainage directly into subarachnoid veins	Hemorrhage risk 10%/year
IV	Type III with venous ectasias of the draining subarachnoid veins	Hemorrhage risk 20%/year
V	Direct drainage into spinal perimedullary veins	High risk of SAH and myelopathy

Abbreviation: SAH, subarachnoid hemorrhage.

Borden Type II fistulas drain into the dural venous sinus but have venous reflux into subarachnoid veins (i.e., cortical venous reflux). An example of a Type II fistula would be a transverse sinus fistula in which blood flows in the transverse sinus but refluxes into the vein of Labbe. These lesions have an annual hemorrhage rate of 6% and up to 20% of Type II fistulas present with hemorrhage.

Borden Type III fistulas have direct drainage into subarachnoid veins or into an isolated venous sinus (i.e., a segment of dural sinus which is trapped between two thrombosed segments). These lesions have an annual hemorrhage rate of 10%, which increases to 20% in the presence of a venous ectasia and about 33% of these patients present with hemorrhage.

The Cognard grading scale is a five-point scale for the classification of dAVF angioarchitecture and is also summarized in ▶ Table 5.6. Cognard Types I and IIa are similar to Borden Type I. The difference between Cognard Types I and IIa is that in Type I there is antegrade flow in the sinus and in Type IIa, there is retrograde flow in the sinus (but no cortical venous drainage). Cognard Types IIb and IIa + b are similar to Borden Type II in that

there is drainage into the dural venous sinus with cortical venous reflux. In Type IIb, there is antegrade venous sinus flow with cortical venous reflux and in Type IIa + b there is retrograde venous sinus flow with cortical venous reflux. Cognard Type III is the same as Borden Type III with direct drainage of the dAVF into a cortical vein and Cognard Type IV is the same as Borden Type III but with venous ectasia. A Cognard Type V fistula is a lesion which drains directly into spinal perimedullary veins.

5.6.5 What the Clinician Needs to Know

- Location and caliber of dominant feeding arteries. Presence of arterial pathologies which can compromise vascular access (i.e., tortuosity, etc.).
- Purported location of the arteriovenous shunt (i.e., transverse sinus, hypoglossal canal, torcular, tentorium, superior sagittal sinus, anterior cranial fossa, etc.).
- Venous drainage pattern (i.e., anterograde drainage in a dural sinus, cortical venous drainage, cortical venous reflux, leptomeningeal venous reflux/drainage).
- The evidence of medullary venous reflux or medullary venous congestion.
- Possible pathways through which the normal brain is achieving its venous drainage.
- The evidence of dural venous sinus thrombosis.

5.6.6 High-yield Facts

- Venous drainage patterns are the primary determinant of dAVF natural history.
- Cortical venous drainage or reflux with venous ectasia is associated with two-times higher rate of hemorrhage compared to dAVFs with cortical venous drainage alone.
- dAVFs with perimedullary venous drainage are associated with high rates of SAH and myelopathy.

Further Reading
[1] Cognard C, Gobin YP, Pierot L, et al. Cerebral dural arteriovenous fistulas: clinical and angiographic correlation with a revised classification of venous drainage. Radiology. 1995; 194(3):671–680
[2] Awad IA, Little JR, Akarawi WP, Ahl J. Intracranial dural arteriovenous malformations: factors predisposing to an aggressive neurological course. J Neurosurg. 1990; 72(6):839–850
[3] Geibprasert S, Pereira V, Krings T, et al. Dural arteriovenous shunts: a new classification of craniospinal epidural venous anatomical bases and clinical correlations. Stroke. 2008; 39(10):2783–2794
[4] Borden JA, Wu JK, Shucart WA. A proposed classification for spinal and cranial dural arteriovenous fistulous malformations and implications for treatment. J Neurosurg. 1995; 82(2):166–179
[5] Gross BA, Du R. The natural history of cerebral dural arteriovenous fistulae. Neurosurgery. 2012; 71(3):594–602, discussion 602–603
[6] Bhogal P, Yeo LL, Henkes H, Krings T, Söderman M. The role of angiogenesis in dural arteriovenous fistulae: the story so far. Interv Neuroradiol. 2018; 24(4):450–454

5.7 Cranial dAVF Characteristics on MRI and CT

5.7.1 Clinical Case

A 76-year-old male with rapid onset dementia (▶ Fig. 5.23).

5.7.2 Description of Imaging Findings and Diagnosis

Diagnosis

dAVF of the superior sagittal sinus with medullary venous congestion and dilatation and subsequent decrease in CSF reabsorption.

5.7.3 Background

Cranial dAVFs have multiple clinical presentations. In general, dAVF symptoms vary by the location of the fistula and the venous drainage patterns. Benign venous drainage patterns are characterized by antegrade flow in the dural venous sinus without cortical venous reflux or venous congestion. These patients typically present with bruit, tinnitus, dizziness, or conjunctival chemosis. Malignant venous drainage patterns are characterized by cortical venous reflux/arterialization and medullary venous reflux/arterialization and can result in hemorrhage, dementia, encephalopathy, seizures, cranial nerve deficits, and mass effect.

Structural imaging with MRI can be extremely useful in not only identifying the presence of a dAVF, but also characterizing the effect of the dAVF on the surrounding parenchyma and thus explaining the patient's neurological presentation. The purpose of this chapter is to identify findings on non-angiographic imaging that not only indicate the presence of a dAVF, but also the presence of a benign versus malignant dAVF.

5.7.4 Imaging Findings

Typical imaging manifestations of dAVFs on conventional cross-sectional MRI include venous thrombosis, engorged intradural vessels adjacent to the meninges or dural sinus walls, and abnormal signal within dural venous sinuses, and asymmetric contrast opacification of the jugular veins.

The identification of clustered vascular flow voids, which robustly enhance close to the dural sinuses or meninges is a direct imaging sign of a dAVF. This commonly has a "salt and pepper" appearance similar to that described in carotid body tumors and should prompt angiographic evaluation. Oftentimes, these salt-and-pepper flow voids are in the presence of a thrombosed venous sinus.

Venous sinus thrombosis is relatively common in dAVFs as many dAVFs are thought to be triggered by venous sinus thrombosis; conversely, sinus narrowing or even occlusion can occur in patients with known dAVF, which is one of the reasons for the spontaneous disappearance or conversion of dAVF with time. Although the presence of an isolated sinus thrombosis is not necessarily a risk factor for aggressive fistula, the presence of a double sinus thrombosis which leaves an isolated intervening segment of sinus patent can portend a poorer prognosis due to the obligate presence of cortical venous reflux and/or cortical venous congestion (▶ Fig. 5.24).

A summary of imaging manifestations of malignant dAVFs is provided in ▶ Table 5.7. Malignant dAVFs often present with

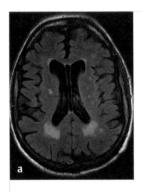 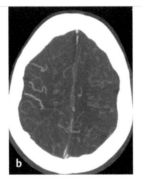 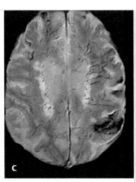

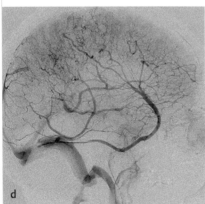 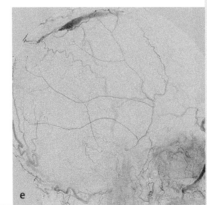

Fig. 5.23 A 76-year-old male with rapid onset dementia secondary to superior sagittal sinus fistula. (a) T2/FLAIR MRI shows moderate hydrocephalus with increased periventricular T2 signal consistent with transependymal flow of CSF. (b) CTA shows multiple dilated transmedullary vessels, most consistent with transmedullary veins. (c) SWI MRI shows multiple T2* hypointense transmedullary veins as well as a focal area of chronic hemorrhage in the left parietal lobe. These veins have deoxyhemoglobin in them and are essentially congested medullary veins, which are unable to drain through normal pathways. (d) Left ICA cerebral angiogram in the venous phase shows multiple corkscrew medullary veins in the left hemisphere. Note the absence of the superior sagittal sinus. (e) Selective injection shows the fistula of an isolated segment of the superior sagittal sinus.

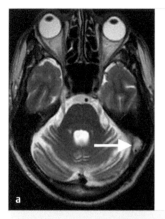
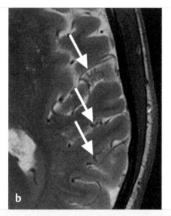
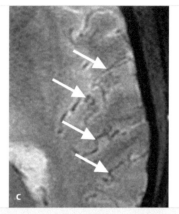
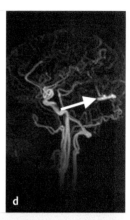

Fig. 5.24 Isolated sinus and ipsilateral cortical venous congestion. (**a**) T2 MRI shows absent flow void in the left transverse sinus consistent with local thrombosis (*arrow*). (**b**) T2 MRI shows increased vascularity overlying the left cerebral hemisphere of unclear etiology (*arrows*). (**c**) SWI MRI shows dilated and tortuous vessels overlying the left hemisphere which are T2* hypointense suggesting presence of deoxyhemoglobin (*arrows*). (**d**) TRICKS MRA shows a fistula in an isolated sinus segment (*arrow*). This resulted in obligate cortical venous reflux and associated cortical venous congestion.

Table 5.7 Imaging Findings of Malignant Dural Arteriovenous Fistulas

Imaging Finding	MRI Characteristics	Clinical Significance
Cluster of dilated vessels adjacent to or within dural sinus	Multiple punctate T2 vascular flow voids, salt, and pepper enhancement on pattern on T1CE	Site of a dural arteriovenous fistula
Venous Sinus Thrombosis	Focal area of blooming artifact on T2* or loss of normal vascular flow void on T2/T1. Sometimes robustly enhancing	Site of dural arteriovenous fistula, can indicate poor natural history if isolated intervening segment is patent
Mass Effect	Displacement of normal structure with surrounding vasogenic edema on T2/FLAIR	Can result in neurological deficit, seizure or headache
Diffuse or patchy cerebral edema	Patchy areas of T2/FLAIR hyperintensity	Reflects chronic venous congestion/hypertension.
Cortical venous reflux/Leptomeningeal venous reflux	T2 flow voids or enhancing engorged sulcal vessels. Leptomeningeal enhancement. Hyperintense venous signal on SWI	Predicts future venous congestion or hemorrhage risk
Medullary venous congestion	Cerebral edema, dilated transmantle T2 flow voids, T2 hypointense flow transmantle veins on SWI	May be associated with encephalopathy, cognitive dysfunction, hydrocephalus and seizure
Hemorrhage	Blooming artifact on T2*	High risk of future hemorrhage, urgent treatment warranted.A23

venous congestive edema, subarachnoid, or intraparenchymal hemorrhage, and dilated corkscrew-like medullary veins (pseudophlebitic pattern).

Cerebral edema from dAVFs can be the result of mass effect from a venous varix or, more commonly, chronic venous hypertension/congestion. In the setting of a large venous varix, the edema (T2/FLAIR hyperintense) is often focal, surrounding the varix itself and sometimes associated with intraluminal thrombosis. Cerebral edema from venous hypertension is more complex as it often occurs in areas remote from the fistula. When edema is bilateral and supratentorial, the fistula is often located in a midline structure such as the superior sagittal sinus or vein of galen/falcotentorial region. If edema involves the brainstem, there is often venous congestion along the median pontomesencephalic vein (▶ Fig. 5.25). Meanwhile, unilateral cerebral edema is often the result of a transverse or sigmoid sinus type fistula with involvement of the vein of Labbe. ▶ Table 5.8 summarizes location-specific findings of cranial dAVFs.

Cortical venous reflux is an important imaging manifestation of a malignant fistula. When engorged vessels (seen as T2 flow voids or enhancing veins on T1-CE) are found within the cerebral sulci they likely represent dilated cortical veins from venous reflux. Leptomeningeal enhancement is a particularly strong indicator of poor natural history and cortical venous reflux. On SWI cortical venous reflux is demonstrated by the presence of hyperintense venous signal from rapid wash-in of oxygenated blood in the setting of arteriovenous shunting (▶ Fig. 5.26). If the hyperintense venous signal on SWI extends to the medullary venous system, this would indicate medullary venous reflux, which is a particularly poor prognostic sign placing the patient at risk for both hemorrhage and impaired CSF hydrodynamics as a substantial proportion of CSF resorption happens at the levels of the medullary veins.

Medullary venous congestion is different from cortical or medullary venous reflux as it is an indicator of poor venous outflow of the medullary venous system in the setting of

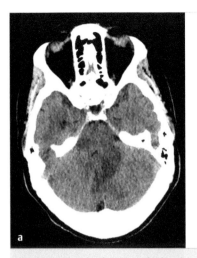
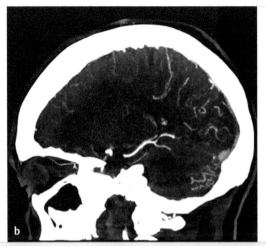
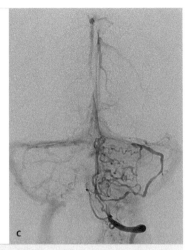

Fig. 5.25 Example of a Cognard III/Borden III fistula. (**a**) Non-contrast CT shows vasogenic edema in the left cerebellar hemisphere and vermis. (**b**) CT angiogram shows multiple dilated a corkscrew cerebellar cortical veins, a finding which is almost pathognomonic for a dural fistula. (**c**) Cerebral angiogram shows a fistula, which drains directly into a cortical vein and is associated with severe venous congestion of the cerebellum.

Table 5.8 Location-specific Structural Imaging Findings of Dural Arteriovenous Fistulas

Fistula Location	Common Imaging Manifestations
Anterior Cranial Fossa/Ethmoidal	Inferior frontal vascular flow voids, Inferior frontal lobe edema. Hemorrhage
Indirect CCF	Asymmetric cavernous sinus enhancement, SOV dilatation, enlarged cavnerous sinus, proptosis, retroorbital edema – watch out for cortical venous reflux through either the basal vein of Rosenthal or the sphenoparietal sinus
Superior Sagittal Sinus	Parenchymal edema or hemorrhage. Intracranial hypertension. Enlarged ventricles. Arterialized flow in cortical veins along SSS course. Isolated sinus in setting of thrombosis
Transverse-Sigmoid Sinus	Commonly asymptomatic-flow voids. Transcalvarial small arteries, salt and pepper appearance. Cerebellar or temporal lobe edema or hemorrhage
Tentorial	Hemorrhage. Diecephalic venous congestion, posterior fossa subarachnoid venous varices
Condylar/Hypoglossal	Salt and pepper appearance at condylar canal/hypoglossal canal. Dilated perimedullary vascular flow voids, brainstem edema.

Abbreviations: CCF, Carotico-cavernous fistula; SSS, Subclavian steal syndrome.

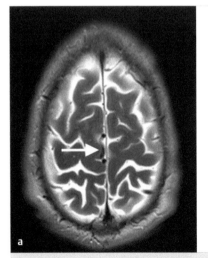
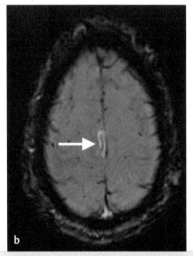
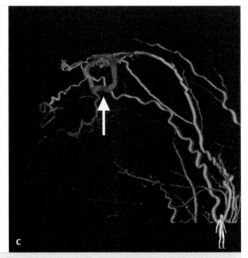

Fig. 5.26 Example of an arterialized vein on SWI. (**a**) Patient with headaches. T2 MRI shows an abnormal vascular flow void overlying the medial right frontal lobe (*arrow*). (**b**) SWI MRI shows this flow void to by hyperintense on SWI suggesting arterialized flow (*arrow*). (**c**) ECA cerebral angiogram shows the fistula in the superior sagittal sinus and the arterialized cortical vein (*arrow*).

venous hypertension in a cortical vein or dural venous sinus. Medullary venous congestion often presents with concomitant cerebral edema and when bilateral, hydrocephalus due to impaired CSF drainage. On imaging, it presents with dilated transmantle T2 flow voids in the cerebral white matter, which enhance on contrast administration. On SWI, these structures are often T2 hypointense due to the presence of deoxyhemoglobin (▶ Fig. 5.23). Occasionally, chronic venous congestion can result in venous ischemia and cortical calcifications (▶ Fig. 5.27).

Hemorrhage in dAVF can be intraparenchymal, subarachnoid, intraventricular, or subdural or multicompartimental. Multi-compartimental bleed in the absence of trauma should prompt for investigation of dAVF (▶ Fig. 5.28). The presence of

hemosiderin staining along the cerebellar or cerebral cortex is an indicator of prior hemorrhage and should prompt treatment.

Lastly, mass effect can result in debilitating neurological symptoms for many patients with dAVFs. Mass effect from venous varices, particularly those which are acutely throm-bosed, can result in headache, seizures, and focal neurological deficits. In the setting of infratentorial dAVFs or dAVFs with reflux into brainstem veins, mass effect can result in cranial neuropathies including facial pain (trigeminal nerve mass effect), facial weakness (facial nerve mass effect), and ocular symptoms (▶ Fig. 5.29). Thus, it is important to consider, which structures are being effected by venous varices seen in dAVFs.

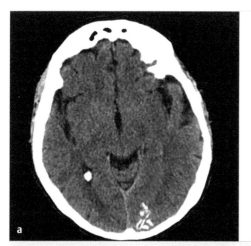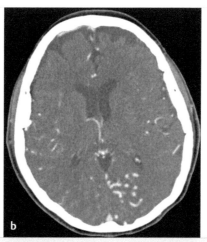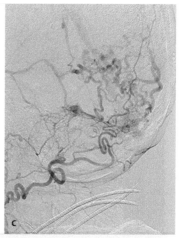

Fig. 5.27 Cortical calcification as a result of chronic venous hypertension. (a) Non-contrast CT shows gyriform calcification of the left medial occipital lobe. (b) CTA shows multiple dilated and tortuous vessels in the region of the calcification, but these vessels themselves are not calcified. (c) Left ECA cerebral angiogram shows a dural arteriovenous fistula, which is draining directly into a cortical vein and has marked cortical venous reflux. We believe that these cortical calcifications were the result of chronic venous ischemia.

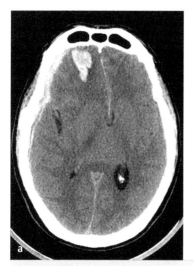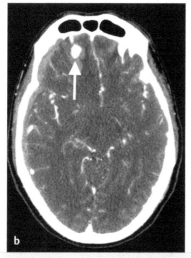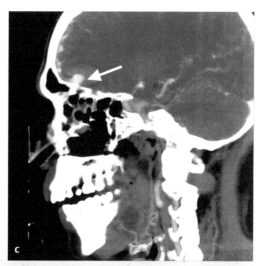

Fig. 5.28 Multi-compartment hemorrhage in dural AV fistula. (a) Non-contrast CT shows intraparenchymal and subdural hemorrhage overlying the right frontal lobe. (b) CTA shows a large venous aneurysm in the right frontal lobe, which is the source of the patient's hemorrhage (*arrow*). (c) Sagittal CTA shows the venous aneurysm (*arrow*) and dilated and tortuous frontal veins. This patient was confirmed to have an ethmoidal fistula.

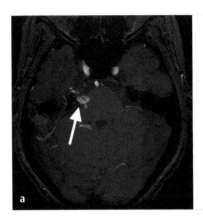 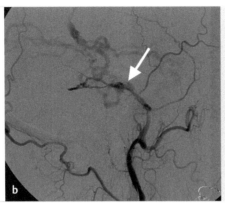

Fig. 5.29 Tooth ache from dAVF-induced venous varix. (**a**) TOF MRA shows a dilated and arterialized lateral pontomesencephalic vein causing mass effect on the right fifth cranial nerve and root entry zone (*arrow*). An AVM or AVF induced venous varix was suspected. (**b**) Lateral right ECA cerebral angiogram shows the large venous varix from a Cognard IV fistula (*arrow*).

5.7.5 What the Clinician Needs to Know

- The presence of isolated venous sinus (i.e., segment of patent venous sinus between two thrombosed segments)
- The presence or absence of cortical venous drainage/venous reflux and medullary venous reflux
- The presence or absence of medullary venous hypertension and associated white matter signal changes
- The evidence of prior hemorrhage as demonstrated by hemosiderin staining
- Mass effect from venous structures including dilated perimedullary/cortical veins and venous varices

5.7.6 High-yield Facts

- Cross-sectional imaging findings suggestive of a malignant dAVF include sulcal vascular flow voids, leptomeningeal enhancement, dilated medullary veins, dilated cortical/sulcal veins, parenchymal edema, hydrocephalus, sulcal hemosiderin deposition, and venous varices.

- The presence of brainstem edema and abnormal vascular flow voids or leptomeningeal enhancement should prompt at least a consideration for the presence of a cranial dAVF.
  Several cases of Cognard V dAVFs have been misdiagnosed as entities such as sarcoidosis or brainstem glioma.
- dAVFs have location specific imaging manifestations summarized in ▶ Fig. 5.8.

Further Reading

[1] Hacein-Bey L, Konstas AA, Pile-Spellman J. Natural history, current concepts, classification, factors impacting endovascular therapy, and pathophysiology of cerebral and spinal dural arteriovenous fistulas. Clin Neurol Neurosurg. 2014; 121:64–75

[2] Gandhi D, Chen J, Pearl M, Huang J, Gemmete JJ, Kathuria S. Intracranial dural arteriovenous fistulas: classification, imaging findings, and treatment. AJNR Am J Neuroradiol. 2012; 33(6):1007–1013

[3] Letourneau-Guillon L, Cruz JP, Krings T. CT and MR imaging of non-cavernous cranial dural arteriovenous fistulas: Findings associated with cortical venous reflux. Eur J Radiol. 2015; 84(8):1555–1563

5.8 Time-resolved (Dynamic) Imaging for Shunting Lesions

5.8.1 Clinical Case

A 35-year-old male with incidental finding on MRI (▶ Fig. 5.30).

5.8.2 Description of Imaging Findings and Diagnosis

Diagnosis

Unruptured brain AVM in the left parietal lobe. Dynamic CTA demonstrates a Spetzler I nidus-type AVM fed by a parietal branch of the left MCA. The AVM has a single superficial cortical draining vein and no dangerous angioarchitectural features.

5.8.3 Background

Conventional angiography is the gold standard for the evaluation of shunting lesions such as brain-AVMs and AVFs due to the fact that it allows for excellent spatial, contrast, and temporal resolution. Over the past decade, there has been growing interest in the use of noninvasive dynamic imaging that allows for the identification of arteriovenous shunting and characterization of basic AVM and AVF angioarchitectural and venous drainage patterns.

5.8.4 Imaging Findings

4D-CTA is a form of dynamic, time-resolved imaging. Optimal time-resolved CTA requires the use of newer 320-row CT scanners, which can provide high resolution (0.5-mm slice thickness) imaging. Unlike a single-phase CTA, 4D-CTA requires serial imaging covering arterial, parenchymal, and venous phases, and typically 20–30 volumes of the brain are obtained, resulting in a temporal resolution of 1 volume every 2 seconds.

4D-CTA has been shown to be sufficient in the diagnosis and surgical classification of brain AVMs. 4D-CTA can identify intranidal aneurysms with a high degree of accuracy, delineate AVM contours prior to radiosurgery, differentiate neoangiogenesis from nidus, and identify feeding arteries and draining vessels. Ultimately, 4D-CTA is a great modality for brain AVM screening and radiosurgical planning.

4D-CTA has been shown to be sufficient in the diagnosis and surgical classification of cranial AVFs. Basic features that can be delineated with current techniques include location of the fistula, presence of cortical venous drainage, direction of flow, and presence of venous ectasias or aneurysms (▶ Fig. 5.30, ▶ Fig. 5.31). Retrograde venous flow in cortical veins, a variable which has been shown to increase the risk of hemorrhage, can be visualized with 4D-CTA.

Time-resolving MR angiographic imaging sequences are known under the acronyms of 4D-TRAK (Philips), TWIST (Siemens), and TRICKS (GE). These sequences obtain a series of images as the contrast bolus is passing through the vascular system at a rate as high as one entire 3D volume per second. Depending on the protocol, upward of 30–40 dynamic images can be obtained following the contrast bolus injection allowing for identification and differentiation between arterial, capillary and venous phases.

Time-resolved MRA has been shown to be effective in the diagnosis and surgical grading of an untreated AVM. It can be helpful in identifying and characterizing feeding arteries, draining veins, and nidus size. However, other imaging features related to brain AVM angioarchitecture that may be equally important in decision making for brain AVMs (intranidal aneurysms, pattern of venous rerouting) cannot be completely characterized as they require either a higher spatial or temporal resolution. Slow-flow AVMs or microAVMs may remain undetected on dynamic MRA for the same reason. Time-resolved imaging has been shown to be very specific but insensitive in the detection of residual AVM after treatment and a negative 4D-MRA does not necessarily indicate a cure. For patients who

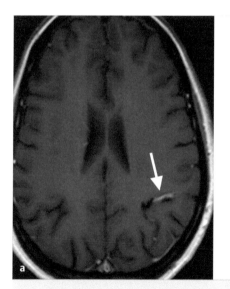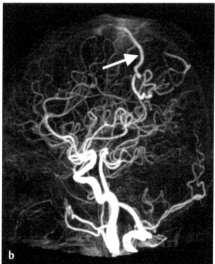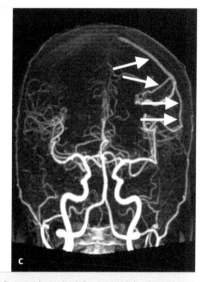

Fig. 5.30 Incidental AVM on 4D-CTA. **(a)** T1 post-contrast MRI demonstrates a focal area of abnormal flow voids in the left parietal lobe (*arrow*). **(b)** and **(c)**. A 4D-CTA was performed which demonstrated an MCA arterial feeder (*arrowheads*) and a focal nidus in the left parietal lobe with early venous opacification (i.e., shunting) into a superficial cortical vein (*white arrow*).

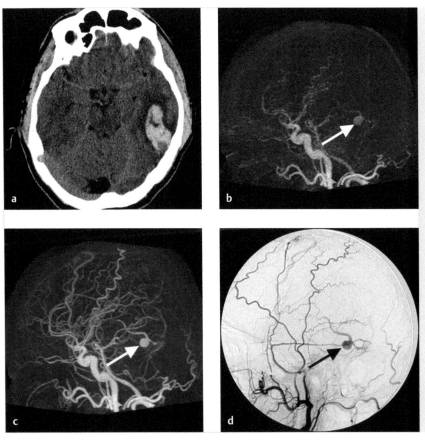

Fig. 5.31 4D-CTA in the evaluation of cranial dAVF angioarchitecture. (**a**) Non-contrast CT shows a patient with a multi-compartmental hemorrhage involving the intraparenchymal and subdural spaces. (**b**) Early-arterial and (**c**). Late-arterial phase 4D-CTAs demonstrate early opacification of a venous aneurysm (*arrow*), the culprit for the hematoma. The parent vein of the venous aneurysm is well see in the late arterial phase. (**d**) Left ECA angiogram clearly shows the AVF with the venous aneurysm (*arrow*) and the parent cortical vein.

have undergone radiosurgery, which gradually occludes the AVM over time, one effective strategy is to perform 4D MRA until the nidus is no longer seen. Once the nidus is no longer apparent on cross-sectional imaging, DSA can be used to verify occlusion status of the AVM.

Time-resolved MRA is also an effective tool for evaluation of cranial dAVFs. It can be helpful in identifying and characterizing feeding arteries, draining veins, and pinpoint the location of the dural arteriovenous shunt but not in characterizing the finer aspects of cranial dAVF angioarchitecture (▶ Fig. 5.32, ▶ Fig. 5.33). Basic features that can be delineated with current techniques include location of the fistula, presence of cortical venous drainage, direction of flow, and presence of venous ectasia. Time-resolved imaging has been shown to be very specific but insensitive in the detection of residual AVF after treatment and a negative 4D-MRA does not necessarily indicate a cure. For patients who have undergone radiosurgery, which gradually occludes the AVF over time, one effective strategy is to perform 4D MRA until shunting is no longer seen. Once the shunt is no longer apparent on cross-sectional imaging, DSA can be used to verify occlusion status of the AVF.

These imaging sequences are not a panacea and will likely not replace cerebral angiography in the diagnostic work-up of an arteriovenous shunting lesion. In MRI, there is a trade-off between spatial and temporal resolution. The higher the spatial resolution, the poorer the temporal resolution and vice versa. Likewise, in 4D-CTA, as temporal resolution increases, spatial

resolution decreases due to trade-offs in image sampling and patient dose. The estimated dose of current 4D-CTA techniques is 5 mSV compared to just 0.6 mSV for single-phase CTA and 2.7 mSV for DSA.

5.8.5 What the Clinician Needs to Know

- Time-resolved MRA techniques are effective in identifying arteriovenous shunting and basic classification (i.e., Spetzler-Martin or Cognard classification) of brain AVMs and AVFs but lack sufficient spatial resolution for detailed AVM angioarchitectural characterization.
- Basic features that can be delineated on 4D-CTA include nidus size, feeding vessels, dural feeders, neoangiogensis, flow-related and intranidal aneurysms, nidus type (compact vs. diffuse), and venous drainage patterns.

5.8.6 High-yield Facts

- Time-resolved CTA techniques provide superior spatial and temporal resolution to time-resolved MRA at the expense of increased dose (5.2 mSv) when compared to single-phase CTA (0.6 mSV) and DSA (2.7 mSV).
- Time-resolved MRA effective for imaging follow-up of treated AVMs and AVFs as it is highly specific; however, sensitivity is limited.

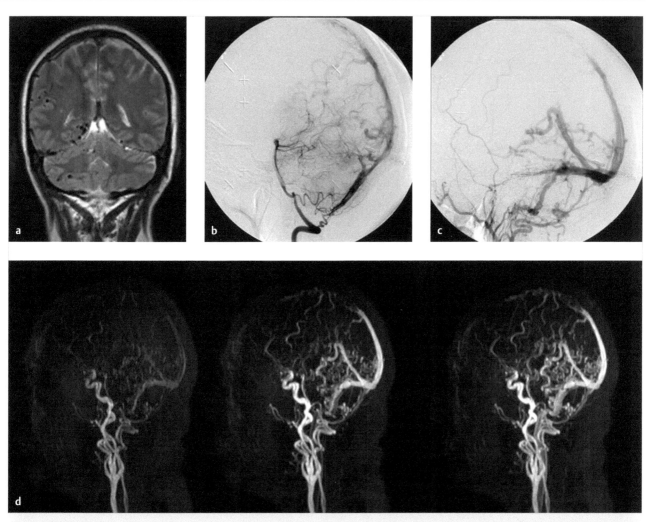

Fig. 5.32 TRICKS MRA for the evaluation of a cranial dAVF. (**a**) Coronal T2 MRI shows multiple abnormal flow voids in the right cerebellar hemisphere and right cerebral hemisphere. (**b**) Early arterial phase vertebral artery DSA shows a fistula supplied by the posterior meningeal artery with cortical venous reflux. (**c**) Venous phase DSA shows a pseudophlebitic pattern in the cerebellum with dilated and tortuous vein. (**d**) Early arterial, mid arterial, and late arterial phase TRICKS MRA (left to right) show arteriovenous shunting in the distal superior sagittal and transverse sinuses, cortical venous reflux in the cerebellar hemispheres, and occipital lobes and a pseudophlebitic pattern.

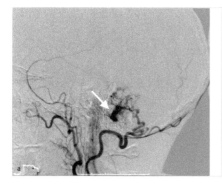

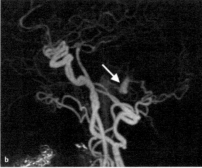

Fig. 5.33 The evaluation of dAVF angioarchitecture with TRICKS. (**a**) DSA demonstrates a dAVF with cortical venous reflux supplied by the posterior division of the MMA and transosseous occipital branches. The site of the fistula is clearly visualized. There is cortical venous reflux as well (*arrow*). (**b**) TRICKS MRA demonstrates the exact same angioarchitectural features with the dAVF with cortical venous reflux supplied by the posterior division of the MMA and transosseous occipital branches. The site of the fistula is clearly visualized (*arrow*).

Further Reading

[1] Tranvinh E, Heit JJ, Hacein-Bey L, Provenzale J, Wintermark M. Contemporary Imaging of Cerebral Arteriovenous Malformations. AJR Am J Roentgenol. 2017; 208(6):1320–1330

[2] Chang W, Wu Y, Johnson K, et al. Fast contrast-enhanced 4D MRA and 4D flow MRI using constrained reconstruction (HYPRFlow): potential applications for brain arteriovenous malformations. AJNR Am J Neuroradiol. 2015; 36(6):1049–1055

[3] Willems PW, Taeshineetanakul P, Schenk B, Brouwer PA, Terbrugge KG, Krings T. The use of 4D-CTA in the diagnostic work-up of brain arteriovenous malformations. Neuroradiology. 2012; 54(2):123–131

[4] Kortman HGJ, Smit EJ, Oei MTH, Manniesing R, Prokop M, Meijer FJ. 4D-CTA in neurovascular disease: a review. AJNR Am J Neuroradiol. 2015; 36(6):1026–1033

[5] Alnemari A, Mansour TR, Bazerbashi M, Buehler M, Schroeder J, Gaudin D. Dynamic Four-Dimensional Computed Tomography Angiography for Neurovascular Pathologies. World Neurosurg. 2017; 105:1034.e11–1034.e18

5.9 Cavernous Carotid Fistulas

5.9.1 Clinical Case

A 56-year-old female with painful exophthalmos and red eye. No prior trauma (▶ Fig. 5.34).

5.9.2 Description of Imaging Findings and Diagnosis

Diagnosis

Non-contrast CT shows slight exophthalmos of the left eye. T2 MRI shows a dilated flowvoid in the left orbit, which represents an enlarged superior ophthalmic vein. TRICKS MRA in the arterial phase shows early opacification of the enlarged superior ophthalmic vein with drainage down the facial vein. This was diagnostic of a carotico-cavernous fistula (CCF).

5.9.3 Background

CCFs are complex shunting lesions between the cavernous carotid artery (CCA), cavernous carotid artery branches or ECA branches, and the cavernous sinus itself. The anatomy and angioarchitecture, especially the presence or absence of cortical venous reflux of these fistulas will define both the natural history and treatment options for these lesions. The evaluation of cavernous carotid fistulas is an exercise in anatomy. Because of this, we will briefly describe the salient anatomic characteristics of cavernous carotid fistulas.

The cavernous sinus is a multi-compartmental extradural venous structure with a number of major tributaries. Veins which typically drain into the cavernous sinus include the superior ophthalmic vein, sphenoparietal sinus, basal vein of Rosenthal through the uncal vein, and petrosal or bridging veins of the pre-pontine and cerebellopontine angle cisterns. Of these veins, the only vein that universally drains into the cavernous sinus is the superior ophthalmic vein. Following the collection of venous supply from the aforementioned veins, the cavernous

sinus then drains into the superior petrosal sinus, inferior petrosal sinus, the pterygoid venous plexus through the foramen ovale, the contralateral cavernous sinus, and the clival venous plexus down to the foramen magnum and into the marginal sinus.

In addition to its complex venous inflow and outflow routes, the cavernous sinus also has a remarkably complex arterial supply from both ICA and ECA branches. The dominant supply from the internal carotid artery is the inferolateral trunk and the meningohypophyseal trunk. Dural branches from the ophthalmic artery such as the recurrent meningeal artery also supply the cavernous sinus. ECA supply to the cavernous sinus includes the artery of the foramen rotundum, which arises off the internal maxillary artery, the MMA, accessory meningeal artery, and clival branches of the ascending pharyngeal artery.

A variety of classification systems exist for CCFs (low-flow and high-flow, traumatic and spontaneous, and direct and indirect, etc.). However, the most commonly used classification system among neurosurgeons is the Barrow Classification. The Barrow Classification system defined four types of CCFs. Type A fistulas are a direct connection between the cavernous segment of the internal carotid artery and the cavernous sinus. These are generally very high-flow fistulas and are the result of blunt or penetrating trauma, iatrogenic complications from neuroendovascular procedures, aneurysm rupture, or the result of a connective tissue disease such as Ehlers-Danlos syndrome. Types B-D are dural shunts and commonly referred to as indirect fistulas. Type B lesions are indirect shunts between the meningeal branches of the cavernous carotid artery and cavernous sinus. Type C lesions are indirect shunts between the meningeal branches of the ECA and the cavernous sinus and Type D lesions are indirect shunts between the cavernous sinus and meningeal branches of the ECA and ICA.

The patient's clinical history is fundamental to the evaluation of a CCF. In patients with slowly progressive ocular symptoms including conjunctival injection or pulsatile exophthalmos, an indirect CCF should be considered. In patients with trauma and rapidly progressive neuro-ophthalmalogic symptoms, a post-traumatic CCF should be considered. Nonetheless, careful

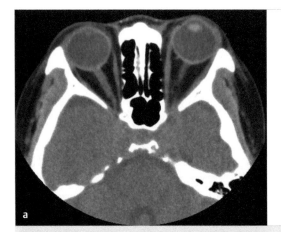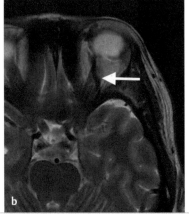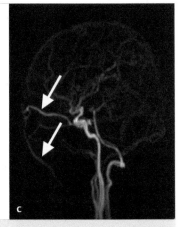

Fig. 5.34 Patient with painful exophthalmos of the left eye due to CCF. (a) Non-contrast CT shows slight exophthalmos of the left eye. (b) T2 MRI shows a dilated flow void in the left orbit, which represents an enlarged superior ophthalmic vein (*arrow*). (c) TRICKS MRA in the arterial phase shows early opacification of the enlarged superior ophthalmic vein (*arrow*) with drainage down the facial vein (*arrowhead*). This was diagnostic of a CCF. There is no cortical venous drainage.

attention should be paid to the cavernous sinus and orbits in all patients presenting with nonspecific ocular symptoms.

5.9.4 Imaging Findings

In the endovascular era, nearly all CCFs will undergo evaluation, characterization, and treatment with a cerebral angiogram or venogram. The goal of noninvasive imaging is to (1) detect the CCF and (2) identify features, which are associated with a poorer prognosis or natural history.

On CT/CTA, key imaging features of CCF include a dilated or ectatic SOV, extra-occular muscle thickening, and periorbital fat stranding (▶ Fig. 5.34). Up to 90% of patients have a dilated contrast filled SOV on CTA. Increased flow in CCFs can also result in cavernous sinus dilatation. CTA can be used to distinguish between direct and indirect fistulas as in indirect fistulas the timing and intensity of contrast enhancement is substantially lower than direct fistulas, which demonstrate fast and exuberate contrast opacification. The presence of a skull-base fracture in the region of the cavernous sinus should also clue one in on the presence of a direct CCF (▶ Fig. 5.35). Regarding natural history, the extent of cortical venous reflux should be established

on CTA imaging. Cortical venous reflux is manifested by the presence of large and dilated cortical veins, which have a similar contrast intensity to the arteries and which are substantially higher in attenuation than other venous structure. Subarachnoid hemorrhage (SAH) or ICH can develop due to a ruptured cortical vein.

MRI and MRA are superior to CT in the detection and characterization of CCFs (▶ Fig. 5.36, ▶ Fig. 5.37). Minimal SOV dilatation, subtle proptosis, and extra-occular muscle thickening are more easily identified on MRI. The CCF itself can be identified by exuberant contrast enhancement of the cavernous sinus and abnormal cavernous sinus vascular flow voids. Time of flight MRA is extremely useful in diagnosis of CCFs. In TOF MRA, arterial flow is hyperintense. The presence of hyperintense signal in the cavernous sinus, petrosal veins, or SOV has a high positive predictive value for a CCF. Cortical venous reflux can be identified by the presence of hyperintense and dilated cortical veins on SWI, dilated, and tortuous vascular flow voids on T2 or enhancing dilated and tortuous venous structures on postcontrast T1 weighted imaging (▶ Fig. 5.36). An ectatic SOV can be detected with high sensitivity on T2, T1CE, and SWI imaging in up to 80% of patients. Chronic venous hypertension can result

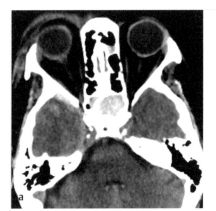
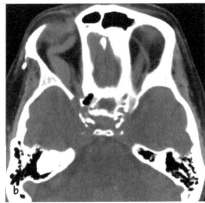
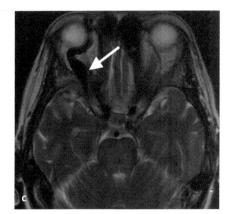
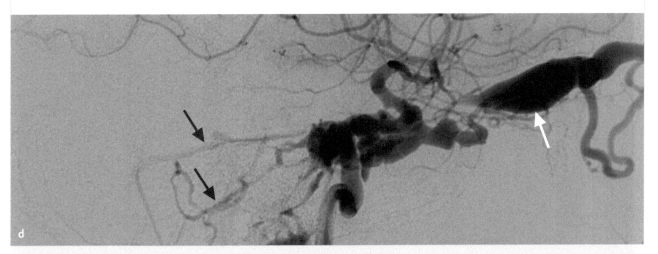

Fig. 5.35 Direct CCF in a patient status post MVA. **(a)** Non-contrast CT following an MVA shows blood in the sphenoid sinuses. There was a small non-displaced fracture in the wall of the sphenoid sinus (not shown). **(b)** 2 months later the patient presented with a painful right eye and a red eye. Repeat CT shows a markedly engorged superior ophthalmic vein. The left superior ophthalmic vein is also mildly dilated. **(c)** T2 MRI shows enlarged flow voids in the right (*arrow*), greater than left, orbit. Imaging findings are classic for a CCF. **(d)** Right ICA cerebral angiogram shows a direct, posttraumatic CCF between the right cavernous carotid artery and the cavernous sinus. There was retrograde cortical venous drainage (*black arrows*) as well as drainage through the right greater than left SOVs (*white arrow*).

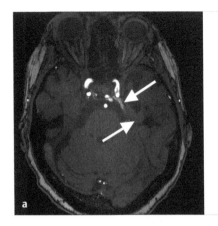
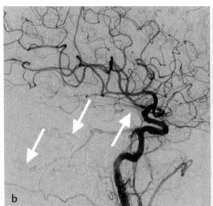

Fig. 5.36 Malignant venous drainage pattern of a CCF seen on TOF MRA. (a) TOF MRA in a patient with a history of pulsatile tinnitus shows arterialization of the cavernous sinus (*arrow*) as well as the superior petrosal vein and petrous vein (*arrowhead*). (b) Left CCA angiogram shows a left sided CCF with drainage into the superior petrosal sinus (*arrowhead*) and then cortical venous drainage in the cerebellum (*arrows*).

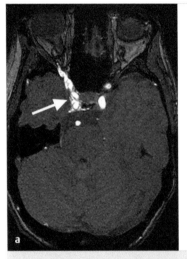
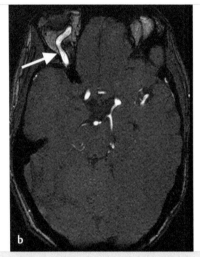
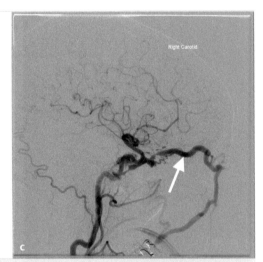

Fig. 5.37 CCF without malignant venous drainage on TOF MRA. (a) TOF MRA shows arterialization of the cavernous sinus (*arrow*). The cavernous sinuses should never be bright on a TOF MRA. (b) TOF MRA also shows arterialization of an enlarged superior ophthalmic vein, a classic imaging finding of a CCF (*arrow*). (c) Right CCA DSA shows the CCF, which drains into a large superior ophthalmic vein (*arrow*) and then into the facial vein.

in venous hemorrhage or congestion demonstrated by T2* blooming artifact and T2 hyperintensity, respectively.

5.9.5 What the Clinician Needs to Know

- Whether there are imaging sequelae of trauma, which could suggest the presence of a direct CCF
- The presence or absence of cortical venous drainage, which can portend a poorer natural history
- The presence of parenchymal venous congestion or intraparenchymal hemorrhage/SAH

5.9.6 High-yield Facts

- Direct CCFs are exceedingly rare the West. However, in Vietnam, Thailand, and China, they are more common. In the presence of acute onset neuro-ophthalmalogic symptoms

and skull-base trauma, a direct CCF should be highly considered.
- Cortical venous reflux of a CCF is associated with high rates of neurological deficit from venous ischemia and parenchymal hemorrhage.
- There should be a low threshold for diagnostic angiography in patients with a suspected CCF.

Further Reading

[1] Dos Santos D, Monsignore LM, Nakiri GS, Cruz AA, Colli BO, Abud DG. Imaging diagnosis of dural and direct cavernous carotid fistulae. Radiol Bras. 2014; 47 (4):251–255

[2] Razek AA, Castillo M. Imaging lesions of the cavernous sinus. AJNR Am J Neuroradiol. 2009; 30(3):444–452

[3] Rahman WT, Griauzde J, Chaudhary N, Pandey AS, Gemmete JJ, Chong ST. Neurovascular emergencies: imaging diagnosis and neurointerventional treatment. Emerg Radiol. 2017; 24(2):183–193

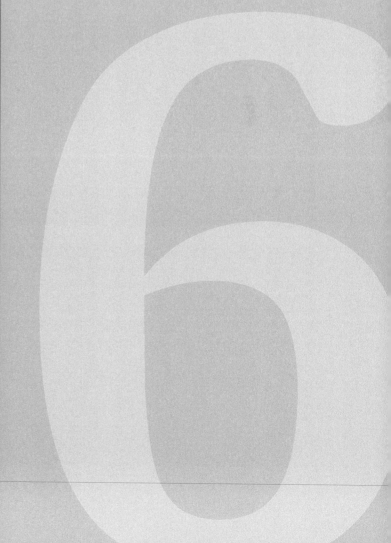

Chapter 6

Pediatric Neurovascular Disease

6 Pediatric Neurovascular Disease

6.1 Pediatric Aneurysms

6.1.1 Clinical Case

A 6-month-old boy, obtunded, with right-sided weakness (▶ Fig. 6.1).

6.1.2 Description of Imaging Findings and Diagnosis

Diagnosis

Giant "partially thrombosed" left MCA aneurysm.

6.1.3 Background

Pediatric intracranial aneurysms are exceedingly rare, comprising just 0.6% of all cerebral aneurysms. The pathogenesis and pathophysiology of pediatric cerebral aneurysms differ substantially from that of adult cerebral aneurysms. These lesions are typically the result of a dissecting disease that can be related to vasculopathy or connective tissue diseases. Other causes include infection, immunodeficiency, or trauma. In fact, previous

(even minor) trauma has been identified as a major predisposing factor for pediatric cerebral aneurysms as up to 40% of all aneurysms are believed to be related to trauma. Unlike in adults, pediatric intracranial aneurysms are more commonly found in males than females. "Classical" saccular aneurysms are relatively less common in the pediatric age group as compared to adults.

Given their different etiology as compared to the adult population, the clinical presentation of these lesions is also different from that of adults. Pediatric cerebral aneurysms can present with compressive effects, focal ischemic deficits, intraparenchymal hemorrhage, seizures, or subarachnoid hemorrhage (SAH). Over 60% of pediatric patients with SAH have a cerebral aneurysm.

6.1.4 Imaging Findings

In a child with suspected SAH, the first diagnostic imaging modality of choice is non-contrast CT. If SAH is identified, MR angiography may be preferred over CT angiography due to the added radiation dose of CTA. However, at many institutions, the presence of SAH on CT prompts multimodality imaging including MR/MRA, CTA, and a diagnostic cerebral angiogram due to the relatively high rate of false-negatives on conventional

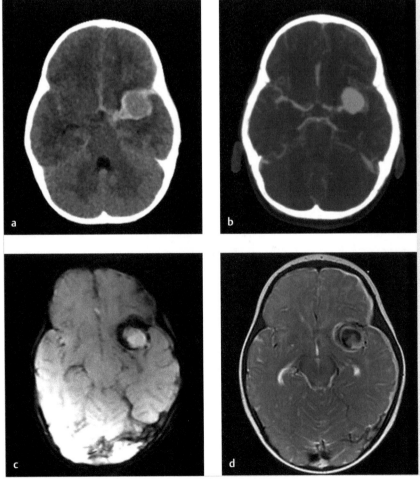

Fig. 6.1 A 6 month-old boy with aneurysmal SAH from thrombosed left MCA aneurysm. (**a**) Non-contrast CT shows the aneurysm in the left sylvian fissure with surrounding vasogenic edema as well as subarachnoid blood in the sylvian and inter-hemispheric fissure. (**b**) CTA confirms the presence of a giant left MCA aneurysm. (**c**) Axial SWI images demonstrate the aneurysm with blooming artifact surrounding the aneurysm reflecting blood products. There is also some thicker blooming artifact along the anterior aspect of the aneurysm consistent with thrombus in the aneurysm sac. (**d**) Axial T2-weighted MRI shows laminated thrombus in the anterior aspect of the aneurysm wall consistent with a giant, partially thrombosed aneurysm.

cross-sectional imaging and the potentially life-threatening consequences of an undiagnosed ruptured aneurysm.

Important factors that must be distinguished on luminal imaging include aneurysm size, location, and morphology that may give clues on underlying etiology. Unlike in the adult population, giant aneurysms are relatively common in the pediatric population with up to 40% of aneurysms in some series. Regarding location, approximately 5–10% of aneurysms are located at the anterior cerebral artery (ACA)/Acom, 25% at the ICA terminus, and about 25% are located in the posterior circulation. This distribution of locations differs substantially from the adult population where 30% of aneurysms are located at the ACA/Acom, 5% are located at the ICA terminus, and 10% located in the posterior circulation. Similar to the adult population, about 20% of aneurysms are located along the MCA.

Larger case series classify aneurysm etiology into four categories: saccular, infectious, dissecting, and traumatic. Understanding aneurysm etiology is important because it dictates both treatment decisions and clinical presentation. The most common type of aneurysm is the "classical" saccular aneurysm, although its proportion (approximately 40–50% of all pediatric aneurysms) is lower as compared to the adult population. These aneurysms can be large and may have intraluminal thrombus within them. Saccular aneurysms are the most likely to rupture into the subarachnoid space. Dissecting or "fusiform" aneurysms comprise 30–40% of all pediatric aneurysms and are particularly common in patients with connective tissue diseases (▶ Fig. 6.2). The number of layers involved in the dissection and perforator involvement by the intramural hematoma will determine their clinical presentation. Dissecting fusiform aneurysms can present with infarction via either reopening of the dissection into the parent artery, perforator occlusion through intramural hematoma progression, or complete vessel occlusion. In rare cases, repeated dissections can present with "growing" partially thrombosed aneurysms. Transmural dissecting aneurysms present with hemorrhage. Infectious aneurysms can be distal "mycotic" aneurysms, typical of those seen in patients with endocarditis, or proximal fusiform aneurysms related to viral infections or immunodeficiencies (HIV, familial candidiasis). These aneurysms can demonstrate mural enhancement secondary to the inflammatory process that is responsible for their pathogenesis and often present with infarction (▶ Fig. 6.3). Traumatic aneurysms are generally located at the skull base or the periphery and associated with adjacent fractures.

There are a number of important factors the radiologist must consider when interpreting a scan in a pediatric patient with a cerebral aneurysm. Close attention to the peri-aneurysmal environment focusing on perianeurysmal edema, wall enhancement/inflammation, mass effect, and infarction in the aneurysm vascular territory is essential. Attention to the remainder of the cerebral vasculature evaluating for the presence of additional aneurysms is important as about 15% of pediatric patients have multiple aneurysms. Intracranial stenosis, particularly of the ICA terminus, should also be ruled out as aneurysms can form secondary to occlusive arteriopathies such as moyamoya disease, sickle cell, or ACTA1 mutations. Cervical arterial tortuosity should be commented on as it could suggest an underlying connective

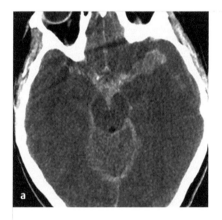
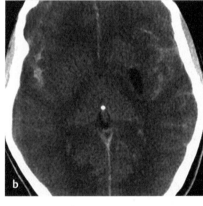
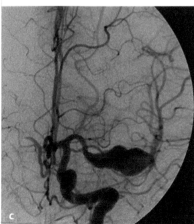
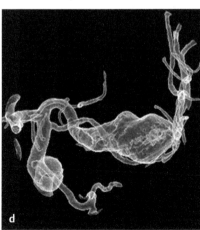

Fig. 6.2 Example of dissecting aneurysm presenting with stroke and hemorrhage. (a) Non-contrast CT demonstrates SAH in the left greater than right sylvian fissure and suprasellar cistern. There is clearly a structural abnormality in the left sylvian fissure. (b) Non-contrast CT also demonstrates a perforator infarct in the left lentiform nucleus. (c) and (d). AP cerebral angiogram and 3D reconstruction demonstrate a large fusiform dissecting type aneurysm involving the entirety of the left MCA segment. The dissecting aneurysm involves the origin of the lateral lenticulostriate supplying the left lentiform nucleus, which is why it presented with both hemorrhage and infarction.

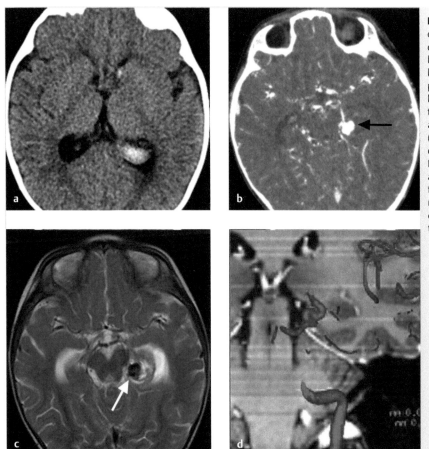

Fig. 6.3 Ruptured traumatic dissecting aneurysm of the left posterior cerebral artery. (**a**) Non-contrast CT demonstrates intraventricular hemorrhage in the frontal horn and atrium of the left lateral ventricle. (**b**) Axial CTA demonstrates a partially thrombosed fusiform aneurysm of the left PCA (*arrow*). (**c**) Axial T2-weighted MRI shows the aneurysm with laminated thrombus and mild associated edema in the adjacent hippocampus (*arrow*). There is also a small amount of mass effect on the left midbrain. (**d**) Fused image of an MRI and angiogram shows the position of the aneurysm at the point where the left PCA goes from its infratentorial location to its supratentorial location. This is a common location for dissecting aneurysms resulting from minor trauma.

tissue disease (Marfan's syndrome, Loeys-Dietz syndrome) and has implications for endovascular management.

6.1.5 What the Clinician Needs to Know

- Aneurysm size and location
- Aneurysm etiology (i.e., saccular, dissecting, traumatic, or infectious)
- Presence of intra-aneurysmal or intramural thrombus
- Presence of aneurysm-associated cerebral edema, mass effect, or infarction
- Tortuosity of cervical vasculature affecting endovascular access
- Aneurysm multiplicity
- Presence of vascular abnormalities (stenoses and tortuosity) elsewhere suggesting underlying moyamoya, sickle cell, or other occlusive arteriopathy

6.1.6 High-yield Facts

- Etiology, as well as morphology, of pediatric aneurysms differs substantially from adult population; more likely to be giant, non-saccular, and located in posterior circulation.

- Pediatric cerebral aneurysms often secondary to connective tissue diseases, infection, or trauma; important to evaluate for additional imaging findings suggestive of an underlying disease process.
- Fusiform and infectious aneurysms are more commonly associated with infarction, whereas saccular are more commonly associated with SAH.
- In pediatric SAH, it is reasonable to consider diagnostic cerebral angiography in lieu of CT angiography.

Further Reading

[1] Gemmete JJ, Toma AK, Davagnanam I, Robertson F, Brew S. Pediatric cerebral aneurysms. Neuroimaging Clin N Am. 2013; 23(4):771–779
[2] Jian BJ, Hetts SW, Lawton MT, Gupta N. Pediatric intracranial aneurysms. Neurosurg Clin N Am. 2010; 21(3):491–501
[3] Kanaan I, Lasjaunias P, Coates R. The spectrum of intracranial aneurysms in pediatrics. Minim Invasive Neurosurg. 1995; 38(1):1–9
[4] Krings T, Choi IS. The many faces of intracranial arterial dissections. Interv Neuroradiol. 2010; 16(2):151–160
[5] Chen L, Yau I, deVeber G, Dirks P, Armstrong D, Krings T. Evolution of a chronic dissecting aneurysm on magnetic resonance imaging in a pediatric patient. J Neurosurg Pediatr. 2015; 15(2):192–196
[6] Krings T, Geibprasert S, terBrugge KG. Pathomechanisms and treatment of pediatric aneurysms. Childs Nerv Syst. 2010; 26(10):1309–1318

6.2 Pediatric Dural Arteriovenous Fistulae

6.2.1 Clinical Case

A 6-year-old boy. Enlarging head circumference since infancy (▶ Fig. 6.4).

6.2.2 Description of Imaging Findings and Diagnosis

Diagnosis

Torcular dural sinus malformation.

6.2.3 Background

Pediatric dural arteriovenous shunts are a rare form of vascular disease in the pediatric population. With less than 200 cases reported in the literature, little is known regarding their natural history. The most widely accepted classification of pediatric dural arteriovenous shunts is that of Lasjuanias et al., which includes three types: (1) dural sinus malformation, (2) infantile dural arteriovenous shunt, and (3) adult type dural arteriovenous shunt. Common clinical manifestations of these lesions include seizure, macrocrania, hydrocephalus, and hemorrhage.

Regarding the classification of these lesions, dural sinus malformations often involve the torcula but can be found anywhere along the dural sinuses and are characterized by giant dural lakes and slow-flow mural arteriovenous shunting that derives its arterial supply from the meningeal branches. These lesions can involve other sinuses or the jugular bulb in which case they are associated with high-flow arteriovenous shunts. Infantile dural arteriovenous shunts are high-flow low-pressure lesions draining into a patent sinus and are not associated with a malformation of the sinus. Adult-type dural arteriovenous shunts develop following thrombosis in the sinus wall or trauma to the sinus.

Little is known regarding the pathogenesis of these lesions. Most of these lesions are considered to be congenital (▶ Fig. 6.5). Dural sinus malformations, as in the case presented here, are thought to result from persistent ballooning of the torcula in utero. This results in sinus wall overgrowth and development of abnormal venous spaces/lakes, which may predispose to the development of arteriovenous shunts. Unlike in the adult population, cerebral sinus thrombosis is considered a rare cause of pediatric dural arteriovenous shunts.

6.2.4 Imaging Findings

A number of imaging techniques can be used to evaluate pediatric dural arteriovenous fistulas (dAVFs) including CTA, MRA/MRI, ultrasound, and conventional angiography. On prenatal and neonatal ultrasounography, dural sinus malformations can be identified by the presence of an enlarged torcular with arterialized flow on Doppler (▶ Fig. 6.5). Occasionally, intraluminal thrombus in the torcula can be seen on intrauterine ultrasound. This may be mistaken for an epidural hematoma. On non-contrast CT, dural sinus malformations classically present with a markedly

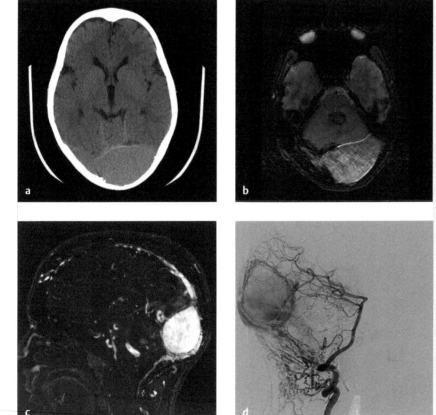

Fig. 6.4 Dural sinus malformation in a 6-year-old boy. (a) Non-contrast CT demonstrates marked dilatation of the torcula and bilateral transverse sinuses. (b) Axial T2* weighted MRI demonstrates high signal in the torcula consistent with arterialized flow. (c) Sagittal MR venogram demonstrates the marked dilatation of the torcula consistent with a torcular dural sinus malformation. (d) Right vertebral artery cerebral angiogram demonstrates dural vascular supply to the torcular dural AVF from posterior meningeal arteries.

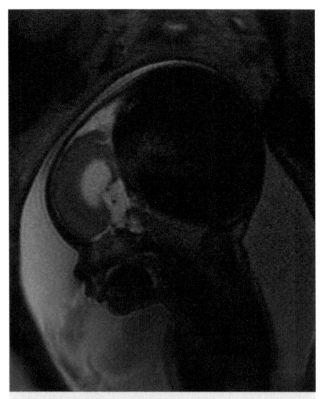

Fig. 6.5 Fetal MRI demonstrating severe dilatation of the torcula and fetal hydrocephalus consistent with a dural sinus malformation.

enlarged torcular. Persistent venous hypertension can result in hydrocephalus as well. In terms of noninvasive neurovascular imaging CTA/V and MRA/V can both be used in evaluation of these lesions. However, given obvious concerns for radiation dose in a patient population that will require multiple sessions of repeat imaging, MRI with MRA/V is preferable.

There are a number of important imaging findings that one must hone in on when evaluating a pediatric patient with a dural arteriovenous shunt. The location of the shunt is important in that it can determine natural history. In general, shunts involving the torcula have a poorer prognosis than those involving either the superior sagittal sinus or transverse sinus (▶ Fig. 6.6). MR venography can be very helpful in evaluating for venous sinus thromboses and stenoses in the draining veins and sinuses. The presence of jugular bulb stenosis is particularly important as it portends a poorer prognosis due to increased rates of venous hypertension and future hemorrhage. MR venograms should also be inspected for the presence of dilated corkscrew pial and medullary veins suggestive of chronic venous hypertension in the setting of cortical venous reflux. On MR angiography, one should evaluate the types of arterial feeders to the fistula with particular attention to the middle meningeal and occipital arteries. MRI may show vasogenic edema in the vascular territory draining the arteriovenous fistula (AVF), if there is chronic venous hypertension. In neonates and infants, this can result in delayed myelination, focal or diffuse venous ischemia, venous infarcts or hemorrhage, severe hydrocephalus, and, in terminal cases, brain calcifications from focal or diffuse melting-brain syndrome (▶ Fig. 6.7).

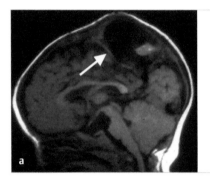
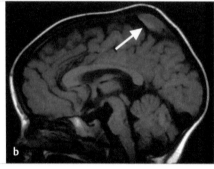

Fig. 6.6 Spontaneously thrombosing dural sinus malformation of the superior sagittal sinus. (a) Sagittal T1-weighted MRI demonstrates marked focal dilatation of the superior sagittal sinus consistent with a superior sagittal sinus dural sinus malformation (*arrow*). (b) Follow-up sagittal T1-weighted MRI performed 3 years later demonstrates spontaneous thrombosis of the dural sinus malformation with otherwise normal development of the brain (*arrow*).

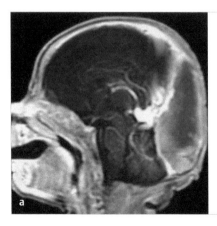
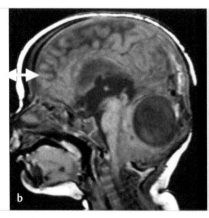

Fig. 6.7 Dural sinus malformation with poor prognosis. (a) Sagittal T1-weighted MRI with contrast demonstrating a large dural sinus malformation of the torcula. (b) Follow-up sagittal T1-weighted MRI shows interval development of superior sagittal sinus thrombosis and marked hydrocephalus, common complications of torcular dural sinus malformations.

Dural sinus malformations are unique in that they are typically slower flowing than other dural arteriovenous shunts. Because of this, they are more prone to undergo spontaneous thrombosis (► Fig. 6.6). This can result in devastating consequences including venous infarction and intraparenchymal hemorrhage. In cases of spontaneous thrombosis of a dural sinus malformation, the radiologist must try to figure out how the brain is draining. If this occurs late in infancy, following cavernous sinus capture of the basal veins and sylvian veins, the cavernous sinus will be the primary venous drainage outlet. If this occurs prior to cavernous sinus capture, cortical and medullary veins will preferentially be used to drain the brain, resulting in venous hypertension and hemorrhage.

Treatment of these challenging lesions therefore is thus comprised of a staged embolization approach that allows the dural sinuses to remodel. A complete obliteration of all shunts in the neonatal period is contraindicated.

6.2.5 What the Clinician Needs to Know

- Classification of the shunt (i.e., dural sinus malformation, infantile dAVF, and adult type dAVF)
- The presence of venous thrombosis or venous stenosis
- The patency of the jugular bulb
- The presence of sylvian vein or basal vein drainage into the cavernous sinus
- The location of arterial feeders
- Imaging evidence of chronic venous hypertension (i.e., dilated corkscrew medullary veins, vasogenic edema)

6.2.6 High-yield Facts

- Dural sinus malformations are characterized by a markedly dilated, "malformed" dural sinus and slow-flow arteriovenous shunts.
- Involvement of the torcular is associated with poorer prognosis as compared to involvement of the transverse sinuses alone.
- Infantile dural arteriovenous shunts are considered congenital and not the result of venous sinus thrombosis.
- Jugular venous stenosis and thrombosis of the draining venous sinus or any other venous outlet obstruction portend a poorer prognosis with higher risk of hemorrhage and venous hypertension.
- Thrombosis of a draining vein prior to cavernous sinus capture of the basal and sylvian veins portends a poorer prognosis.
- Venous hypertension signs include dilated corkscrew medullary veins and vasogenic edema.

Further Reading

[1] Barbosa M, Mahadevan J, Weon YC, et al. Dural Sinus Malformations (DSM) with Giant Lakes, in Neonates and Infants. Review of 30 Consecutive Cases. Interv Neuroradiol. 2003; 9(4):407–424

[2] Yang E, Storey A, Olson HE, et al. Imaging features and prognostic factors in fetal and postnatal torcular dural sinus malformations, part I: review of experience at Boston Children's Hospital. J Neurointerv Surg. 2017

[3] Yu J, Lv X, Li Y, Wu Z. Therapeutic progress in pediatric intracranial dural arteriovenous shunts: A review. Interv Neuroradiol. 2016; 22(5):548–556

[4] Krings T, Geibprasert S, Terbrugge K. Classification and endovascular management of pediatric cerebral vascular malformations. Neurosurg Clin N Am. 2010; 21(3):463–482

6.3 Pediatric Pial Arteriovenous Fistula

6.3.1 Clinical Case

A 2-day old boy with multiorgan failure.

6.3.2 Description of Imaging Findings and Diagnosis

Diagnosis

Pial arteriovenous fistula with cerebral atrophy (▶ Fig. 6.8).

6.3.3 Background

Pediatric pial arteriovenous fistulas are extremely rare intracranial vascular malformations comprising less than 2% of all arteriovenous malformations. To date, less than 200 cases of these lesions have been reported in the literature and their exact incidence is unknown. These lesions usually become symptomatic in childhood, although some of them may be diagnosed prenatally. Neonates with large shunts may present with congestive heart failure, whereas infants present with increased head circumference and focal neurological deficits. Beyond childhood, these lesions can present with headaches, seizures, and focal neurological deficits. Because these lesions consist of high-flow direct shunts between a pial artery and a cortical vein, prognosis is often poor with conservative management due to problems of venous congestion, mass effect of the pouches (▶ Fig. 6.9), or arterial steal from normal brain parenchyma. Natural history data are missing and these shunts cannot be sub grouped into criteria set out in the ARUBA trial or other natural history studies of brain vascular malformations.

Greater than 90% of pial AVFs are diagnosis before the age of 5. There is a male predominance (M:F = 2:1), similar to that seen in vein of Galen malformations.

Multiplicity of these pial arteriovenous fistulas is a strong predictor for a congenital origin (hereditary hemorrhagic telangiectasia [HHT]).

6.3.4 Imaging Findings

Pial AVFs may be identified on prenatal ultrasound as a dilated high flow shunt with pial dilated arteries and veins without an intraparenchymal nidus. Prenatal diagnosis has not been found to be associated with patient prognosis in most large series of pial AVFs. The key to diagnosis of these lesions is the identification of a dilated pial artery connecting directly into an ectatic and dilated draining vein. At the site of the arteriovenous connection, the vein is usually markedly dilated (▶ Fig. 6.10). Most lesions are located supratentorially with the vast majority of lesions located in the frontal or temporal lobes.

There are a number of important angioarchitectural characteristics that should be relayed to the treating physician in interpreting scans of pial AVF patients. On the arterial side, identification of the arterial feeder, its maximum diameter and the presence of feeding arterial aneurysms or stenoses is important. It is interesting to point out that arterial pathology in these lesions is rare with less than 5% of patients having arterial stenosis or aneurysms. Many lesions will have multiple arterial feeders converging on a single venous pouch.

The neuroradiologist must pay special attention to the venous side, however, as this is what will likely influence the presentation and natural history of the lesion. Venous ectasia is present in up to 90% of patients and should be commented on (▶ Fig. 6.8, ▶ Fig. 6.9, ▶ Fig. 6.10). The presence of pial venous stenosis, seen in 40% of patients, is also important as anything that limits venous outflow is a risk factor for hemorrhage.

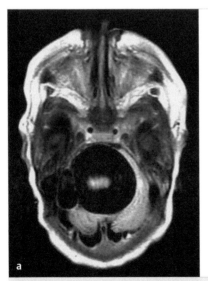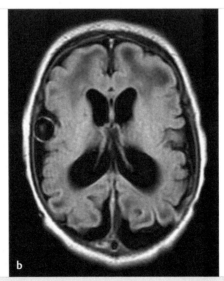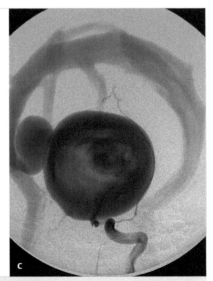

Fig. 6.8 A 1-day-old boy with pial arteriovenous fistula, multiorgan failure, and cerebral atrophy. (a) and (b). Axial T1-weighted MRI demonstrates large venous pouch in the posterior fossa and right sylvian fissure. There are marked brain atrophy likely secondary to chronic venous congestion. (c) AP projection of a left ICA angiogram demonstrating the pial arteriovenous fistula. Note the fact that there is arterialization of venous flow in the bilateral transverse sinuses. This is likely the cause of the patient's cerebral atrophy as the patient has likely suffered from poor cerebral venous drainage during his entire in utero life.

Patency of the dural venous sinuses is important as the presence of dural venous sinus thrombosis can substantially increase the rupture rate of the fistula. Dural venous sinus thrombosis is present in up to 20% of patients. False venous aneurysms are a potential bleeding source and should be identified (▶ Fig. 6.9).

Approximately 40% of patients will have multiple AVFs. By convention, multiple arterial feeders converging on to a single draining vein would comprise a single AVF. AVF multiplicity is defined as multiple distinct arteries feeding different draining veins with distinct fistulous points. AVF multiplicity, or, the presence of an AVF with a concomitant AVM should prompt an investigation for HHT or a *RASA1* mutation. Nearly 30% of pial AVF patients have such a mutation.

Hemorrhage from pial AVFs is not rare. There are three distinct patterns of hemorrhage: (1) at the site of the fistula – usually associated with a venous pseudoaneurysm, (2) regional venous hemorrhage due to local venous hypertension from pial venous reflux, and (3) remote venous hemorrhage secondary to global venous hypertension with sinus congestion and pial reflux.

"Melting brain syndrome" is a rare manifestation of these lesions. It is related to a progressive brain apoptosis related presumably to arterial steal from normal brain parenchyma and subsequent brain death. When present, it is usually located in the territory of the fistula (i.e., where the steal occurs). Because there is typically no subpial drainage associated with these AVFs, medullary venous congestion is rare.

6.3.5 What the Clinician Needs to Know

- The location of pial AVF, presence or absence of multiplicity, and number of arterial feeders
- The presence of venous thrombosis or venous outflow stenosis including draining pial veins and dural venous sinuses
- The presence of venous pseudoaneurysm
- The presence of additional brain AVMs or AVFs that could prompt investigation for HHT or *RASA1*
- The imaging evidence of chronic medullary venous hypertension (i.e., dilated corkscrew medullary veins, vasogenic edema) or pial venous reflux

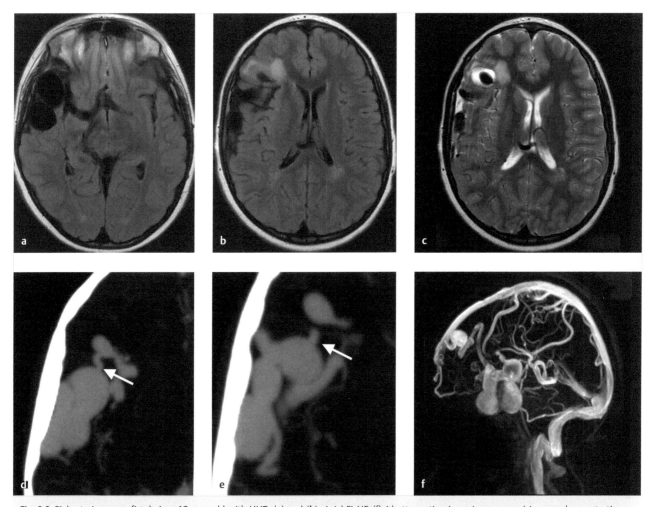

Fig. 6.9 Pial arteriovenous fistula in a 12-year-old with HHT. (**a**) and (**b**). Axial FLAIR (fluid attenuation inversion recovery) images demonstrating marked venous dilatation overlying the right temporal lobe, characteristic of venous ectasia. Note the edema surrounding one ectatic vein, which appears partially thrombosed on Axial FLAIR and T2-weighted imaging (**c**). (**d**) and (**e**) are CTA images of the pial AVF demonstrating the site of arteriovenous fistula with a transition in the size of the feeding artery and draining vein (*arrow*). (**f**) Sagittal MRV demonstrating the venous ectasia and course of the three large draining veins. Note the venous ectasia of the frontal vein draining into the superior sagittal sinus.

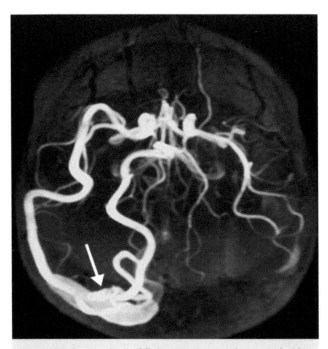

Fig. 6.10 Pial AVF on time of flight MRA. Direct pial AVF supplied by the right PCA and MCA with drainage into the transverse sinus and an occipital sinus. Arterialization of the draining vein is clearly present. The AV shunt is likely where the PCA and MCA branches converge (*arrow*).

- The imaging evidence of melting brain syndrome
- Arterial aneurysms or stenosis

6.3.6 High-yield Facts

- Pial arteriovenous fistula are characterized by a direct connection between a pial artery and an enlarged cortical vein.
- There is no intraparenchymal nidus.
- Risk factors for hemorrhage include draining venous stenosis, dural venous sinus thrombosis, and venous pseudoaneurysm.
- Locoregional effects of the fistula can include hemorrhage or, in case of significant arterial steal from normal brain parenchyma, melting brain syndrome.
- AVF multiplicity or the presence of additional brain AVMs suggests a diagnosis of HHT or *RASA1* mutations.

Further Reading

[1] Weon YC, Yoshida Y, Sachet M, et al. Supratentorial cerebral arteriovenous fistulas (AVFs) in children: review of 41 cases with 63 non choroidal single-hole AVFs. Acta Neurochir (Wien). 2005; 147(1):17–31, discussion 31

[2] Hetts SW, Moftakhar P, Maluste N, et al. Pediatric intracranial dural arteriovenous fistulas: age-related differences in clinical features, angioarchitecture, and treatment outcomes. J Neurosurg Pediatr. 2016; 18(5):602–610

[3] Krings T, Ozanne A, Chng SM, Alvarez H, Rodesch G, Lasjaunias PL. Neurovascular phenotypes in hereditary haemorrhagic telangiectasia patients according to age. Review of 50 consecutive patients aged 1 day-60 years. Neuroradiology. 2005; 47(10):711–720

[4] Krings T, Chng SM, Ozanne A, Alvarez H, Rodesch G, Lasjaunias PL. Hereditary hemorrhagic telangiectasia in children: endovascular treatment of neurovascular malformations: results in 31 patients. Neuroradiology. 2005; 47(12):946–954

6.4 Pediatric Venous Occlusive Disease

6.4.1 Clinical Case

A 17 month-old girl with 5-day history of vomiting, dehydration, and decreased level of consciousness.

6.4.2 Description of Imaging Findings and Diagnosis

Diagnosis

Extensive dural venous sinus thrombosis involving the superior sagittal sinus and straight sinus.

6.4.3 Background

Cerebral venous sinus thrombosis is one of the most common causes of childhood and neonatal stroke. More than 40% of all pediatric cerebral venous sinus thromboses cases are in neonates. In general, i.e., for all age groups, common risk factors for cerebral venous sinus thrombosis include sepsis, mastoiditis, nephrotic syndrome, tumor, oral contraceptive agents, anemia, dehydration, chemotherapy, and meningitis.

The clinical presentation of cerebral venous sinus thrombosis is highly variable and depends on the age of the patient and extent and location of the venous thrombus and its extent to the cortical veins and their outflow options. Neonates and infants may present with a wide range of symptoms ranging from irritability to coma. Likewise, older children and teenagers may present with severe headache, focal neurological deficits, or coma, depending on a variety of factors.

There is a wide spectrum of venous sinus thrombosis brain injury. The primary mechanism of brain injury is due to venous congestion. Venous congestion can result in venous infarction (either cortical, subcortical, or deep) or primary hemorrhage (intraventricular, intraparenchymal, or extra-axial).

6.4.4 Imaging Findings

Because of the protean clinical manifestations of cerebral venous sinus thrombosis, most cases are first identified on nonvascular imaging including cranial ultrasound (in the neonate), CT, and MRI. On non-contrast CT, the typical finding is a linear hyperdensity at the expected location of a cerebral vein (▶ Fig. 6.11, ▶ Fig. 6.12). On MRI, signs of cerebral venous sinus thrombosis include high signal on sagittal T1 in the methemoglobin stage of blood degradation, loss of normal flow voids on axial T2-weighted images, loss of flow voids or hyperintense signal on FLAIR, blooming on GRE or SWI, and filling defects on spin echo contrast enhanced T1-weighted sequences (▶ Fig. 6.13). It is important to point out that in the acute phase on MRI, the thrombus is isointense to the brain on T1-weighted imaging and low signal on T2-weighted imaging and can be missed. However, in the subacute phase, the thrombus is readily apparent on T1-weighted imaging when it is of high signal (▶ Fig. 6.13). The sensitivity and specificity for the identification of cerebral venous sinus thrombosis are 80 and 90%, respectively.

Angiographic imaging for evaluation of dural venous sinus thrombosis consists of CT venography and MR venography. Thrombus is found in the superficial venous system in about 90% of cases and in the deep venous system in 40%. Multiple sinuses are involved in about 50% of cases. On CT, thrombosis can be easily identified as the lack of filling of the venous structures in the venous phase. Because of radiation concerns, however, MR venography is now the imaging modality of choice in evaluating the dural venous sinus. MR venography can be performed using a gadolinium bolus technique with image acquisition timed for the venous phase or using non-contrast techniques such as time of flight or phase contrast MR venography. One common pitfall of all venography techniques is the fact that they are all T1 weighted and thus, it is possible to mistake a very hyperintense thrombus for a patent sinus.

The sequelae of cerebral venous sinus thrombosis are extremely important to comment on. The natural history and clinical/imaging sequelae of pediatric cerebral venous sinus thrombosis differ from that seen in adults. In the acute phase, hemorrhagic infarct or venous ischemia (with restricted diffu-

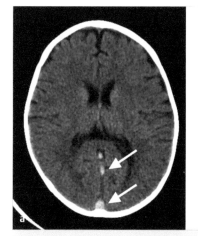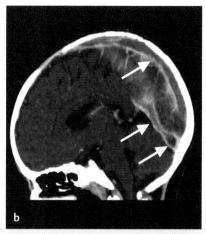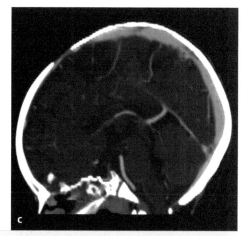

Fig. 6.11 A 17-month-old girl with 5-day history of vomiting, dehydration, and decreased level of consciousness due to extensive venous sinus thrombosis. **(a)** Axial non-contrast CT scan demonstrates a hyperdense superior sagittal sinus and straight sinus (*arrows*). **(b)** Sagittal CT venogram demonstrates extensive thrombosis of the superior sagittal sinus and the straight sinus (*arrows*). **(c)** CT venogram after 6 months of oral anticoagulation shows recanalization of the occluded dural venous sinuses.

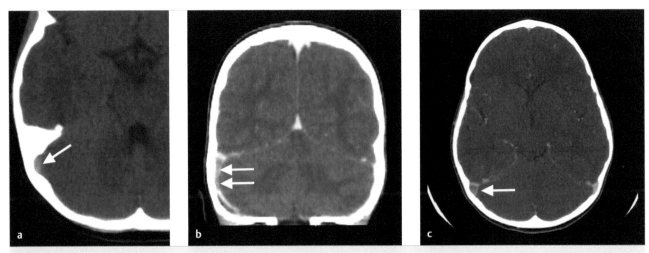

Fig. 6.12 A 6-year-old girl who developed transverse sinus thrombosis following episode of otomastoiditis (*arrow*). (**a**) Non-contrast head CT demonstrates hyperdensity of the right transverse sigmoid junction (*arrow*). (**b**) Coronal and (**c**). Axial reconstruction of a CT venogram shows focal thrombus in the right transverse-sigmoid junction (*arrow*).

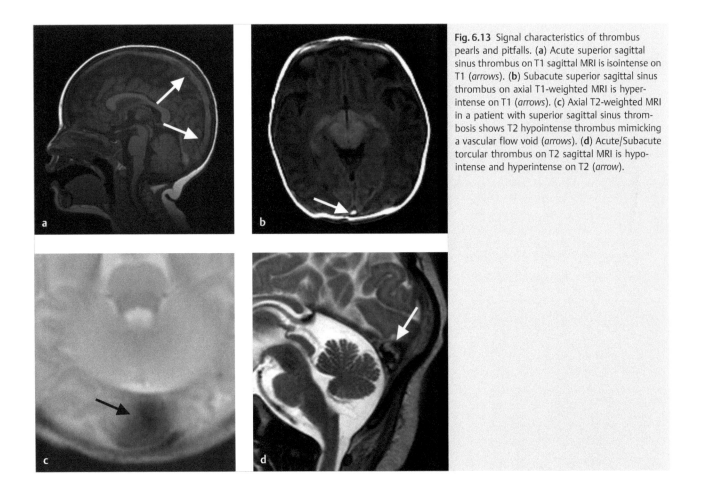

Fig. 6.13 Signal characteristics of thrombus pearls and pitfalls. (**a**) Acute superior sagittal sinus thrombus on T1 sagittal MRI is isointense on T1 (*arrows*). (**b**) Subacute superior sagittal sinus thrombus on axial T1-weighted MRI is hyperintense on T1 (*arrows*). (**c**) Axial T2-weighted MRI in a patient with superior sagittal sinus thrombosis shows T2 hypointense thrombus mimicking a vascular flow void (*arrows*). (**d**) Acute/Subacute torcular thrombus on T2 sagittal MRI is hypointense and hyperintense on T2 (*arrow*).

sion) can occur, similar to adults. The location of the ischemic insult or hemorrhage will be lobar and in a non-arterial distribution, if a superficial cortical vein or superficial venous sinus is involved. In the setting of a deep vein thrombosis, deeper structures including the thalami and basal ganglia will be involved. Long-lasting thrombosis or occlusion of a dural venous sinus can lead to additional problems including melting brain syndrome and cerebral white matter dysmaturation; particularly, if the patient is a neonate or infant. Chronic but recanalized thrombus can result in chronic venous hypertension and pseudotumor cerebri with papilledema and mild tonsillar prolapse (▶ Fig. 6.14). Adult-type dural arteriovenous fistulae

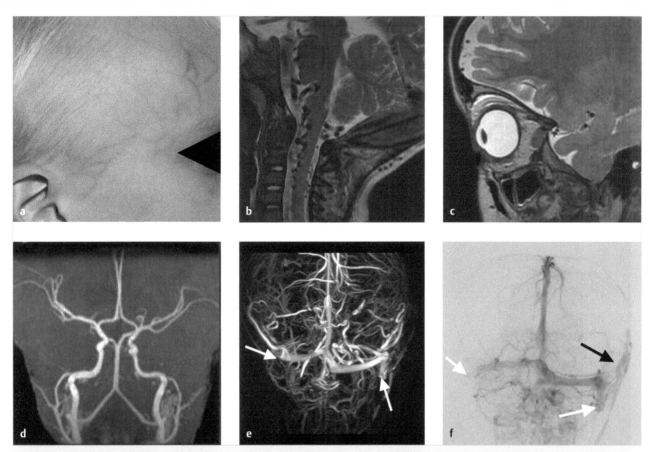

Fig. 6.14 A 4-year-old boy with chronic headaches increasing in frequency and macrocephaly. Noted to have prominent scalp veins at birth. Optic nerve swelling present on eye exam. (**a**) Photograph of the prominent scalp veins. (**b**) Sagittal T2-weighted MRI shows innumerable prominent vascular flow voids in the posterior fossa as well as prominent vascular flow voids along the upper cervical spine. Findings were initially concerning for a shunting vascular malformation. (**c**) Sagittal T2-weighted MRI shows flattening of the optic disc due to elevated intracranial pressure. (**d**) TOF MRA shows the fact that none of the prominent vascular flow voids had arterialized flow, suggesting the absence of a vascular malformation. (**e**) MRV demonstrates occlusion of the bilateral sigmoid sinuses (*arrows*) and lack of flow in the internal jugular veins. (**f**) Venous phase of a left vertebral artery cerebral angiogram shows no antegrade flow in the bilateral sigmoid sinuses (*white arrows*). There is a large emissary vein draining to a facial vein which is the cause of the prominent scalp veins (*black arrow*).

have been reported to form in the setting of dural venous sinus thrombosis in children as well.

6.4.5 What the Clinician Needs to Know

- Location, age, and extent of thrombus
- Presence of venous ischemia or hemorrhagic infarct
- Potential outflow alternatives through superficial venous collaterals
- Any recanalization of the venous channels
- Imaging findings suggestive of intracranial hypertension including tonsillar prolapse, optic nerve atrophy, or flattening of optic disc
- Signs of white matter dysmaturation or melting brain syndrome

6.4.6 High-yield Facts

- Most cases of cerebral venous sinus thrombosis can be identified using standard non-contrast MRI sequences with loss of

flow voids, high-signal thrombus on T1, and blooming artifact on T2* weighted sequences.
- MR venography is preferred imaging modality for diagnosis of cerebral venous sinus thrombosis.
- Venous hemorrhagic infarcts are relatively common and involve deep gray matter structures in deep venous thrombosis and are lobar in location for superficial thrombosis.
- Chronic imaging sequelae include white matter dysmaturation, pseudotumor cerebri findings, and, in rare cases, melting brain syndrome.

Further Reading

[1] Patel D, Machnowska M, Symons S, et al. Diagnostic Performance of Routine Brain MRI Sequences for Dural Venous Sinus Thrombosis. AJNR Am J Neuroradiol. 2016; 37(11):2026–2032
[2] Ritchey Z, Hollatz AL, Weitzenkamp D, et al. Pediatric Cortical Vein Thrombosis: Frequency and Association With Venous Infarction. Stroke. 2016; 47(3): 866–868

6.5 Vein of Galen Malformation

6.5.1 Clinical Case

A 1-day-old boy with abnormal fetal MRI scan and cranial ultrasound.

6.5.2 Description of Imaging Findings and Diagnosis

Diagnosis

Mural type vein of Galen malformation.

6.5.3 Background

Vein of Galen arteriovenous malformations (VOGM) are shunts that form in utero between the choroidal arteries and the precursor of the vein of Galen, the median prosencephalic vein of Markowski. These lesions are quite rare, and found in approximately 1/25,000 deliveries. While many VOGMs are identified in utero, a substantial proportion are still diagnosed early in the neonatal or infant period with children presenting with congestive heart failure from the high-flow shunt. Other common clinical presentations of VOGM include multisystem organ failure, macrocrania, hydrocephalus, seizure, and, much rarer, intracranial hemorrhage. These lesions have a slight male predominance.

6.5.4 Imaging Findings

There are a number of imaging findings one has to consider when evaluating a VOGM patient (▶ Table 6.1). Identification of the lesion itself is relatively straightforward given the marked dilatation of the midline venous structure referred to as the "vein of Galen" and prominent dilated choroidal feeding vessels surrounding the malformation bilaterally. However, detailed evaluation of the lesion angioarchitecture is important for treatment planning purposes. The two ends of the spectrum of VOGM are choroidal and mural types. Choroidal VOGMs are supplied by all choroidal arteries (anterior and posterior) as

well as the pericallosal arteries, which then feed into an interposed network or nidus before emptying into the venous pouch. This is the most common lesion. Mural VOGMs consist of a single direct AV fistula within the wall of the median vein of the prosencephalon (▶ Fig. 6.15). This lesion is rarer and better tolerated. Intermediate types are possible and often encountered. A combination of 3D time of flight MRA and high-resolution T2-weighted imaging can be used to determine the arterial feeders and angioarchitecture of the lesion. When the vessels converge on the wall of the venous pouch, the lesion is a mural (or fistulous) type, and when they converge on a vascular network just prior to the pouch, the lesion is of a choroidal type.

In addition to studying the arterial feeders, special attention should be paid to the venous drainage of both the brain and the VOGM. The venous drainage of the VOGM is always toward the median vein of the prosencephalon and then into the inferior aspect of the superior sagittal sinus through the persistent falcine sinus. According to Lasjaunias and most imaging studies, in the vast majority of cases, NO communication exists between the malformation itself and the deep venous system, although more recent studies using high quality MR venography have identified a subset of patients in which the internal cerebral veins do, in fact, have a connection with the VOGM. In most VOGM patients, the deep venous system of the normal brain thus generally drains into the lateral perimesencephalic vein and into the superior petrosal sinus, forming the classical typical "epsilon" shape of drainage pattern. The straight sinus is absent in almost all cases. A number of persistent embryonic sinuses remain present in these patients (presumably related to the arterialization of the sinuses) including the persistent falcine sinus, occipital sinus, and marginal sinus. Patency of the dural venous sinuses, presence of dural venous sinus thrombosis, and maturation/patency of the jugular bulbs should be described as any narrowing or occlusion can result in pial venous reflux or dural venous congestion, further exacerbating problems related to high intracranial pressure. Relaying information regarding the presence or absence of cavernous sinus capture is important as this represents an important pathway for draining normal brain. Cavernous sinus capture can be implicated in the presence of dilated cavernous sinus, ophthalmic,

Table 6.1 Important Imaging Findings

Brain Parenchyma	Arterial Side	Venous Side
		Venous outflow obstruction (sinus stenosis or thrombotic occlusion)
Status of myelination	Pattern of arterial feeders	
Presence of brain atrophy	Presence of secondarily recruited vessels (i.e., subependymal network)	Status of jugular bulb maturation
Periventricular white matter ischemia	Type of VOGM	Persistent embryonic sinuses
Encephalomalacia	Rule out a mimic lesion	Cavernous sinus capture (prominent ophthalmic veins, enlarged facial veins)
DWI abnormalities from steal (i.e., not in an arterial distribution)	Recruiting thalamoperforator lesions	Pseudophlebitic pattern
Calcifications in striatum, deep and subcortical white matter		Venous reflux
Hydrocephalus		
Tonsillar ectopia and syringomyelia		

Abbreviations: VOGM, Vein of Galen malformation; DWI, diffusion weighted imaging.

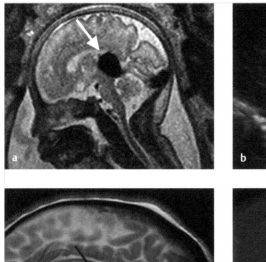
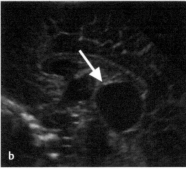
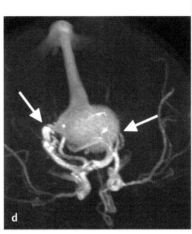

Fig. 6.15 Prenatally diagnosed mural-type vein of Galen malformation. (**a**) T2-weighted fetal MRI scan demonstrates dilatation of the prosencephalic vein and torcula, consistent with a vein of Galen malformation (*arrow*). (**b**) Sagittal ultrasound demonstrates a dilated vein of Galen confirming the prenatal diagnosis (*arrow*). (**c**) Sagittal T2-weighted MRI demonstrates the dilated vein of Galen and a couple vessels along the anterior wall of the vein with no intervening nidus (*arrows*). (**d**) 3D-TOF MR angiogram demonstrates direct arteriovenous shunts (*arrows*) along the wall of the prosecenphalic vein consistent with a mural-type vein of Galen malformation.

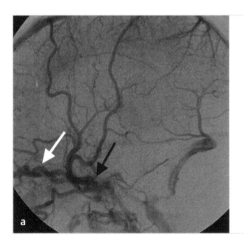
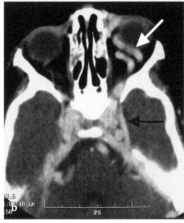

Fig. 6.16 Example of cavernous capture. (**a**) Lateral left ICA cerebral angiogram demonstrating drainage of normal brain parenchyma into the cavernous sinus (*black arrow*) with dilatation of the left superior ophthalmic vein (*white arrow*). This is a result of cavernous capture of the deep venous system, which is allowing the vein of Galen malformation patient's brain to drain through the cavernous sinus system rather than the Galenic system. (**b**) CT angiogram demonstrating cavernous sinus capture with dilatation of the lateral ponto-mesencephalic vein, cavernous sinus (*black arrow*), and left superior ophthalmic vein (*white arrow*). This is a characteristic imaging finding of cavernous sinus capture in the setting of a vein of Galen malformation.

or intraorbital veins. Most importantly though, the presence of a sphenoparietal sinus connecting to the cavernous sinus indicates that the brain has found alternate pathways of drainage indicating a positive prognosis (▶ Fig. 6.16).

VOGMs can result in substantial neurological deficits beyond the neurological injury induced by congestive heart failure (which would typically manifest itself in the neonatal period). Arterial steal can be present in the first days after birth with blood flow shunted to the high-flow shunt thus leading to brain hypoperfusion distant from the shunt. Imaging findings include dilated MCA branches (that do not contribute to the shunt but are dilated due to hypoxemia related autoregulation). In cases of severe arterial steal, DWI abnormalities will appear that were previously referred to as signs of "melting brain" but that are now

believed to be related to progressive hypoxemia due to high-flow shunting (▶ Fig. 6.17). If not symptomatic through cardiac manifestations or arterial steal in the first weeks of life, children may become symptomatic due to venocongestive problems. Hydrocephalus and macrocrania are among the most common imaging and clinical manifestations at this stage. It was previously presumed that hydrocephalus was related to compression of the aqueduct by the enlarged venous pouch; however, this is not the case. In fact, hydrocephalus in a VOGM is the result of a high venous pressure in the dural sinus, which impedes drainage of CSF in the presence of immature arachnoid granulations (▶ Fig. 6.18). The majority of CSF is reabsorbed through the transmedullary veins, which means that in cases of arterialization of these veins (which invariably occurs in VOGM), the CSF

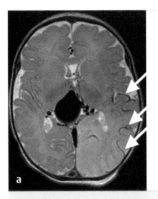 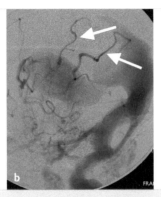 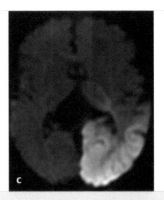 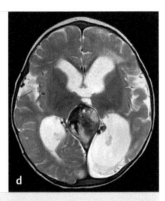

Fig. 6.17 Example of arterial steal in the setting of a vein of Galen malformation. (**a**) T2-weighted MRI demonstrates the enlarged prosencephalic vein with multiple surrounding vascular flow voids consistent with a vein of Galen malformation. In addition, there is dilatation of distal MCA branches overlying the left cerebral hemisphere (*arrows*) and high T2 signal in the left parieto-occipital lobe. The hypertrophied pial arteries and associated underlying signal abnormality is a classic imaging manifestation of arterial steal. (**b**) Left ICA cerebral angiogram demonstrates slow filling of the left MCA vessels that were seen in (**a**) (*arrows*). These vessels are maximally dilated in order to provide blood flow to the temporooccipital lobe. (**c**) Axial DWI MRI obtained preoperative shows restricted diffusion in the left parietooccipital lobe related to progressive hypoxemia from high flow shunting. (**d**) Axial T2-weighted MRI obtained postoperatively shows thrombus formation in the vein of Galen and encephalomalacia in the now infarcted left temporo-occipital lobe. The patient had an episode of intraoperative hypotension. Because the vessels were maximally vasodilated pretreatment, the hypotensive insult resulted in infarction of the supplied territory.

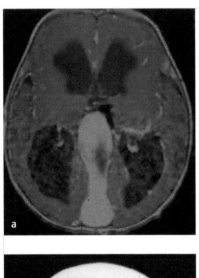 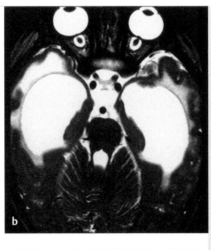

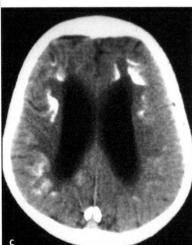 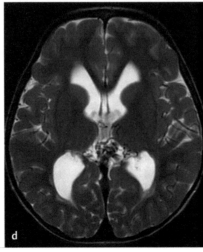

Fig. 6.18 Imaging manifestations of vein of Galen malformation complications. (**a**) T1 contrast enhanced MRI shows dilatation of subependymal and intramedullary veins consistent with medullary venous congestion. This is the underlying cause of the patients' hydrocephalus as well. (**b**) FIESTA MRI of the brain demonstrating severe hydrocephalus, dilatation of the optic nerve sheaths, and flattening of the posterior sclera from increased intracranial hypertension. (**c**) Non-contrast CT of the head demonstrating diffuse parenchymal calcifications consistent with the so-called melting brain syndrome. (**d**) Axial T2-weighted MRI showing a choroidal type vein of Galen malformation with hydrocephalus and transependymal flow of CSF.

will not be reabsorbed or can only be reabsorbed against an "arterialized" pressure, which will increase the backpressure in the ventricles thus leading to hydrocephalus. Increased intracranial pressure and venous congestion can result in serious complications including white matter dysmaturation, intracranial hemorrhage (if the backflow results in outflow obstruction of the brain), or venous ischemia.

It is important to distinguish a VOGM from other vein of Galen-related pathologies. For example, the vein of Galen aneurysmal dilatations are commonly mistaken for VOGM. However, these lesions are related to pial (NOT choroidal) arteriovenous shunts which drain into the deep venous system with an acquired dilatation of the vein of Galen secondary to stenosis at the venodural junction or straight sinus. This is different from a true VOGM in that the dilated vein is the vein of Galen itself and not the prosencephalic vein and thus drains both normal brain and the AVM. Dural arteriovenous shunts can drain into the vein of Galen (falcotentorial shunts) but they appear later in life and have only secondarily induced pial shunts. Vein of Galen varices represent a dilatation of the vein of Galen in the absence of an AV shunt. The dilatations persist for a few days after birth but then disappear. They can also be the result of aberrant but normal variant deep venous drainage.

6.5.5 What the Clinician Needs to Know

- Angioarchitecture including arterial feeders and VOGM type (choroidal versus mural)
- Pathway for the drainage of normal deep venous system
- Types of persistent embryonic sinuses
- The degree of hydrocephalus
- The extent and severity of cerebral white matter changes

- The presence of cerebral atrophy and sequelae of melting brain syndrome
- The patency of dural venous sinuses and maturation status of the jugular bulbs
- The presence of venous ischemia or hemorrhagic infarct

6.5.6 High-yield Facts

- In choroidal VOGMs, the choroidal arteries converge in a vascular plexus before draining into the promesencephalic vein.
- In mural VOGMs, arteries converge on the wall of the promesencephalic vein to form direct AV fistulas.
- Hydrocephalus is a result of venous hypertension.
- Venous outflow narrowing or occlusion can exacerbate white matter disease and result in a higher rate of venous ischemia or hemorrhagic infarct.
- Chronic imaging sequelae include white matter dysmaturation or pseudotumor cerebri findings.

Further Reading

[1] Alvarez H, Garcia Monaco R, Rodesch G, Sachet M, Krings T, Lasjaunias P. Vein of galen aneurysmal malformations. Neuroimaging Clin N Am. 2007; 17(2):189–206

[2] Lasjaunias PL, Chng SM, Sachet M, Alvarez H, Rodesch G, Garcia-Monaco R. The management of vein of Galen aneurysmal malformations. Neurosurgery. 2006; 59(5) Suppl 3:S184–S194, discussion S3–S13

[3] Geibprasert S, Krings T, Armstrong D, Terbrugge KG, Raybaud CA. Predicting factors for the follow-up outcome and management decisions in vein of Galen aneurysmal malformations. Childs Nerv Syst. 2010; 26(1):35–46

[4] Saliou G, Dirks P, Sacho RH, Chen L, terBrugge K, Krings T. Decreased Superior Sagittal Sinus Diameter and Jugular Bulb Narrowing Are Associated with Poor Clinical Outcome in Vein of Galen Arteriovenous Malformation. AJNR Am J Neuroradiol. 2016; 37(7):1354–1358

[5] Brinjikji W, Krings T, Murad MH, Rouchaud A, Meila D. Endovascular Treatment of Vein of Galen Malformations: A Systematic Review and Meta-Analysis. AJNR Am J Neuroradiol. 2017; 38(12):2308–2314

6.6 Pediatric Arterial Acute Ischemic Stroke

6.6.1 Clinical Case

A 12-year-old girl with headaches, vomiting, left homonymous hemianopsia, and left-sided weakness following minor trauma (▶ Fig. 6.19).

6.6.2 Description of Imaging Findings and Diagnosis

Diagnosis

Right PCA distribution infarction affecting the mesial right temporal lobe, occipital lobe, and thalamus. There is a dissecting aneurysm of the right posterior cerebral artery.

6.6.3 Background

Pediatric acute ischemic stroke is a major cause of neurological morbidity and mortality worldwide with an estimated annual incidence of 2–13 per 100,000 children. Clinical diagnosis of stroke in children is not straightforward as patients may present with nonspecific symptoms such as seizures, altered mental status, headaches, or lethargy. For this reason, neuroimaging is essential for the diagnosis of stroke and differentiation from stroke mimics such as tumor, Todd's paresis, demyelination, or hemiplegic migraine (▶ Fig. 6.20).

Stroke in the pediatric population is divided into two age-range categories. Perinatal stroke is defined as stroke occurring in the first 28 days of life, whereas childhood stroke is defined as stroke occurring from 29 days to 18 years. Common causes of perinatal arterial ischemic stroke include asphyxia from complicated delivery, infection, dehydration, congenital heart disease, and placental vasculopathy. In older children, the common causes are congenital heart disease in 30% of patients while arteriopathies account for 50% (i.e., dissection, transient cerebral arteriopathy, moyamoya disease, sickle cell, vasculitis, and fibromuscular dysplasia). Other common causes include hypercoagulable states and drug abuse. In general, perinatal stroke is a one-time event, whereas, in the older population, recurrence rates range from 15 to 50%, depending on etiology.

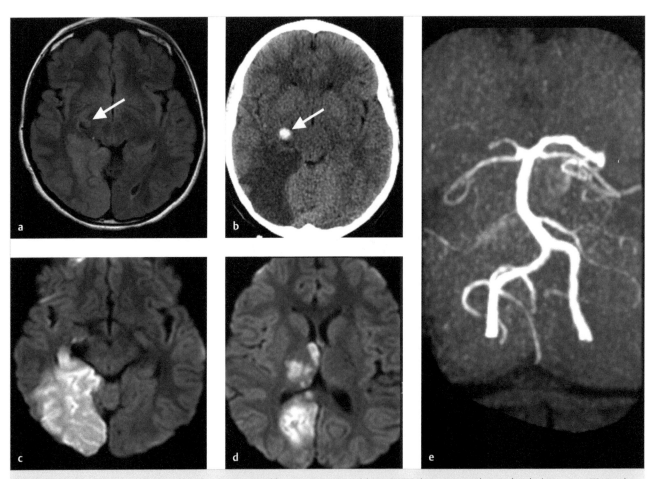

Fig. 6.19 Right PCA territory infarction secondary to dissection/dissecting aneurysm. (**a**) FLAIR MRI shows increased cortical and white matter T2 signal as well as gyral swelling. There is a well-circumscribed aneurysm of the right P2 (*arrow*). (**b**) Non-contrast CT shows a wedge shaped hypodensity in the right PCA territory and a hyperdense partially thrombosed dissecting aneurysm (*arrow*). (**c**) and (**d**). DWI MRI demonstrates infarction of the right mesial temporal lobe, occipital lobe, and thalamus. (**e**) Coronal MIP image from TOF MRA demonstrates loss of signal in the distal right PCA secondary to the dissecting aneurysm.

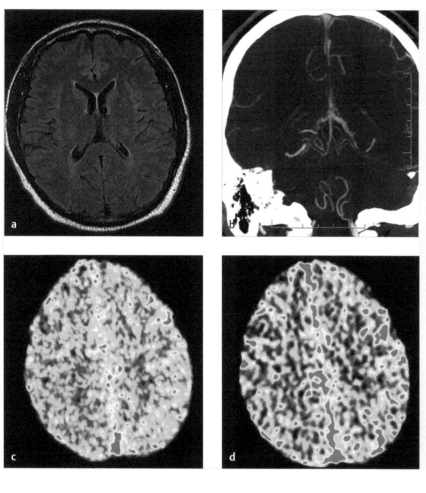

Fig. 6.20 Familial hemiplegic migraine as a stroke mimic. (**a**) FLAIR MRI demonstrates no signal abnormality. (**b**) CTA demonstrates a paucity of pial vessels overlying the entirety of the right hemisphere. (**c**) CBV map demonstrates reduced cerebral blood volume in the right cerebral hemisphere. (**d**) CBF map demonstrates reduced cerebral blood flow in the right cerebral hemisphere. The patient's symptoms resolved after a few hours. Repeat CTP (not shown) shows the restoration of normal CBV and CBF in the right cerebral hemisphere.

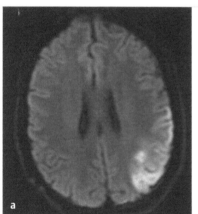
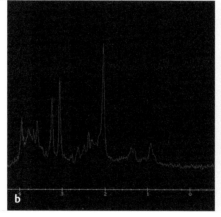

Fig. 6.21 A 17-year-old male with MELAS syndrome. (**a**) DWI MRI shows restricted diffusion in the left parietal cortex with relative sparing of the white matter. (**b**) MR spectroscopy in this patient showed elevated lactate in all regions of the brain, consistent with a mitochronial encephalopathy.

6.6.4 Imaging Findings

Imaging approaches for stroke evaluation differ by age group. In cases suspicious for neonatal stroke (0–28 days of life), MRI is generally the preferred imaging modality in both the acute and subacute phase with standard sequences being DWI, GRE or SWI, 3D TOF, and axial T1 and T2 sequences. MRV can be considered to rule out cerebral venous sinus thrombosis. In patients beyond the neonatal age, again MRI is the preferred imaging modality. In the hyperacute phase, the aforementioned MR imaging protocol is ideal. Additional sequences focused on determining stroke

etiology can be added including MRA of the neck to evaluate for dissection, perfusion weighted imaging to evaluate for perfusion defects, and pre- and post-gadolinium vessel wall imaging (VWI) to evaluate for stroke etiologies such as vasculitis, transient cerebral arteriopathy (which may be related to varicella immunocomplex-vasculitis), and moyamoya (▶ Fig. 6.21).

When MR is available, CT is generally avoided in the setting of acute stroke, simply due to concerns regarding cumulative radiation dose in the pediatric population. Furthermore, CT is not as sensitive in the acute phase and provides little information regarding potential stroke etiologies.

Imaging appearance of stroke on CT and MRI by time from onset is summarized in ▶ Table 6.2. The basic factors that should be reported by the neuroradiologists include infarct location, presumed etiology, type (large vessel occlusion – perforator – embolic – hemodynamic – hypoxic – venous) distribution, size, and age. The presence of a substantial perfusion-diffusion or diffusion-FLAIR mismatch should be reported as it could prompt intervention such as intra-arterial therapy or IV-tPA. Likewise, it is important to identify the presence of a large vessel occlusion, which can be easily identified on MRA.

Because stroke recurrence rates are so highly dependent on the stroke etiology, the most important job for neuroradiologists is to attempt to determine the etiology. Venous thrombosis is a common cause of childhood ischemic stroke and was described in a previous chapter. Arteriopathic causes including dissection, focal cerebral arteriopathy, moyamoya disease, sickle cell, vasculitis (▶ Fig. 6.21), and fibromuscular dysplasia should be evaluated. In evaluating the intracranial and extracranial circulation, synthesizing VWI, TOF MRA, and MRI findings may be necessary to come up with an accurate diagnosis. MRA, VWI, and MRI imaging findings for arteriopathic causes of childhood stroke are summarized in ▶ Table 6.3.

Lastly, one must consider hereditary causes of stroke in infancy and childhood, particularly mitochondrial diseases such as Mitochondrial encephalomyopathy, lactic acidosis, and stroke-like episodes (MELAS) and *POLG1* mutations (▶ Fig. 6.22). In general, infarcts related to these processes are multifocal and predominantly involve the parieto-occipital and parieto-temporal regions, and in case of MELAS have a predominance for the cortex of metabolically active regions (▶ Fig. 6.22).

6.6.5 What the Clinician Needs to Know

- The location, size, type, etiology, and distribution of infarct
- The presence of perfusion-diffusion mismatch for FLAIR-DWI mismatch
- The presence of large vessel occlusion
- The age of infarct and signs of old infarct
- The status of intracranial and cervical vessels, which may shed light on stroke etiology
- Hemorrhagic conversion or risk thereof (increased permeability or loss of blood brain barrier in the early phase of ischemia)

Table 6.2 Imaging Findings of Stroke on CT and MRI

	Early Hyperacute	Acute	Subacute	Chronic
CT	Loss of GW differentiation and hypoattenuation of deep nuclei or cortex	Marked hypoattenuation, gyral swelling with or without mass effect	Decreased swelling, petechial hemorrhage, CT fogging	Encephalomalacia
MRI				
DWI	Restricted diffusion	Restricted diffusion	T2 shine through	T2 shine through
T1	Normal	Low signal	Low signal in infarct, cortical high T1 signal for petechial hemorrhage	Low signal
T2/FLAIR	Loss of normal flow voids	High signal	High signal	High signal or encephalomalacia
Post-Contrast	Intravascular enhancement at occlusion location	No enhancement	Enhancement of infarcted parenchyma	Enhancement up to 12 weeks

Table 6.3 VWI Findings

	MRA Appearance	VWI Appearance	MRI Brain Appearance
Dissection	Focal narrowing with or without post-stenotic dilatation. Occasional double lumen sign.	Intrinsic T1 hyperintensity in vessel wall	Infarcts in vascular territory of dissection
Focal/Transient Cerebral Arteriopathy	Unilateral stenosis at carotid T or proximal M1, non-progressive, may reverse	Robust circumferential enhancement	Basal ganglia infarct
Primary CNS Vasculitis	Multifocal bilateral stenoses of proximal and distal vessels	Multifocal regions of circumferential enhancement	Multifocal cerebral infarcts
Moyamoya	Unilateral or bilateral carotid T occlusion/stenosis; prominent lenticulostriate collaterals	Negative vessel wall remodeling, minimal to no vessel wall enhancement	Watershed distribution infarcts, Ivy sign, absent M1 flow voids
Fibromuscular Dysplasia/Connective Tissue Disease	String of beads, multifocal dissections	Nothing specific, unless dissection	Infarcts in vascular territory of dissection
Varicella Vasculopathy	Vascular narrowing in one (often M1) arterial distribution	Circumferential wall enhancement	Infarcts in vascular territory of disease process

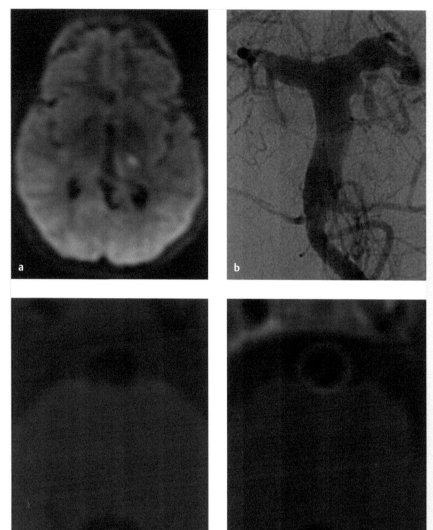

Fig. 6.22 Patient presented with sudden onset right arm tingling and weakness and subsequently developed right face and neck tingling and right arm weakness. Following an extensive infectious disease work-up including serology, sputum samples, and a lumbar puncture, the CSF polymerase chain reaction (PCR) for Varicella Zoster Virus (VZV) was positive. (**a**) MRI demonstrates a punctate thalamoperforator infarct in the left thalamus. (**b**) Conventional angiogram shows fusiform dilatation of the basilar artery and bilateral PCAs consistent with a vasculopathy. (**c**) and (**d**). Pre- and Post-gadolinium MRI showed concentric enhancement of the basilar artery consistent with an inflammatory/infectious vasculitis.

6.6.6 High-yield Facts

- Stroke etiology in perinatal period is rarely arteriopathic; usually related to birth trauma, cardiac disease, or metabolic derangement.
- Most common cause of stroke in childhood are vascular diseases (50%) followed by cardiac causes.
- Because stroke recurrence is high if etiology is vascular, it is important to perform comprehensive vascular imaging with TOF MRA and VWI.
- Transient cerebral arteriopathy is a well-described unilateral inflammatory arteriopathy involving the carotid terminus and is often characterized by basal ganglia infarction.

Further Reading

[1] Lee S, Mirsky DM, Beslow LA, et al. International Paediatric Stroke Study Neuroimaging Consortium and the Paediatric Stroke Neuroimaging Consortium. Pathways for Neuroimaging of Neonatal Stroke. Pediatr Neurol. 2017; 69:37–48

[2] Mirsky DM, Beslow LA, Amlie-Lefond C, et al. International Paediatric Stroke Study Neuroimaging Consortium and the Paediatric Stroke Neuroimaging Consortium. Pathways for Neuroimaging of Childhood Stroke. Pediatr Neurol. 2017; 69:11–23

[3] Moharir M, Deveber G. Pediatric arterial ischemic stroke. Continuum (Minneap Minn). 2014; 20 2 Cerebrovascular Disease:370–386

6.7 Pediatric Spinal Vascular Malformation

6.7.1 Clinical Case

A 6-year-old boy with progressive lower extremity weakness.

6.7.2 Description of Imaging Findings and Diagnosis

Diagnosis

Spinal arterial metameric syndrome (SAMS) with a spinal vascular malformation involving the vertebral body, epidural space, dura, cord, and paraspinal tissues of the mid thoracic spine.

6.7.3 Background

Spinal vascular malformations have an estimated incidence of one in 1 million patients with an even lower incidence in the pediatric population. It is thought that many spinal vascular malformations in the pediatric population are congenital and the result of a genetic defect such as HHT, *RASA1* mutation, or SAMS. Among patients < 2 years old with spinal vascular malformations, over 60% are estimated to have HHT or (SAMS). Among patients 2–18, approximately 25% have HHT or SAMS.

There are a variety of classification systems used in characterization of spinal vascular malformations. Spinal vascular malformations are classified as follows in this text: (1) dural AVFs, (2) glomus or nidus-type arteriovenous malformations (AVM) (including those of the conus), (3) juvenile or metameric AVM, (4) perimedullary AVF, (5) epidural AVF, (6) filum terminale AVFs, and (7) paraspinal AVFs. Dural and epidural AVFs are exceedingly rare in the pediatric population.

Spinal vascular malformations can result in symptoms either from chronic venous congestion, vascular steal, subarchnoid hemorrhage, or hematomyelia from rupture of arterial or venous aneurysms. Among patients < 2 years of age, myelopathic symptoms are the most common presentation (60%) followed by hemorrhage (25%). In the remainder of the pediatric population, myelopathic symptoms and hemorrhage are found in 90 and 70% of patients, respectively. To date, every spinal vascular malformation reported to be associated with HHT has been a perimedullary AVF.

6.7.4 Imaging Findings

Spinal vascular malformations are generally categorized by a combination of the location of the arteriovenous shunt, the nature of its feeding artery, as well as the angioarchitecture of the shunt itself (i.e., nidus-type vs. direct fistula). Glomus or nidus-type AVMs are characterized by an intramedullary nidus. Juvenile or metameric AVMs are also known as SAMS or Cobb's syndrome and are vascular malformations which involve an entire metamere, often involving bone, dural, cord, and the overlying skin (▶ Fig. 6.23). Perimedullary AVFs represent a direct arteriovenous fistula between an anterior or posterior spinal artery and a spinal vein without an intervening nidus. Paraspinal AVFs are direct arteriovenous shunts in the paraspinal tissues.

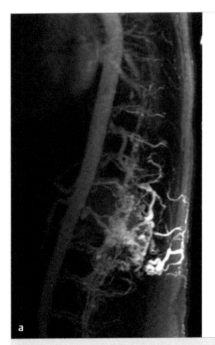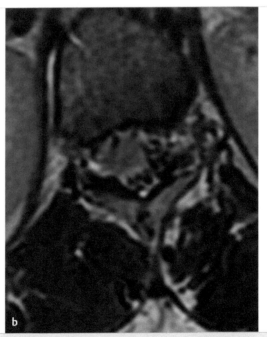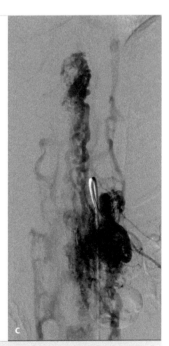

Fig. 6.23 A 6-year-old boy with progressive lower extremity weakness. (**a**) Sagittal maximum intensity projection of a gadolinium bolus MRA demonstrates a vascular malformation involving the osseous, epidural, cord, and paraspinal soft tissues from T7-T9. (**b**) Axial T2-weighted MRI demonstrates innumerable vascular flow voids in the thecal sac as well as in the paraspinal soft tissues consistent with a spinal vascular malformation. In addition there is elevated signal in the cord consistent with myelopathy. (**c**) Conventional spinal angiogram shows a large spinal vascular malformation involving both intradural and extradural tissues from T7-T9. Spinal vascular malformations which involve osteo-epidural, spinal and paraspinal tissues are characteristic of SAMS or Cobb's syndrome.

Most spinal vascular malformations can be identified on conventional MRI by the presence of prominent and tortuous vascular T2 flow voids within the thecal sac, which enhance with contrast. Useful T2 sequences to evaluate flow voids include standard Constructive Interference Steady State (CISS)/ FIESTA and single slab 3D TSE sequence with slab selective, variable excitation pulse (SPACE) sequences. In cases of paraspinal, osteo-epidural, or metameric/SAMS-type vascular malformations, flow voids will also be identified in the paraspinal tissues and the bone (▶ Fig. 6.24). It is important to identify how the vascular malformation is affecting the spinal cord as well. Dilated veins and large venous varices can cause compressive myelopathy. There is almost always some degree of local T2 hyperintensity related to venous congestion. When severe, local myelomalacia can be present. In cases of severe venous congestion, T2 hyperintensity can extend far below the lesion to the level of the conus. Venous congestion of the cauda equina nerve roots can be identified by nerve root thickening and enhancement. As already mentioned, a sizeable proportion of spinal vascular malformations are associated with hemorrhage (▶ Fig. 6.25). Spinal SAH can be identified as linear high-signal intensity on T1/T2 within the thecal sac. Sometimes, hemorrhage can be seen layering in the dependent most portions of the thecal sac. Local hemorrhage can result in hemosiderin staining of the cord.

While digital subtraction angiography (DSA) is certainly the gold standard in characterization of spinal vascular malformations, gadolinium bolus spine MRA is extremely useful. Spinal MRA can aid the angiographer by providing information regarding the potential location of the arterial feeders so that a more focused exam can be performed, limiting contrast, and radiation dose. In addition, spinal MRA can be very helpful in characterizing the angioarchitecture of the lesion and thus classifying the spinal vascular malformation. Identification of large venous varices or angiographic weak points such as spinal arterial aneurysms is important, particularly in lesions which have bled.

6.7.5 What the Clinician Needs to Know

- Extent and location of cord edema from venous congestion
- The presence, location, and extent of hematomyelia and spinal SAH
- Angioarchitecture and location (perimedullary vs. intramedullary) of the spinal vascular malformation and lesion classification
- Any imaging findings supporting a diagnosis of SAMS, HHT, or *RASA1*
- The presence of compressive myelopathy from vascular structures

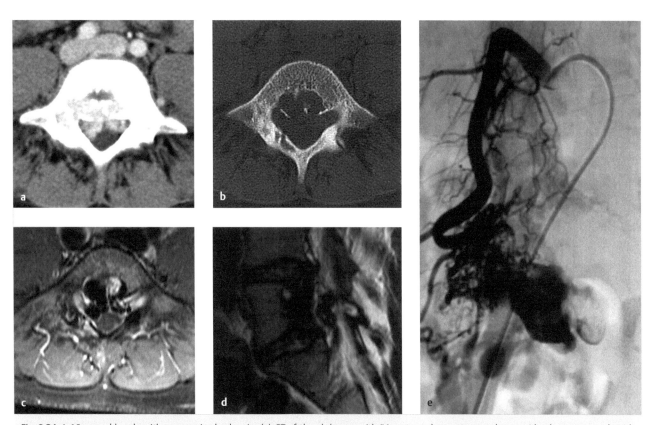

Fig. 6.24 A 16-year-old male with progressive back pain. (a) CT of the abdomen with IV contrast demonstrates a large epidural venous pouch with mild mass effect on the thecal sac. (b) Bone window CT images show scalloping of the posterior margin of the vertebral body with a thin sclerotic rim. (c) Axial T1 post-contrast MRI of the spine shows large vascular flow voids scalloping the posterior margin of the vertebral artery. (d) These are also present on the sagittal T2-weighted MRI. (e) Selective spinal angiography shows a large feeding artery supplying the osteo-epidural shunt with a large epidural venous pouch. There was no intradural venous drainage.

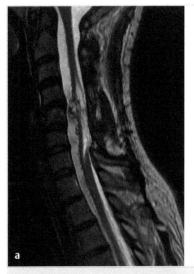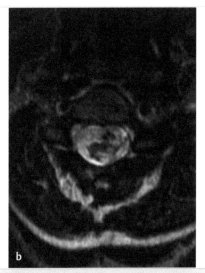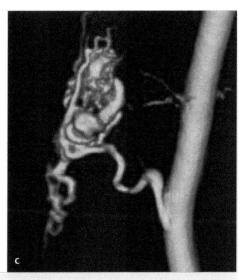

Fig. 6.25 A 14-year-old male with a nidus-type spinal vascular malformation who presented with bilateral upper and lower extremity sensory changes and severe weakness. (**a**) and (**b**) Sagittal and axial T2-weighted images show myelomalacia from C3-C7 from prior hemorrhage of a cervical nidus-type arteriovenous malformation. Multiple flow voids are seen in the cord itself as well as along the cord surface. There is no associated cord edema. This is a typical imaging finding for a cervical spinal arteriovenous malformation. (**c**) 3D reconstruction of a catheter angiogram demonstrates the arteriovenous malformation with a large intranidal aneurysm, the cause of the hematomyelia.

- The presence of angiographic weak points such as aneurysms.
- Level at which the arterial feeder arises on spinal MRA

- Spinal MRA is useful in assessing lesion angioarchitecture and in guiding subsequent conventional angiography.

6.7.6 High-yield Facts

- Spinal vascular malformations in children are much more likely to present with hematomyelia/hemorrhage than those in adults.
- Most spinal vascular malformations in children are intradural.
- Among children < 2 years old, the majority of patients have HHT or SAMS.

Further Reading

[1] Davagnanam I, Toma AK, Brew S. Spinal arteriovenous shunts in children. Neuroimaging Clin N Am. 2013; 23(4):749–756

[2] Cullen S, Krings T, Ozanne A, Alvarez H, Rodesch G, Lasjaunias P. Diagnosis and endovascular treatment of pediatric spinal arteriovenous shunts. Neuroimaging Clin N Am. 2007; 17(2):207–221

Chapter 7

Venous Occlusive Diseases

7

7 Venous Occlusive Diseases

7.1 Deep Venous Thrombosis

7.1.1 Clinical Case

A 45-year-old female, loss of consciousness (▶ Fig. 7.1).

7.1.2 Description of Imaging Findings and Diagnosis

Diagnosis

Restricted diffusion in the bilateral thalami and basal ganglia with extensive venous sinus thrombosis affecting superior sagittal sinus and the deep venous system.

7.1.3 Background

Deep cerebral venous thrombosis is a subset of cerebral vein thrombosis with similar risk factors and epidemiology. Presentation is often substantially more severe than superficial venous thrombosis and includes nausea, vomiting, headache, focal neurological deficit, loss of consciousness, neuropsychiatric symptoms, or seizures. Treatment is generally systemic anticoagulation, even in the presence of hemorrhage. Compared to dural venous sinus thrombosis (DSVT), deep cerebral vein thrombosis carries a much poorer prognosis.

7.1.4 Imaging Findings

Diagnosis of deep cerebral vein thrombosis is difficult because of the unspecific presentation and the wide variety of differential diagnoses. Typical imaging findings on non-contrast CT include edema of deep structures including the bilateral thalami and basal ganglia with or without hemorrhage and hyperdense clot in the internal cerebral veins and straight sinus (▶ Fig. 7.2). Occasionally, the parasagittal cortex can be involved. Unilateral venous thrombosis is rare, but not unheard of. On MRI, T2-weighted images demonstrate hyperintense swelling of the deep gray structures with possible high T1 signal or hemosiderin deposition indicating hemorrhage. Clot can be identified as linear hyperintense material filling the veins. Acute clot is T2 hypointense and can mimic vascular flow voids. SWI or GRE imaging can be very helpful in confirming the presence of thrombus by identifying blooming artifact. Diffusion weighted imaging (DWI) confirms the presence of predominantly vasogenic edema in the affected regions. Vascular imaging is useful in confirming the diagnosis. MR and CT venography will demonstrate the lack of

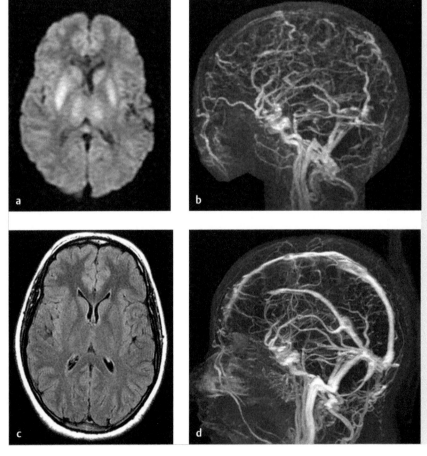

Fig. 7.1 Deep cerebral venous thrombosis. (**a**) Axial DWI MRI shows restricted diffusion in the bilateral thalami and basal ganglia. This was confirmed on apparent diffusion coefficient (ADC) as well (not shown). (**b**) Gadolinium bolus MRV shows no contrast filling of the superior sagittal sinus and deep cerebral venous system. Six months post-anticoagulation, follow-up FLAIR (fluid attenuation inversion recovery) MRI (**c**) shows resolution of the T2 signal in the deep structures and (**d**) MRV shows recanalization of the entirety of the cerebral venous system.

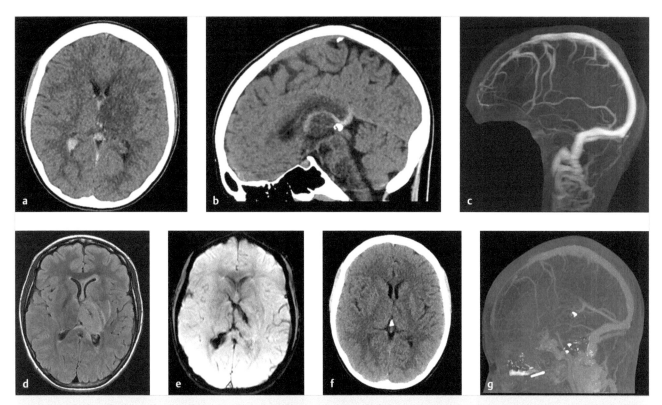

Fig. 7.2 Internal cerebral vein thrombosis resulting in unilateral venous ischemia and intraventricular hemorrhage. (**a**) Non-contrast head CT demonstrates hyperdense deep venous system as well as blood products in the lateral ventricles. (**b**) Sagittal non-contrast CT showing hyperdense internal cerebral vein and vein of galen and unilateral thalamic edema. (**c**) Gadolinium bolus MRV shows absent filling of the deep venous system. (**d**) Axial FLAIR MRI shows unilateral thalamic edema. (**e**) Axial SWI MRI shows hypointense blooming artifact of a thalamostriate vein and the deep venous system as well as blood products in the right lateral ventricle. (**f**) Axial non-contrast CT scan 4 months later demonstrates near complete reversal of the thalamic hypodensity and (**g**) sagittal gadolinium bolus MRV shows recanalization of the deep venous system.

flow in the deep cerebral veins. It is important for neuroradiologists to comment on extension of thrombus into the dural venous sinuses as well.

The preferred treatment of deep venous thrombosis is anticoagulation therapy. Follow-up imaging is essential in these patients to document resolution of the thrombus. Oftentimes, there is complete recanalization of the occluded vein after several weeks of therapy. This is often accompanied by resolution of parenchymal injury on T2 and DWI (▶ Fig. 7.1).

Differential considerations are manifold and include artery of Percheron infarct (which should demonstrate cytotoxic rather than vasogenic edema on DWI and be confined to the thalamotuberal regions) and bithalamic glioma. In the setting of an artery of Percheron infarct, multiple small patchy infarcts are seen in both thalami rather than the contiguous T2 signal and edema seen in a deep venous thrombosis (▶ Fig. 7.3). Bithalamic gliomas are exceedingly rare. It is important to point out that occasionally, deep cerebral venous thrombosis affects only one hemisphere. Other differential considerations include infectious diseases such as West-Nile Virus encephalitis, CJD,

or Japanese Virus Encephalitis; or toxic-metabolic disorders (including acute Wilson Crisis, Carbon Monoxide Poisoning, Leigh Syndrome, etc.) (▶ Fig. 7.3). Clinical history as well as meticulous imaging interpretation are important to make the diagnosis.

7.1.5 What the Clinician Needs to Know

- Extent and location of thrombus including involvement of the superficial venous system
- The presence of edema in deep gray matter structures and reversibility on follow-up imaging
- Hemorrhage
- A broad range of differential diagnoses

7.1.6 High-yield Facts

- Deep cerebral vein thrombosis classically presents with diffuse bithalamic swelling but a unilateral presentation is not unheard of.

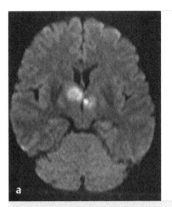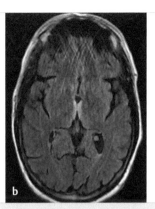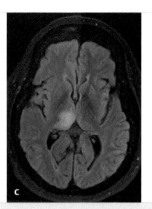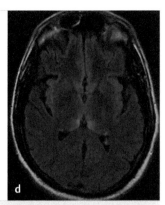

Fig. 7.3 Deep venous thrombosis mimics. (**a**) Artery of Percheron infarct with patchy areas of restricted diffusion in the bilateral thalami. (**b**) Wernickes encephalopathy with T2 hyperintensity in the bilateral medial thalami and along the mammillothalamic tracts. (**c**) Thalamic glioma with expansion of the right thalamus. This was distinguished from a unilateral ICV thrombus due to the absence of blooming artifact in the ICV and a normal venogram. (**d**) Patient with West Nile Virus infection with T2 hyperintensity of the bilateral pulvinars.

- Thrombus is hyperdense on CT and T1 hyperintense on MRI. Blooming artifact is present on GRE/SWI.
- CT/MR venography can be confirmatory.
- After several weeks of anticoagulation therapy, revascularization of the occluded vein and reversal of parenchymal imaging findings can occur.

Further Reading

[1] Steven A, Raghavan P, Altmeyer W, Gandhi D. Venous Thrombosis: Causes and Imaging Appearance. Hematol Oncol Clin North Am. 2016; 30(4):867–885

[2] Lin N, Wong AK, Lipinski LJ, Mokin M, Siddiqui AH. Reversible changes in diffusion- and perfusion-based imaging in cerebral venous sinus thrombosis. J Neurointerv Surg. 2016; 8(2):e6

7.2 Cortical Vein and Dural Venous Sinus Thrombosis

7.2.1 Clinical Case

A 55-year-old male with left-sided headache and garbled speech (▶ Fig. 7.4).

7.2.2 Description of Imaging Findings and Diagnosis

Diagnosis

Left temporal lobe edema and hemorrhage secondary to cortical vein thrombosis (CVT).

7.2.3 Background

DSVT is a relatively common cause of infarction and hemorrhage in the young- and middle-aged population. Its prevalence is higher in females. Common risk factors include oral contraceptive use, pregnancy, trauma, coagulation disorders, infection, dehydration, and compressive mass. In about 10% of cases, the cause is unknown. Clinical presentation of DSVT can include headaches, decreased levels of consciousness, altered vision, elevated intracranial pressure, seizures, coma, and death. The pathophysiology of DSVT is related to venous hypertension from poor venous outflow as well as impaired CSF resorption, which can be exacerbated if thrombosis affects the arachnoid granulations as well. Cerebral venous infarction and hemorrhage can occur in up to 50% of cases.

CVT often accompanies DSVT. Isolated CVT is, however, rare. Isolated CVT can present with localized subarachnoid hemorrhage (SAH) with or without parenchymal involvement, edema, or venous infarct.

7.2.4 Imaging Findings

Any of the dural venous sinuses can be affected by DSVT, including the cavernous sinus. In general, findings of DSVT are first identified on non-contrast CT where one can identify hyperdensity of the sinus in the form of a cordlike hyperattenuation with or without underlying cortical edema or peripheral venous hemorrhage (▶ Fig. 7.5). It is important to note that the distal superior sagittal sinus or one of the transverse sinuses may be congenitally absent, thus mimicking dural sinus thrombosis on MRV or CTV. CT venography has a sensitivity of 95% for identifying DSVT with common imaging findings being a filling defect in the sinus, gyral enhancement, and prominent intramedullary veins.

On MRI, conventional spin echo sequences demonstrate loss of the normal flow void of the dural sinuses. In the acute phase,

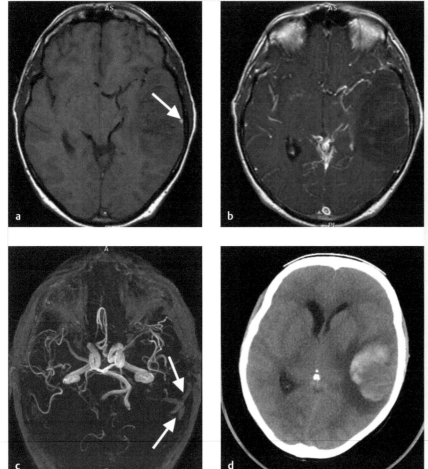

Fig. 7.4 CVT of the vein of Labbe. A 55-year-old male with left-sided headache and garbled speech. Patient was initially misdiagnosed with a GBM based on imaging. (a) Non-contrast T1-weighted MRI demonstrates marked edema in the left temporal lobe. Note the focal T1 hyperintensity in the vein of Labbe on the left (*arrow*). (b) Post-contrast T1-weighted MRI demonstrates faint enhancement of the lesion. (c) 3D TOF MRA shows a linear area of hyperintensity in the left vein of Labbe (*arrows*) consistent with thrombus seen in panel A. (d) Non-contrast CT demonstrates hemorrhage within the area of venous ischemia in the Labbe territory.

clot is isointense on T1 and hypointense on T2. The clot becomes hyperintense on T1 in the subacute phase (▶ Fig. 7.4). SWI or GRE can identify clot by the presence of blooming artifact. Conventional MRI sequences can be very sensitive and specific in identifying DSVT. MRV will demonstrate lack of flow.

Isolated CVT is a commonly missed diagnosis. There is wide variability in the number, size, and location of cortical veins. Each individual hemisphere can have variations in the size and location of Labbe, Trolard, and the superficial middle cerebral vein, not to mention the smaller cortical veins. Non-contrast CT is usually normal, but occasionally an isolated hyperdense cortical vein can be identified. Because the anatomy of the cerebral venous system is inconstant, MRV, and CTV are not usually helpful unless there is extension of the thrombus into a dural sinus. On MRI, SWI or GRE will demonstrate blooming at the site of the thrombosed vein, T1 hyperintensity, and T2/FLAIR

hypointensity. While the T2 and T1 signal changes normalize over time, blooming artifact on T2* weighted imaging can persist for several months. Most common secondary findings include local edema and petechial hemorrhage or hematoma.

In addition to evaluating for direct signs of CVT or DSVT, the radiologist should inspect for secondary signs and sequelae. Identification of cortical infarction in a non-arterial location supports the diagnosis of venous thrombosis. Heterogeneous or gyriform cortical or peripheral hemorrhage along with cortical edema are important to identify (▶ Fig. 7.6). Although the majority of the T2 hypersignal is NOT restricting on DWI (given its vasogenic nature), there may be cortical or gyriforme DWI restriction, which is related to compression of the leptomeningeal perforators due to the compressive vasogenic edema. Follow-up imaging is necessary to document resolution of the thrombus as well as any long-term sequelae, including venous sinus stenosis and development of dural arteriovenous fistulae.

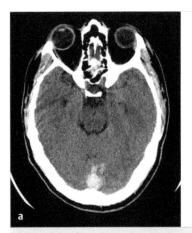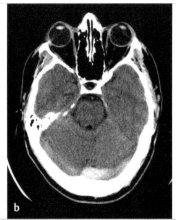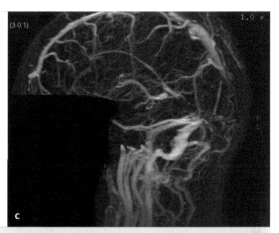

Fig. 7.5 A 26-year-old female recently post-partum with severe headache. (a) and (b). Non-contrast CT demonstrating hyperdense thrombus in the superior sagittal sinus and bilateral transverse sinuses. Attenuation of the thrombus was 85HU. (c) Sagital MIP MRV demonstrating absent filling of the distal superior sagittal sinus and proximal bilateral transverse sinuses.

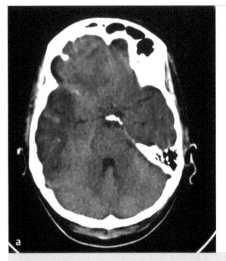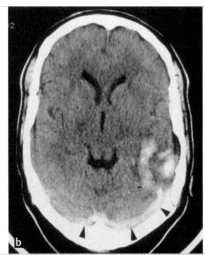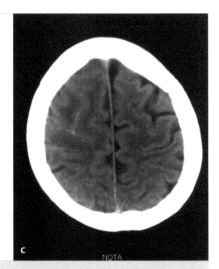

Fig. 7.6 Typical parenchymal imaging findings of DSVT on non-contrast CT. (a) Patient with right transverse sinus thrombosis affecting the vein of Labbe as well has marked edema in the right temporal lobe as well. There is some sulcal hemorrhage. (b) Patient with left transverse sinus thrombosis has hemorrhage and edema in the posterior left temporal lobe. (c) Axial non-contrast CT demonstrating sulcal SAH, which can be seen in patients with isolated CVT or superior sagittal sinus thrombosis.

There are a few pitfalls to diagnosis of DSVT. Hypoplasia or atresia of the transverse sinus is a relatively common normal anatomic variant (▶ Fig. 7.7). In most patients, the right transverse sinus is larger than the left. There are a few complimentary imaging findings, which can help one determine if a sinus is congenitally small. First, one should inspect the ipsilateral jugular foramen. If the ipsilateral jugular foramen is small then the transverse sinus is likely hypoplastic. Another trick is the so-called Gibraltar Sign, named after the Rock of Gibraltar which has a gradual, asymmetric slope. The bony groove for the superior sagittal sinus often slopes to one side (usually the right). The direction which the bony groove slopes is usually the side of the

dominant sinus. Arachnoid granulations are commonly overcalled as thrombus. However, these are usually well-defined focal filling defects within the sinus, are located in the lateral aspects of the transverse sinus, and have CSF signal intensity (▶ Fig. 7.8).

7.2.5 What the Clinician Needs to Know

- Extent and location of thrombus
- The presence of edema, hemorrhage, or infarct related to the thrombus
- The extension of thrombus to deep venous system

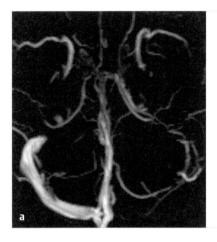
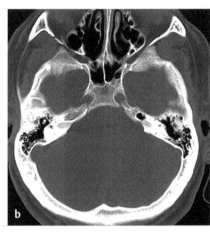

Fig. 7.7 Congenitally hypoplastic sinus. (**a**) MR venogram demonstrates absent filling of the left transverse sinus. The question now is whether the sinus is thrombosed or hypoplastic. (**b**) Non-contrast CT demonstrates a large osseous groove for the sigmoid sinus on the right and a very tiny groove on the left. In addition, the inclination for the groove of the superior sagittal sinus is to the right supporting the idea that the right sinus is the dominant one.

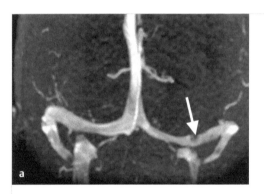
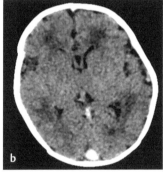

Fig. 7.8 Mimics for DSVT. (**a**) Arachnoid granulation creating the appearance of a filling defect in the left transverse sinus. The circular/rounded appearance is what suggests the present of the arachnoid granulation (*arrow*). (**b**) Young child with a dense superior sagittal sinus and straight sinus. Hematocrit was 60. (**c**) Phase-contrast MRV demonstrates narrowing of the left transverse sinus in a woman with headache. (**d**) Venous phase of a left ICA angiogram shows stenosis of the left transverse sinus. The patient was later diagnosed with pseudotumor cerebri.

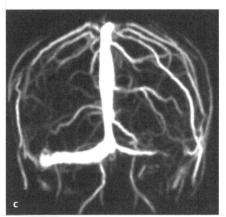
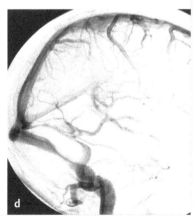

7.2.6 High-yield Facts

- Normal anatomy (i.e., non-dominant transverse sinus or arachnoid granulations) are a common cause of over diagnosis in DSVT.
- MRI with GRE/SWI, T1, and T2/FLAIR-weighted sequences is necessary to diagnose CVT.
- Secondary imaging findings such as local vasogenic edema, non-arterial distribution infarct, and petechial/peripheral

hemorrhage should clue one in on the diagnosis of venous thrombosis.

Further Reading

[1] Boukobza M, Crassard I, Bousser MG, Chabriat H. MR imaging features of isolated cortical vein thrombosis: diagnosis and follow-up. AJNR Am J Neuroradiol. 2009; 30(2):344–348

[2] Bonneville F. Imaging of cerebral venous thrombosis. Diagn Interv Imaging. 2014; 95(12):1145–1150

7.3 Venous Stenosis and Pseudotumor Cerebri

7.3.1 Clinical Case

A 30-year-old obese female with history of headaches with pressure behind her eyes (▶ Fig. 7.9).

7.3.2 Description of Imaging Findings and Diagnosis

Diagnosis

Bilateral transverse sinus stenosis, optic nerve flattening, empty sella, typical imaging findings of pseudotumor cerebri.

7.3.3 Background

Pseudotumor cerebri, also known as idiopathic intracranial hypertension, is a relatively rare, but reversible cause of headache. Common signs and symptoms include headache, pulsatile bruit, visual symptoms, and, in children, posterior fossa signs such as imbalance. The disease is predominantly seen in females (10:1 = F:M) and is 20 times more common in the obese population than in the general population. Approximately, 20–40% of the pseudotumor population develop significant vision loss from papilledema.

An understanding of the pathophysiology of pseudotumor cerebri remains elusive. There are some data to suggest that CSF overproduction in the choroid plexus is the primary cause of the disease. However, others have recently suggested that the elevated ICPs may also be related to impaired resorption of CSF at the level of the arachnoid granulation-venous sinus interface due to either dysfunction of the arachnoid granulation or increased pressure in the cerebral venous system from a venous stenosis resulting in an impaired gradient for the flow of CSF from the granulation to the vein. Others have suggested that the disease is the result of an impairment in glymphatic system clearance of CSF. It is possible that the disease is the result of a combination of factors leading to elevated intracranial pressure.

Diagnostic criteria for pseudotumor are the modified Dandy criteria including symptoms and signs attributable only to elevated ICP, elevated ICP > 25 cm H_2O, normal CSF composition, and no evidence of hydrocephalus, mass, or structural lesion.

7.3.4 Imaging Findings

Regions of interest in the MRI evaluation of pseudotumor cerebri include the orbits, skull base, and transverse sinus. Orbital findings include bilateral dilated optic nerve sheaths, flattening of the optic nerve head, and a DWI bright spot at the optic nerve head. In the skull base, one can identify an empty sella (CSF filling the sella and flattening of the pituitary gland) and possible bony remodeling as well as dilatation of Meckel's cave. These aforementioned findings are only 40–50% sensitive in identifying pseudotumor (▶ Fig. 7.9, ▶ Fig. 7.10).

Evaluation of the transverse sinuses should be performed using both post-contrast T1-weighted sequences and MR venography. On post-contrast T1, total effacement of the transverse sinuses bilaterally can be seen with herniation of the temporo-occipital brain tissue into the space that the transverse sinus occupied. This finding is present in over 80% of pseudotumor

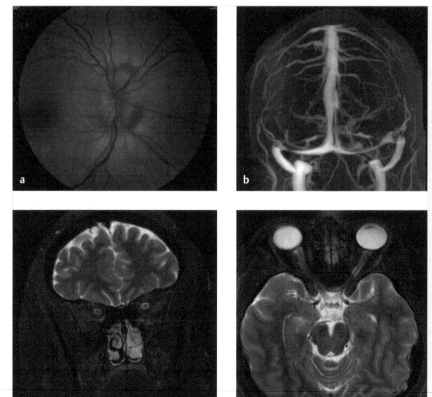

Fig. 7.9 Typical imaging findings in pseudotumor cerebri. (**a**) Fundoscopic exam demonstrates optic disc edema. (**b**) Gadolinium bolus MRV demonstrates bilateral transverse sinus stenoses. (**c**) Coronal T2-weighted MRI with fat saturation demonstrates dilatation of the bilateral optic nerve sheaths. This finding was also present on the axial T2-weighted MRI in (**d**).

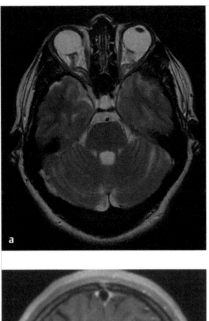
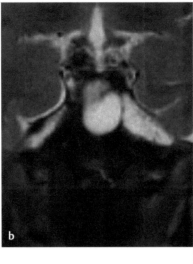
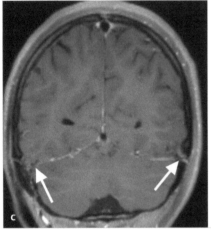
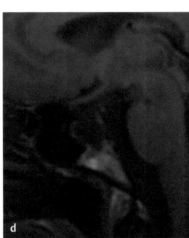

Fig. 7.10 Typical non-angiographic imaging manifestations of pseudotumor cerebri. (a) T2-weighted MRI demonstrates dilatation and kinking of the bilateral optic nerve sheaths. (b) Coronal FIESTA-weighted MRI shows dilatation of both Meckel's caves. (c) Coronal T1 post-gad MRI shows narrowing of the bilateral transverse sinuses secondary to herniation of temporal lobe tissue into the transverse sinus groove (*arrows*). (d) Sagittal T1-weighted MRI shows an empty sella.

patients and in only 7% of controls. Bilateral transverse sinus stenosis, identified on MRV, is present in over 90% of pseudotumor patients and only 3% of controls. These two imaging findings in combination are extremely useful in the imaging diagnosis of pseudotumor (▶ Fig. 7.9, ▶ Fig. 7.10).

In evaluating the venous sinuses, the radiologist must determine whether there is chronic thrombus within the sinus as this can have implications for the prevention of future pathology. Signs of chronic thrombus include blooming artifact on susceptibility weighted imaging, wall thickening on high resolution T2-weighted images, and iso- or hyperintense thrombus on T1-weighted images. It is also important to distinguish a stenotic transverse sinus from a congenitally small sinus. Secondary signs of a congenitally small sinus include a small ipsilateral jugular bulb, small bony groove in the occipital bone in the region of the transverse sinus and angulation of the groove of the superior sagittal sinus toward the opposite transverse sinus.

7.3.5 What the Clinician Needs to Know

- The presence of imaging findings suggesting elevated ICP (i.e., optic disc flattening, empty sella, dilated optic nerve sheaths, dilated Meckel's cave)

- The presence of reversible causes suggest elevated ICP (i.e., transverse sinus stenosis, DSVT)
- The presence of a hypoplastic transverse sinus

7.3.6 High-yield Facts

- Bilateral transverse sinus stenosis is present in over 90% of pseudotumor patients and less than 3% of controls.
- Coronal T1-weighted images at the level of the transverse sinus shows effacement of the bilateral transverse sinuses and herniation of temporo-occipital tissue into the region the transverse sinuses previously occupied.
- Elevated intracranial pressure also presents with optic nerve sheath distention, optic disc flattening, and partially empty sella.

Further Reading

[1] Degnan AJ, Levy LM. Pseudotumor cerebri: brief review of clinical syndrome and imaging findings. AJNR Am J Neuroradiol. 2011; 32(11):1986–1993
[2] Morris PP, Black DF, Port J, Campeau N. Transverse Sinus Stenosis Is the Most Sensitive MR Imaging Correlate of Idiopathic Intracranial Hypertension. AJNR Am J Neuroradiol. 2017; 38(3):471–477

7.4 Cavernous Sinus Thrombosis

7.4.1 Clinical Case

A 74-year-old diabetic male with difficulty seeing out of the left eye.

7.4.2 Description of Imaging Findings and Diagnosis

Diagnosis

Invasive sinusitis with resultant cavernous sinus thrombosis, exophthalmos, and stenosis of the left ICA.

7.4.3 Background

Cavernous sinus thrombosis is the least common type of DSVT affecting approximately 4/1,000,000 per year. The disease is most commonly infectious in nature and more commonly seen in the pediatric and immunosuppressed population than in the adult population. Accounting for less than 1% of all types of DSVT, the most common presenting symptoms are cranial nerve III palsy, chemosis, periorbital swelling, and exophthalmos. Risk factors include sinus, dental or facial infection, sinus compression by a tumor, and procoagulable conditions. It is idiopathic in 25% of cases.

7.4.4 Imaging Findings

Cavernous sinus thrombosis is very difficult to detect and diagnose as there are no reliable imaging findings. Non-contrast CT may demonstrate high-density thrombus but this is present in less than 25% of cases. CTV may show a distended cavernous sinus with a filling defect. On MRI, there will be an absent flow void on T1- and T2-weighted images. Asymmetry of the cavernous sinus including is a common anatomical variation, which makes diagnosis of a unilateral filling defect an unreliable indicator for thrombosis of the cavernous sinus. Signal characteristics of the thrombus are variable and can be T2 iso-hyperintense and T1 iso-hyperintense. Subacute thrombus is hyperintense on all pulse sequences. The thrombus can enhance if chronic or if the thrombosis is related to a thrombophlebitis. However, the presence or absence of contrast enhancement is not a reliable indicator of the disease (▶ Fig. 7.11, ▶ Fig. 7.12). Restricted diffusion of the cavernous sinus is a common finding.

MR venography is helpful in confirming the diagnosis. Typical imaging findings include reduced filling of one side of the cavernous sinus compared to the other. MRV may also demonstrate dilatation or thrombosis of the ipsilateral superior ophthalmic vein. There is often thrombosis of draining and tributary veins of the cavernous sinus. Jugular vein and sigmoid sinus involvement can be seen in up to 30% of patients.

Important secondary and associated findings to comment on include internal carotid artery narrowing and arterial wall enhancement, which can suggest an inflammatory or infectious etiology. This can occasionally result in cerebral infarction or aneurysm formation within the cavernous sinus (▶ Fig. 7.11, ▶ Fig. 7.12). Because cavernous sinus thrombosis is often associated with infection, there can be extension of the infectious process to the pituitary gland with pituitary abscess. Orbital cellulitis with fat stranding in the orbital fat as well as optic neuritis with high T2 signal and diffusion restriction of the optic nerve.

7.4.5 What the Clinician Needs to Know

- The extension of thrombus beyond cavernous sinus into various tributaries of the cavernous sinus
- Any imaging findings suggestive of the etiology of cavernous sinus thrombosis including mass, sinus infection, orbital cellulitis, or other facial infection
- Sequelae of cavernous sinus thrombosis including ICA narrowing or aneurysmal dilatation, cerebral infarct, pituitary abscess, optic neuritis, SOV thrombosis

7.4.6 High-yield Facts

- Cavernous sinus thrombosis can be identified as a distended cavernous sinus with iso/hyperintense thrombus on T1/T2-weighted imaging. Diffusion restriction of the cavernous sinus is present in up to 75% of cases.
- Cavernous sinus thrombosis is often the result of infection involving the face, sinuses or orbits, thus there can be extension of the infectious process to adjacent structures including the ICA, pituitary gland, and skull base.
- Cavernous sinus thrombosis can result in both arterial infarcts and venous infarcts affecting the ICA and the cavernous sinus tributaries, respectively.

Further Reading

[1] Razek AA, Castillo M. Imaging lesions of the cavernous sinus. AJNR Am J Neuroradiol. 2009; 30(3):444–452
[2] Press CA, Lindsay A, Stence NV, Fenton LZ, Bernard TJ, Mirsky DM. Cavernous Sinus Thrombosis in Children: Imaging Characteristics and Clinical Outcomes. Stroke. 2015; 46(9):2657–2660

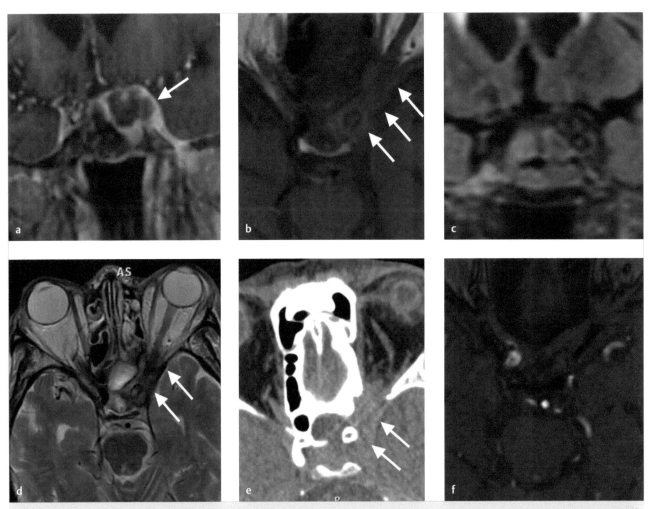

Fig. 7.11 Typical imaging findings of cavernous sinus thrombosis. (**a**) Coronal post-gadolinium T1-weighted MRI shows an expansile filling defect in the left cavernous sinus (*arrow*). (**b**) Axial T1-weighted MRI shows the mildly T1 hyperintense filling defect in the left cavernous sinus consistent with subacute thrombus, which is extending into the orbit through the left superior orbital fissure (*arrows*). This finding is also present on the coronal FLAIR MRI in (**c**). (**d**) Axial T2-weighted MRI shows the thrombotic lesion in the left cavernous sinus which is T2 iso-hypointense (*arrows*). In addition, there is some mild left exophthalmos. (**e**) Non-contrast CT shows increased soft-tissue density in the left cavernous sinus (*arrows*). (**f**) Time of flight MRA demonstrates absence of flow in the left cavernous ICA.

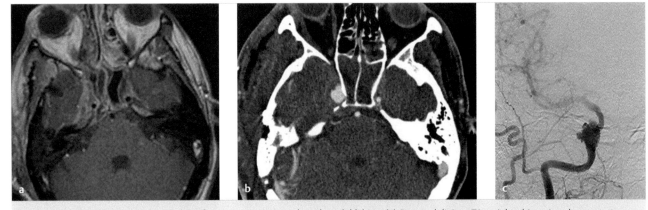

Fig. 7.12 Inflammatory aneurysm resulting from cavernous sinus thrombosis/phlebitis. (**a**) Post-gadolinium T1-weighted imaging demonstrates marked enhancement of the cavernous sinus and the cavernous sinus wall as well as inflammation of the bilateral ethmoid sinuses. Findings are consistent with cavernous sinus phlebitis. (**b**) CTA demonstrates aneurysmal dilatation of the right ICA as well as poor filling of the bilateral cavernous sinuses. (**c**) Right ICA angiogram confirms the presence of an inflammatory aneurysm of the right cavernous ICA, likely the result of the cavernous sinus infection/thrombophlebitis.

7.5 Venous Causes of Pulsatile Tinnitus

7.5.1 Clinical Case

A 48-year-old female with pulsatile tinnitus and a retrotympanic vascular mass.

7.5.2 Description of Imaging Findings and Diagnosis

Diagnosis

Dehiscent jugular bulb with diverticulum.

7.5.3 Background

Tinnitus is a relatively common complaint in the general neurology and ENT clinic. The definition of tinnitus is the conscious perception of sound that arises or seems to arise in the ear of an affected individual in the absence of a genuine physical source of sound. Less than 10% of tinnitus patients suffer from pulsatile tinnitus, which is tinnitus in which the sound is rhythmic and often objective (i.e., can be detected by the clinician). Two plausible sources of pulsatile tinnitus include the acceleration of blood flow and changes in blood flow resulting in disruption of laminar flow or disturbance of sound conduction in the middle ear leading to loss of the masking effect of internal sounds.

Pulsatile, objective tinnitus is usually unilateral. A cause can be identified in about 70% of cases. Arterial causes of pulsatile tinnitus include (1) vascular stenoses from fibromuscular dysplasia, dissection, atherosclerosis, etc.; (2) aneurysms of the petrous ICA; and (3) variations of ICA anatomy including persistent stapedial artery, carotid-cochlear dehiscence, or aberrant ICA. Dural arteriovenous fistulae are a classic cause of pulsatile tinnitus and may be picked up on by the patient when they notice that if they compress the ipsilateral carotid, the tinnitus resolves. Vertebro-vertebral fistulae and carotid-cavernous fistulae are other arteriovenous causes of pulsatile tinnitus. Tympanic and jugular paragangliomas or other hypervascularized tumors are a rare but notable cause of pulsatile tinnitus. Venous pathology, which can cause pulsatile tinnitus, includes intracranial hypertension from venous stenosis, high riding jugular bulb with sigmoid plate dehiscence, transverse-sigmoid or jugular bulb diverticulae, and prominent emissary veins.

7.5.4 Imaging Findings

Imaging evaluation of pulsatile tinnitus often includes an MRA/MRV of the head and neck as well as a high-resolution temporal bone CT. In this chapter, we focus on the venous side to allow the neuroradiologists to develop a solid differential diagnoses for venous causes of pulsatile tinnitus. A high riding jugular bulb without sigmoid plate dehiscence is an important cause of pulsatile tinnitus (▶ Fig. 7.13). The definition of a high riding jugular bulb is an asymmetrically large jugular bulb with its roof higher than the internal auditory canal or basal turn of the cochlea. The normal superior boundary of the jugular bulb is below the floor of the hypotympanon (defined as the line connecting the tympanic annulus and base of the cochlear promontory). This is best diagnosed on MRV or high-resolution temporal bone CT. In the index case, the patient presented with a dehiscent jugular bulb (seen on temporal bone CT) and a jugular bulb diverticulum on MRV. Dehiscent jugular bulbs are present when the jugular plate positioned between the jugular bulb and middle ear is absent. The result of this is bulging of part of the jugular bulb into the middle ear cavity as seen in the otoscopic view. The mechanism of tinnitus is abnormal conduction of the pulsatile venous flow to the inner ear as well as turbulent flow in the jugular bulb and diverticulum. MRI may demonstrate heterogeneous flow in the jugular bulb, which can clue one in on the diagnosis.

Sigmoid sinus wall abnormalities are increasingly recognized as a cause of pulsatile tinnitus. Common sigmoid sinus wall abnormalities include venous diverticulae and sigmoid plate dehiscence. A sigmoid sinus diverticulum is defined as a focal outpouching of the normal semicircular sigmoid sinus groove expanding into the mastoid air cells or temporal bone cortex. These can cause pulsatile tinnitus due to turbulent flow. They are best diagnosed on MRV/CTV and high-resolution temporal bone CT. Sigmoid plate dehiscence is another relatively common

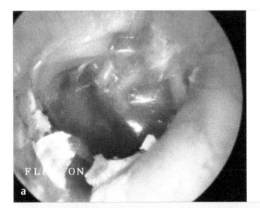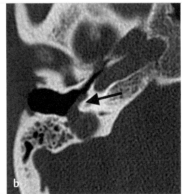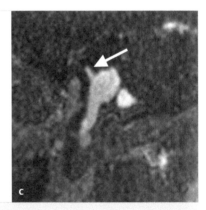

Fig. 7.13 Jugular bulb diverticulum with retrotympanic vascular mass. (a) Otoscopic examination demonstrates a blue retrotympanic mass. (b) Skull base CT with a bone kernel demonstrates a dehiscent sigmoid plate with the anteriorly pointing diverticulum posterior to the tympanic membrane (arrow). (c) Sagittal gadolinium bolus MR venogram demonstrates a high riding jugular bulb with an anteriorly projecting diverticulum (arrow).

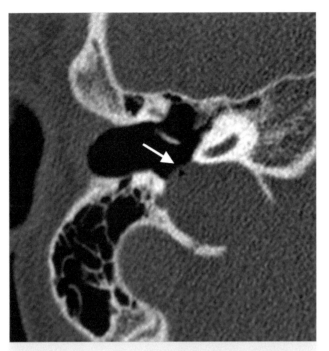

Fig. 7.14 Air on sinus sign. Axial non-contrast CT demonstrates a dehiscent sigmoid plate with air abuting the right sigmoid sinus (*arrow*).

cause of pulsatile tinnitus. This is defined as dehiscence of the sigmoid plate at the site of the mastoid air cells with an "air-on-sinus" sign (▶ Fig. 7.14).

Patients with idiopathic intracranial hypertension also often present with pulsatile tinnitus. These patients can present with transverse sinus stenosis and sigmoid sinus wall abnormalities including dehiscent sigmoid plate and venous diverticulum. Data from case-control studies suggest that these findings are more present in IIH patients than controls; however, there is no consistent relationship between the prevalence of these findings in IIH patients with and without pulsatile tinnitus. Nonetheless, it is important to comment on the presence of these findings, as well as venous sinus stenosis in patients with pulsatile tinnitus, with and without IIH. Venous stenosis is thought to result in pulsatile tinnitus due to the turbulent jet of flow as blood exits the stenotic venous segment during each pulsatile cycle (▶ Fig. 7.15).

Emissary veins are connections between dural venous sinuses and the extracranial venous system. Emissary veins that have been viewed as common culprits in causing pulsatile tinnitus include the posterior condylar emissary vein and the mastoid emissary vein. Mastoid emissary veins course from the mid sigmoid sinus to join the vertebral venous plexus and posterior condylar emissary veins course from the lower end of the sigmoid sinus to the vertebral venous plexus, and traverse through the condylar canal in the occipital condyle (▶ Fig. 7.16).

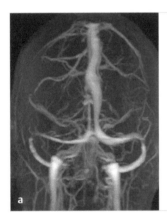
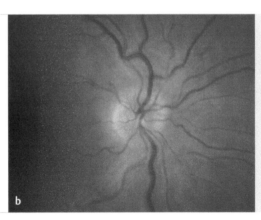

Fig. 7.15 A 54-year-old female with pulsatile tinnitus. (**a**) MRV shows bilateral transverse sinus stenoses. (**b**) Ophthalmoscopic exam shows findings consistent with papilledema.

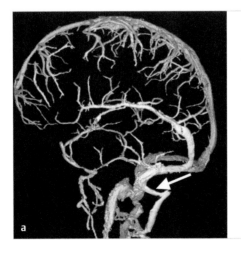
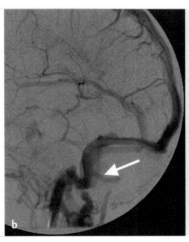

Fig. 7.16 A 43-year-old female with pulsatile tinnitus in the right ear. (**a**) and (**b**). 3DRA and 2D-DSA (digital subtraction angiography) images show emissary veins arising from the right sigmoid sinus, which course along the superficial tissues of the occiput and posterior auricular region (*arrows*). Prominent emissary veins, while often a normal variant of no clinical significance, can occasionally present with pulsatile tinnitus.

7.5.5 What the Clinician Needs to Know

- In setting of vascular retrotympanic mass and pulsatile tinnitus, does the cause appear to be arterial or venous? This is essential to avoid surgical misadventures.
- Relationship of venous structure causing pulsatile tinnitus to middle and inner ear structures.
- The presence of imaging findings suggestive of idiopathic intracranial hypertension (described in section 7.4).

7.5.6 High-yield Facts

- Pulsatile tinnitus is associated with a definite structural cause in up to 70% of patients. Imaging evaluation often includes MRA, MRV, and high-resolution temporal bone CT.

- Common venous causes of pulsatile tinnitus include venous diverticulum, dehiscent jugular bulb/sigmoid plate, high riding jugular bulb, and ipsilateral transverse sinus stenosis.
- Patients with idiopathic intracranial hypertension are more likely to have sigmoid plate dehiscence and venous diverticulae, but their association with pulsatile tinnitus in this population is unclear.

Further Reading

[1] Lansley JA, Tucker W, Eriksen MR, Riordan-Eva P, Connor SEJ. Sigmoid Sinus Diverticulum, Dehiscence, and Venous Sinus Stenosis: Potential Causes of Pulsatile Tinnitus in Patients with Idiopathic Intracranial Hypertension? AJNR Am J Neuroradiol. 2017; 38(9):1783–1788

[2] Reardon MA, Raghavan P. Venous Abnormalities Leading to Tinnitus: Imaging Evaluation. Neuroimaging Clin N Am. 2016; 26(2):237–245

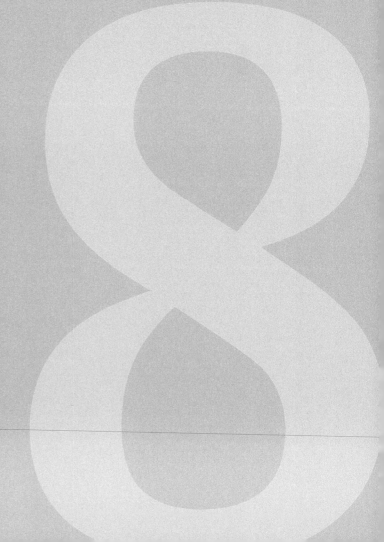

Chapter 8

Angiographically Occult Vascular Lesions

8 Angiographically Occult Vascular Lesions

8.1 Cavernous Malformations

8.1.1 Clinical Case

A 55-year-old female with seizure.

8.1.2 Description of Imaging Findings and Diagnosis

Diagnosis

Cavernous malformation of the mesial left temporal lobe.

8.1.3 Background

Cavernous malformations are relatively common lesions seen in up to 1% of MRI scans. On histology, these lesions are characterized as a mulberry-like mass of dilated and thin-walled capillaries surrounded by hemosiderin. There is no normal brain within a cavernous malformation. Common presenting symptoms include headache, seizures, and focal neurological deficits. Symptoms usually present when these lesions bleed or present with intracavernomatous thrombosis. Natural history studies of cavernous malformations have found that risk factors for hemorrhage include brainstem location, prior hemorrhage, and focal neurological deficit. Age, gender, and number of lesions are not risk factors.

In most cases, cavernous malformations are single and sporadic. However, there is a subset of patients with autosomal dominant familial cavernomatosis who present with multiple lesions. Cavernomas can be associated with developmental venous anomalies in 10–30% of cases depending on the series and have been reported to occur following radiation therapy. The fairly heterogeneous predisposing factors of cavernoma formation point to cavernomas being a veno-occlusive disease with repeated episodes of venular thrombosis causing growth and/or rupture of the cavernoma.

8.1.4 Imaging Findings

Because symptomatic cavernoma patients often present with acute presentations, CT is sometimes the first imaging modality to pick up on these lesions. On non-contrast CT, cavernous malformations are usually characterized by a well-defined region of hyperdensity/hemorrhage with or without calcification. MRI is the imaging test of choice for detection and characterization of CCM.

All imaging protocols for the evaluation or detection of CCMs should use T2* imaging with susceptibility weighted imaging. While gradient echo T2* imaging (GRE) is more sensitive than conventional T2- and T1-weighted sequences, SWI is three times more sensitive than GRE. Higher field strength increases the diagnostic yield of SWI in detecting CCMs, but can be prone to more artifacts. On T1- and T2-weighted images, CCMs often have a heterogeneous signal intensity (mixed hyper and hypointensity) depending on the age of the hemorrhagic products (▶ Fig. 8.1, ▶ Fig. 8.2). This bubbly heterogeneous signal creates a mulberry like appearance on MRI. T1 contrast enhanced MRI is helpful as well, especially in evaluating for the presence or absence of an adjacent developmental venous anomaly. When reporting an MRI in a CCM patient, the radiologist should report on the signal characteristics, size, and location of the lesion, number of lesions, and the presence or absence of a DVA (▶ Fig. 8.2, ▶ Fig. 8.3). Signal characteristics can be characterized using the Zambramski classification (▶ Table 8.1), which helps in aging the hemorrhages within the lesions. One important finding that should be commented on is whether or not the cavernoma reaches the surface of the brain or brainstem or whether there is brain tissue between the cavernoma and the subarachnoid space. This is important for operative planning

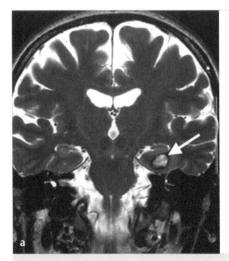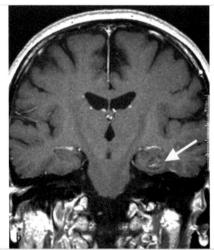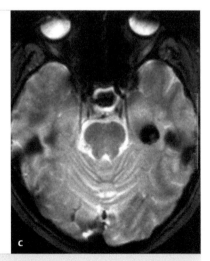

Fig. 8.1 A 55-year-old female with seizure secondary to hippocampal cavernoma. (a) Coronal T2-weighted MRI demonstrates a popcorn-like lesion in the mesial left temporal lobe with intrinsic T2 hyperintensity and a peripheral rim of hemosiderin/T2 hypointensity (*arrow*). (b) Coronal T1 post-contrast MRI shows mild internal enhancement of the lesion (*arrow*). (c) Axial T2*-weighted MRI shows blooming artifact of the lesion from hemosiderin deposition.

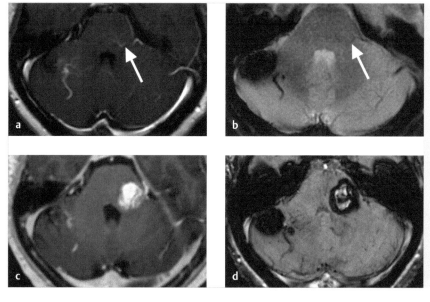

Fig. 8.2 De novo cavernoma inside a DVA in a cancer patient. (**a**) Axial T1 post-contrast MRI demonstrates a developmental venous anomaly of the left pons and right cerebellar hemisphere. Note the kinking/90 degree turn taken by the left pontine DVA (*arrow*). (**b**) T2*-weighted MRI shows a cavernous malformation in a radical of the cerebellar DVA but no cavernous malformation in the pons. The pontine DVA is faintly visualized as well (*arrow*). (**c**) Twelve years later the patient was undergoing neuroimaging for staging of breast carcinoma. A T1 hyperintense and enhancing lesion was noted in the left pons and thought to be consistent with a metastatic lesion. (**d**) SWI demonstrated peripheral hemosiderin deposition and mild internal hemosiderin deposition. The lesion was thought to represent a cavernous malformation which formed in a DVA. The patient had no other metastatic lesions during her metastatic work-up.

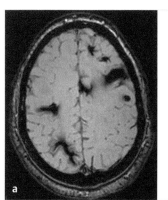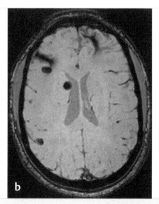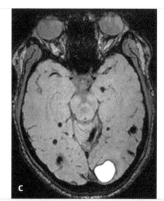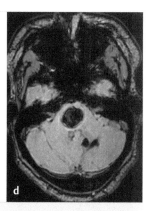

Fig. 8.3 A 17-year-old patient with familial cavernomatosis. (**a–d**). Multiple T2* susceptibility-weighted images demonstrate innumerable foci of T2*blooming consistent with cavernous malformations located throughout both cerebral hemispheres and the posterior fossa.

Table 8.1 Zambramski Classification

Type	T1	T2	T2*	Other
I. Subacute Hemorrhage	Hyperintense	Mixed Signal	May Bloom	
II. Most common type, popcorn lesion.	Mixed signal centrally	Mixed Signal centrally	Low signal rim with blooming	Popcorn appearance
III. Chronic hemorrhage	Hypointense centrally	Hypointense centrally	Low signal rim with blooming	
IV. Multiple punctate hemorrhages	Not seen	Not seen	Multiple black dots with blooming	May be difficult to distinguish from other causes of multiple microhemorrhage

purposes as lesions which reach the surface of the brain are slightly safer to resect due to the lack of any need to dissect through normal neural tissues to reach the lesion.

There is growing interest in using advanced imaging techniques to study the venous angioarchitecture surrounding CCMs. Studies using SWI at 7 T have found abnormal venous structures typical of developmental venous anomalies in over 90% of sporadic CCMs suggesting that most of these lesions are related to local perturbations in venular drainage. Other studies using high-resolution CTA/CTV have found that DVAs with stenoses or kinks are more likely to harbor CCMs than those without such narrowings (▶ Fig. 8.2). Interestingly, the association between DVAs and CCMs is not present in the familial version of these lesions where a mutation in the *KRIT* gene points towards a venous endothelial defect as the root cause for cavernoma formation.

There has also been emerging interest in the use of tractography and quantitative susceptibility mapping in evaluating these lesions. Because many of the most worrisome CCMs are located in the brainstem, DTI can help in operative planning and determining optimal surgical approach for brainstem entry zones. The relationship between the CCM and major fiber tracts such as the corticospinal tract and medial lemniscus/medial longitudinal fasciculus is particularly important to comment on for operative planning. For supratentorial lesions, the relationship between the CCM and corticospinal tracts is important to comment on. An important caveat is that susceptibility effects with signal loss surrounding the cavernoma may underestimate the spatial proximity between the lesion and the studied fiber tracts.

There are some new quantitative imaging techniques on the horizon, which may prove useful in the evaluation of CCMs. Quantitative susceptibility mapping is a SWI-based technique which allows for the quantification of iron concentration. CCMs which have bled are associated with higher iron concentration than stable lesions. This is useful in determining, which lesions have bled in the past. Quantitative perfusion techniques such as dynamic contrast-enhanced quantitative perfusion has been shown to be an effective tool in studying brain vascular permeability. Studies have shown that CCMs with higher permeability indices may have a more aggressive clinical course.

8.1.5 What the Clinician Needs to Know

- Size, signal characteristics, location, and multiplicity of CCMs
- Relationship of the CCM to adjacent DVAs

- The evidence of prior or recent thrombosis within or bleeding outside of the CCM
- The relationship of the CCM with white matter tracts in the brainstem for operative planning purposes

8.1.6 High-yield Facts

- Sporadic CCMs are more commonly associated with DVAs than those in patients with familial cavernomatosis.
- SWI is the most sensitive imaging modality for detecting CCMs and their associated DVAs.
- Quantitative imaging suggests that bleeding CCMs have higher iron concentration and increased vascular permeability.

Further Reading

[1] Akers A, Al-Shahi Salman R, A Awad I, et al. Synopsis of Guidelines for the Clinical Management of Cerebral Cavernous Malformations: Consensus Recommendations Based on Systematic Literature Review by the Angioma Alliance Scientific Advisory Board Clinical Experts Panel. Neurosurgery. 2017; 80(5):665–680

[2] Dammann P, Wrede KH, Maderwald S, et al. The venous angioarchitecture of sporadic cerebral cavernous malformations: a susceptibility weighted imaging study at 7 T MRI. J Neurol Neurosurg Psychiatry. 2013; 84(2):194–200

[3] Mokin M, Agazzi S, Dawson L, Primiani CT. Neuroimaging of Cavernous Malformations. Curr Pain Headache Rep. 2017; 21(12):47

[4] Klostranec JM, Krings T. Neuroimaging of cerebral cavernous malformations. J Neurosurg Sci. 2015; 59(3):221–235

[5] Su IC, Krishnan P, Rawal S, Krings T. Magnetic resonance evolution of de novo formation of a cavernoma in a thrombosed developmental venous anomaly: a case report. Neurosurgery. 2013; 73(4):E739–E744, discussion E745

8.2 Symptomatic Developmental Venous Anomaly

8.2.1 Clinical Case

A 50-year-old male with subacute onset right arm chorea.

8.2.2 Description of Imaging Findings and Diagnosis

Diagnosis

Symptomatic left lentiform nucleus and caudate nucleus DVA with venous congestion and chronic hemorrhage.

8.2.3 Background

Developmental venous anomalies are the most commonly detected vascular malformations on cross-sectional imaging. The estimated prevalence of these lesions is 10% in modern series using contrast enhanced MRI. DVAs must be considered as nonpathological variations of venous drainage patterns and thus represent "don't touch" lesions. DVAs are categorized as deep or superficial by the territory of brain which they drain. Deep DVAs drain normal subcortical areas of the superficial medullary veins into the deep venous collectors while superficial DVAs drain deeper medullary regions into the cortical veins. Essentially, what one is seeing when they see a DVA on imaging is larger than normal medullary veins which represent a fusion of multiple individual smaller medullary veins into a dilated venous collector whose normal bilateral outflow (into the deep and superficial system) has been "plugged" on one end.

What causes the DVA to form remains a mystery. One theory is that early, in utero, venular occlusion causes the DVA to form as an early adaptation to a thrombosed medullary veins. Another theory is that there is regression or normal medullary veins, which causes the DVA to form as an early adaptation to the regressed medullary veins. There has been some doubt cast on the in utero theory in recent years by studies, which show that the prevalence of DVAs increases in early childhood years, the time during which venous development is still taking place.

Theories aside, despite their overwhelmingly benign nature, DVAs can occasionally present with symptoms. DVAs undergo the same age-related changes as the normal venous system and over time can thrombose and stenose causing upstream venous congestion and associated venous infarct and hemorrhage. As mentioned in section 8.1, some studies now suggest that over 90% of all sporadic CCMs are associated with DVAs. Arteriovenous shunting within DVAs has also been reported but is exceedingly rare.

8.2.4 Imaging Findings

DVAs are characterized as a cluster of small venous radicles that converge to a larger collecting vein forming a caput medusa or palm tree appearance. The collector vein then proceeds to drain into the superficial or deep venous system. The most common locations for DVAs are the frontoparietal region and the cerebellar hemispheres; however, they can be located anywhere in the cerebrum, cerebellum, or brainstem. About 10% of DVA patients have multiple lesions.

On non-contrast CT, the collecting vein of the DVA may be mildly hyperdense or isodense to the cortex or markedly hyperdense if thrombosed. CT venography with thin sections can be useful in identifying the classic palm tree appearance. MRI is by far the best imaging modality for identifying and characterizing these lesions. Non-contrast T2-weighted and T1-weighted MRI may demonstrate flow voids produced by the DVA collecting vein and larger venous radicles. These will regularly enhance on post-contrast T1-weighted image. Post-contrast 3D T1-weighted sequences are useful for assessing the venous angioarchitecture of these lesions, particularly in identifying venous stenoses. The lesions are also well seen on SWI where one can see susceptibility artifact in the shape of a caput medusa or palm tree.

Perfusion imaging of DVAs has been gaining interest. Bolus perfusion-weighted imaging is the most useful imaging modality for assessing perfusion abnormalities in the region of a DVA. ASL is less sensitive. One recent study found that over 90% of DVAs have some perfusion abnormality in the draining territory including increased CBF, CBV, MTT, and T_{max} with a higher rate of perfusion abnormalities in larger DVAs. There is evidence to suggest that symptomatic DVAs are associated with higher rates of perfusion abnormalities.

While most DVAs are asymptomatic and in many cases, radiologists consciously forgo the mention of their presence in order to reduce patient and provider anxiety, there are instances in which these lesions may be clinically significant and symptomatic. Because the DVA is draining normal brain, any impairment in venous drainage from the DVA will result in venous hypertension and impaired brain perfusion. Impairment in venous drainage can result from thrombosis or stenosis of the venous collector. Venous stenoses are common in superficial DVAs where the collector vein pierces the dura to drain into the venous sinus. Thromboses can result from hypercoagulable states. Stenoses of larger DVAs can be best identified on MR venography or 3D-T1CE-weighted sequences while thrombosis can be best seen on SWI (blooming) and T1-weighted images (hyperintense clot). Venous congestion in the venous territory of the DVA can be identified as a wedge-shaped region of hyperintensity on T2/FLAIR (fluid attenuation inversion recovery) weighted images without contrast enhancement, diffusion restriction, or mass effect (▶ Fig. 8.4, ▶ Fig. 8.5). Calcifications can also be seen and typically occur in the cerebellar white matter, basal ganglia, and caudate nucleus and result from old hemorrhages or longstanding cerebral ischemia and venous hypertension. In the worst-case scenario, DVA thrombosis can result in acute venous hemorrhage. Chronic low-grade congestion can result in gliosis of the draining territory (▶ Fig. 8.6).

About 10% of DVAs are associated with a cavernoma in one of the venous radicles of the DVA (▶ Fig. 8.7). In general, it is thought that DVA-associated cavernomas are the result of recurrent microhemorrhages. The trigger for microhemorrhages is generally thought to be local venous hypertension resulting from local thrombosis, stenosis, or changes in DVA angioarchitecture. Cavernoma-associated DVAs demonstrate longer mean transit times in the draining territory of the DVA than DVAs not associated with cavernomas. Severe medullary venous tortuosity, medullary venous stenosis, or sharp angles between the radicular vein and the dominant medullary venous drainage are

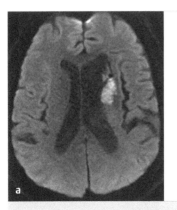 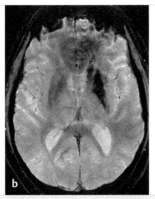 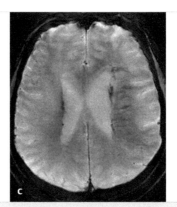 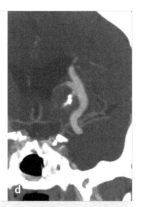

Fig. 8.4 A 50-year-old male with subacute onset right arm chorea. (**a**) Axial DWI MRI demonstrates restricted diffusion in the left caudate. (**b**) Axial T2*-weighted MRI shows susceptibility artifact in the lentiform nucleus and caudate. (**c**) Axial T2*-weighted MRI at the level of the lateral ventricles demonstrates linear T2* blooming artifact in the left hemispheric deep white matter. The T2* blooming artifact in (**b**) and (**c**) are thought to be secondary to a combination of venous congestion, hemorrhage, and calcification. (**d**) CT angiogram demonstrates a large DVA draining the left caudate and lentiform nucleus. The mechanism of stroke in this patient was likely due to thrombosis of DVA radicles draining the caudate and deep cerebral white matter.

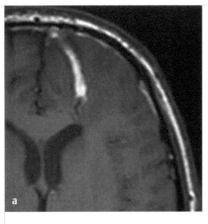 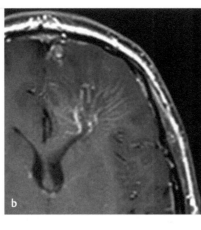

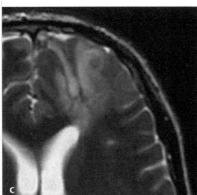 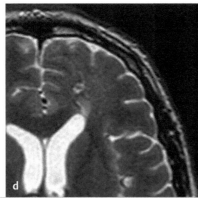

Fig. 8.5 Reversible venous congestion from DVA. (**a**) Axial T1-weighted MRI shows a T1 bright signal in the collector vein of a left frontal DVA. (**b**) Axial post-contrast T1-weighted MRI shows all the venous radicles of the left frontal DVA. (**c**) Axial T2-weighted MRI shows the thrombosed collector vein and T2 signal in the area drained by the DVA consistent with venous congestion. (**d**) Follow-up T2-weighted MRI obtained after 2 months of anticoagulation shows marked improvement in venous congestion and resolution of the thrombus.

associated with a higher prevalence of CCMs associated with DVAs. Most DVA-associated CCMs are Zambramski type 4 lesions, only apparent on T2* weighted imaging.

DVAs can also be associated with mechanical compression of neural structures resulting in symptoms. The draining collector vein can occasionally compress the ventricles, bone, or cranial nerves. This is more common in posterior fossa DVAs where the

draining vein can compress the aqueduct or the trigeminal, facial, or vestibulocochlear nerve.

There has also been some literature to suggest that DVAs may be associated with cortical migration anomalies. This is likely due to the fact that there is a relationship between the development of the cerebral venous system and cortical migration processes. It is important to identify this association in patients with epilepsy.

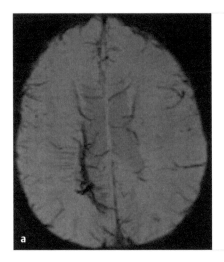
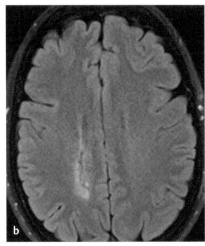

Fig. 8.6 Gliosis forming inside a DVA. (**a**) Axial SWI MRI shows a large DVA in the left cerebral hemisphere. (**b**) Axial FLAIR MRI shows bright T2 signal in the territory drained by the DVA consistent with gliosis.

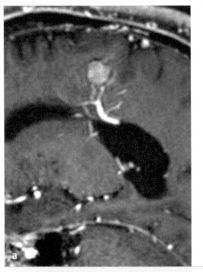
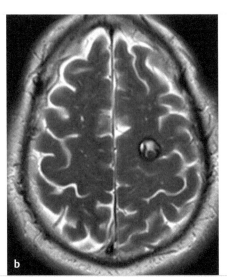
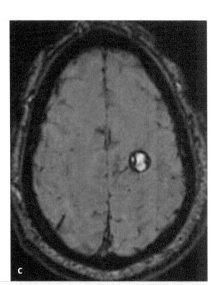

Fig. 8.7 Cavernoma forming inside a DVA. (**a**) Sagittal post-contrast T1-weighted MRI demonstrates a DVA draining the deep left hemispheric white matter into a subependymal vein. There is a cavernoma inside one of the venous radicles. (**b**) Axial T2-weighted MRI shows a popcorn-like lesion in the left hemispheric white matter with a hemosiderin ring consistent with a cavernoma. (**c**) Axial SWI MRI shows the cavernoma closely associated with a radicle of the DVA.

8.2.5 What the Clinician Needs to Know

- If DVA is incidental and not associated with any parenchymal abnormality there is usually no need to describe the finding in detail.
- It is important to identify presence of DVAs near a cavernous malformation or other lesion such as a tumor because it can affect operative planning.
- Findings of venous hypertension, ischemia, or hemorrhage related to the DVA.
- The presence of cortical migration abnormality associated with the DVA in epilepsy patients.

8.2.6 High-yield Facts

- DVAs are best identified on SWI and post-contrast T1-weighted images.

- DVAs can be symptomatic from venous congestion or mass effect. Venous congestion manifested by high T2/FLAIR signal in adjacent brain parenchyma, hemorrhage, cavernoma, and perfusion abnormalities.
- DVAs can be associated with cortical migration anomalies.
- DVAs drain normal brain parenchyma and should not be resected surgically.

Further Reading

[1] Pereira VM, Geibprasert S, Krings T, et al. Pathomechanisms of symptomatic developmental venous anomalies. Stroke. 2008; 39(12):3201–3215

[2] Linscott LL, Leach JL, Jones BV, Abruzzo TA. Developmental venous anomalies of the brain in children – imaging spectrum and update. Pediatr Radiol. 2016; 46(3):394–406, quiz 391–393

8.3 Capillary Telangiectasia

8.3.1 Clinical Case

A 50-year-old male with facial pain (▶ Fig. 8.8).

8.3.2 Description of Imaging Findings and Diagnosis

Diagnosis

Incidental pontine capillary telangiectasia.

8.3.3 Background

Capillary telangiectasias are benign vascular malformations that are usually incidental and asymptomatic. These lesions are thought to be congenital in nature. Histologically, they are composed of multiple thin-walled capillary channels interspersed within normal brain parenchyma. They are found in approximately 0.5% of the population and represent "do not touch lesions." It is important for the radiologist to accurately identify these lesions so they are not mistaken for more sinister pathologies such as metastases.

8.3.4 Imaging Findings

Capillary telangiectasias can generally only be identified on T1 post-contrast MRI and T2*-weighted sequences such as SWI and GRE. On post-contrast imaging, they have a faint, brush like enhancement without any associated mass effect. On SWI/GRE images, they often demonstrate blooming corresponding to the area of enhancement due to slow flow and increased concentration of deoxyhemoglobin (▶ Fig. 8.8). Occasionally, there may be some signal intensity changes on T1- or T2-weighted images but the vast majority of lesions are isointense to brain. In the center of the capillary telangiectasia, there is often a focus of more robust enhancement, which is thought to represent a draining vein. The most common location for these lesions is the pons, but they can also be seen in the supratentorial brain (▶ Fig. 8.9).

In rare cases, capillary telangiectasias can be part of mixed vascular malformation associated with both DVAs and cavernomas. This is thought to be the result of venous congestion in the DVA resulting in dilated upstream capillary beds as well as formation of a cavernous malformation. These lesions can bleed and grow and occasionally require surgical intervention. It is thought that cavernous malformations and capillary telangiectasia are part

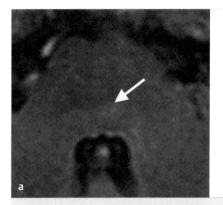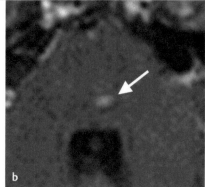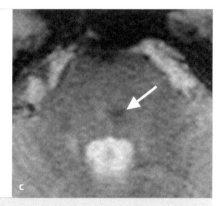

Fig. 8.8 Incidental pontine capillary telangiectasia. (**a**) Axial T2 FLAIR MRI demonstrates a subtle FLAIR hyperintensity in the left pons (*arrow*). (**b**) Post-contrast T1-weighted MRI demonstrates faint enhancement of the lesion (*arrow*). (**c**) Axial T2* GRE MRI shows subtle blooming in the area of the enhancing T2 hyperintense lesion (*arrow*).

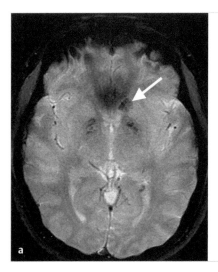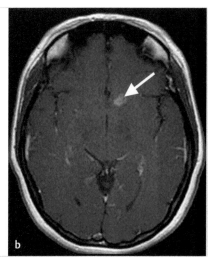

Fig. 8.9 Supratentorial capillary telangiectasia. (**a**) Axial T2*-weighted image shows faint blooming artifact in the inferior left frontal lobe (*arrow*). (**b**) Axial post-contrast T1-weighted MRI shows faint fluffy enhancement in the area of blooming artifact consistent with a capillary telangiectasia (*arrow*).

of a spectrum as both lesions are characterized by the presence of dilated capillary beds.

Capillary telangiectasias can occasionally be symptomatic. Giant telangienctasias are defined as those lesions which measure > 2 cm in maximum diameter and have been shown to be associated with symptoms. Large lesions are more likely to have T1 or T2 signal changes and prominent draining veins. Lesions located in the temporal lobes have been found to be associated with epilepsy while lesions in the brainstem have been found to be associated with cranial nerve deficits. If symptoms localize to the location of a capillary telangiectasia, the radiologist must identify the association.

8.3.5 What the Clinician Needs to Know

- When incidental, capillary telangiectasias have a benign natural history and require no further follow-up.
- Association between capillary telangiectasia and cavernous malformation or DVA as these lesions can grow, rupture, and cause morbidity.

- Localization of the capillary telangiectasia with the patient's symptoms, which happens very rarely.

8.3.6 High-yield Facts

- Capillary telangiectasias classically are located in the pons and have faint brush like enhancement with associated susceptibility artifact.
- Nearly all of these lesions are asymptomatic and incidental.
- Giant capillary telangiectasias can occasionally result in symptoms including cranial nerve deficits and seizures.

Further Reading

[1] Sayama CM, Osborn AG, Chin SS, Couldwell WT. Capillary telangiectasias: clinical, radiographic, and histopathological features. Clinical article. J Neurosurg. 2010; 113(4):709–714

[2] Pozzati E, Marliani AF, Zucchelli M, Foschini MP, Dall'Olio M, Lanzino G. The neurovascular triad: mixed cavernous, capillary, and venous malformations of the brainstem. J Neurosurg. 2007; 107(6):1113–1119

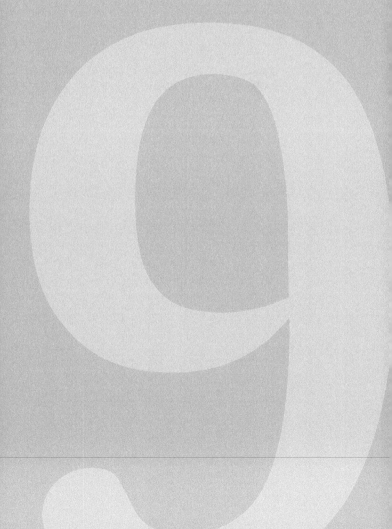

Chapter 9

Small Vessel Disease

9 Small Vessel Disease

9.1 ABRA/Amyloid Spectrum

9.1.1 Clinical Case

A 67-year-old male with memory impairment and encephalopathy.

9.1.2 Description of Imaging Findings and Diagnosis

Infiltrative mass in the left temporal lobe with faint leptomeningeal enhancement. Multifocal bilateral T2* white matter and gray matter hypointense lesions consistent with microhemorrhage. Biopsy revealed a diagnosis of amyloid-beta related angiitis (ABRA) (▶ Fig. 9.1).

9.1.3 Background

Amyloid angiopathy is a relatively common cause of lobar hemorrhage in the elderly population. It is the result of deposition of amyloid in the media and adventitia of cortical and leptomeningeal vessels. This process results in vascular fragility and resultant multicompartmental, predominantly lobar hemorrhage. Screening studies using SWI and GRE imaging have found that up to 15% of asymptomatic elderly patients have imaging findings compatible with amyloid angiopathy. It is found in up to 50% of patients over the age of 90 on autopsy. Approximately 90% of the Alzheimer population have amyloid angiopathy. There is no association between amyloid angiopathy and systemic amyloidosis.

Among patients with amyloid angiopathy is a subset of patients with an inflammatory response to amyloid deposition. ABRA is characterized as a transmural granulomatous inflammatory vasculitis that is angiodestructive. CAA-related inflammation (CAA-RI) is characterized by an inflammatory reaction surrounding CAA-affected vessels without angiodestruction. Both ABRA and CAA-RI are treated with immunosuppressive agents including steroids and cyclophosphamide while CAA is not. Thus, the importance of making the distinction between these entities.

9.1.4 Imaging Findings

Typical findings in cerebral amyloid angiopathy include superficial lobar hemorrhages, multiple microhemorrhages seen on T2*-weighted imaging primarily located in the gray-white junction of the cerebrum and cerebellum, convexal subarachnoid, or subpial hemorrhage seen on CT, FLAIR (fluid attenuation inversion recovery), or T2*-weighted imaging, cortical superficial siderosis located supratentorially, and leukoaraosis without involvement of the subcortical U fibers (▶ Fig. 9.2 and ▶ Fig. 9.3). Hemorrhagic lesions in CAA can be unilateral or bilateral, cerebral or cerebellar, and single or multiple. Lobar hemorrhage is the most common imaging finding seen in 60% of patients and has a sensitivity and specificity of 63 and 93% in distinguishing it from CAA-RI and ABRA. Occasionally, CAA can present as an infiltrative mass-like process resembling a glioma, but the presence of peripheral microhemorrhages at the gray-white junction should lead one to consider a diagnosis of CAA (▶ Fig. 9.1 and ▶ Fig. 9.2).

ABRA and CAA-RI have very similar imaging manifestations and are nearly impossible to distinguish from one another on imaging. Typical findings in ABRA and CAA-RI include leptomeningeal enhancement with infiltrative white matter abnormalities, which can occasionally mimic a low-grade glioma (▶ Fig. 9.1). Lobar hemorrhage is rare. Both of these entities commonly present with subcortical and cortical microhemorrhages on SWI, which is key to distinguishing them from neoplasms and other vasculopathies. The sensitivity and specificity of leptomeningeal enhancement in identifying CAA-RI and ABRA are 70 and 93%, respectively (▶ Fig. 9.1). The identification of leptomeningeal enhancement is essential in guiding biopsies as well.

9.1.5 What the Clinician Needs to Know

- The presence of lobar hemorrhage(s) in setting of multiple microhemorrhages on SWI is highly suggestive of CAA.
- Leptomeningeal enhancement along with cortical/subcortical microhemorrhages should prompt a diagnosis of CAA-RI or ABRA. The leptomeninges should be biopsied in these cases.

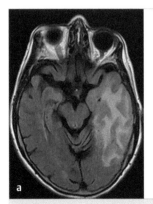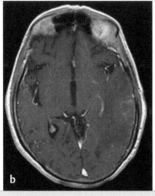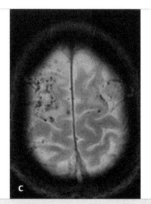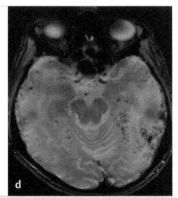

Fig. 9.1 A 67-year-old female presenting with memory impairment and encephalopathy secondary to ABRA. (a) Axial T2/FLAIR MRI shows marked edema in the left temporal lobe. (b) Axial post-contrast T1 weighted MRI shows leptomeningeal enhancement over the left temporal lobe. (c) and (d) Axial GRE T2*-weighted MRI images show multiple microhemorrhages in both gray and white matter. Based on this constellation of findings, a diagnosis of ABRA was suspected and ultimately made on biopsy (not shown).

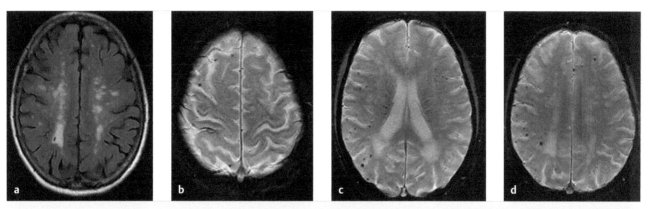

Fig. 9.2 A 74-year-old male with dementia. (**a**) Axial T2/FLAIR MRI shows multiple bilateral deep white matter FLAIR hyperintensities, most consistent with small vessel ischemic disease. (**b**) Axial T2*-weighted MRI shows bilateral foci of blooming artifact consistent with microhemorrhages. Note the sulcal/cortical subarachnoid hemorrhage (SAH) overlying the right post-central gyrus. (**c**) and (**d**). Additional slices from axial T2*-weighted MRI show a number of additional microhemorrhages, consistent with a diagnosis of amyloid angiopathy.

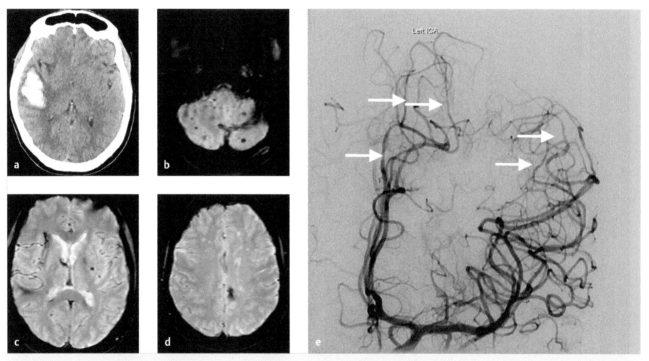

Fig. 9.3 Amyoid angiopathy presenting with lobar hemorrhage. (**a**) Axial non-contrast CT demonstrates a lobar hemorrhage in the right temporal lobe. (**b-d**). Axial T2* GRE images demonstrate multiple punctate microhemorrhages. Findings are consistent with amyloid angiopathy. (**e**) Diagnostic cerebral angiogram demonstrates multifocal vascular narrowing in the distal anterior cerebral artery (ACA) and MCA territories. Such findings are not uncommon among patients with amyloid angiopathy, but are nonspecific (*arrows*).

- Serial imaging is helpful in determining whether therapeutic agents are achieving their desired effect, especially in CAA-RI and ABRA.

9.1.6 High-yield Facts

- Diffuse lobar vasogenic edema or mass-like nonenhancing white matter T2 hyperintensities may mimic low-grade glioma, but the presence of microhemorrhage on SWI should suggest CAA-RI or ABRA, which should prompt the radiologist to contact the treating neurologist about the possibility of these entities and their excellent response to steroids.
- Lobar hemorrhage has a high sensitivity and specificity in distinguishing CAA from CAA-RI/ABRA.

- Leptomeningeal enhancement has a high sensitivity and specificity in distinguishing CAA-RI/ABRA from CAA. While the latter does not respond to steroids, the former two entities show a dramatic and rapid improvement.

Further Reading

[1] Salvarani C, Hunder GG, Morris JM, Brown RD , Jr, Christianson T, Giannini C. Aβ-related angiitis: comparison with CAA without inflammation and primary CNS vasculitis. Neurology. 2013; 81(18):1596–1603

[2] Salvaranti C, Morris JM, Giannini C, Brown RD, Christianson T, Hunder GG. Imaging Findings of Cerebral Amyloid Angiopathy, AB-Related Angiitis (ABRA) and Cerebral Amyloid Angiopathy-Related Inflammation: A Single-Institution 25-Year Experience. Baltimore Medicine. 2016; 95:1–7

9.2 Susac's Syndrome

9.2.1 Clinical Case

A 45-year-old female with encephalopathy, sensorineural hearing loss, and vision loss (▶ Fig. 9.4).

9.2.2 Description of Imaging Findings and Diagnosis

Diagnosis

Multiple T2 hyperintense/T1 hypointense lesions of the corpus callosum with associated retinal branch occlusions. Findings consistent with Susac's syndrome.

9.2.3 Background

Susac's syndrome is a rare autoimmune small vessel vasculitis. Clinical presentation of Susac's syndrome includes an acute or subacute encephalopathy, sensorineural hearing loss, and vision distortion from branch retinal artery occlusions. In only 10% of cases are all three symptoms present at the same time. The disease is usually self-limiting, fluctuating, and monophasic; however, a substantial proportion of patients have long-lasting neurological deficits. The disease typically affects young women (~40 years old) and has a 3:1 F:M ratio. Because Susac's syndrome is an autoimmune disease, most cases are treated with immunosuppressive agents along with antithrombotic agents. In rare cases, cochlear implants can be considered.

While the exact cause of Susac's syndrome has yet to be identified, there is some evidence to suggest that anti-endothelial cell antibodies play a key role in the pathogenesis of the disease. These autoantibodies predominantly affect small arteries and arterioles resulting in thrombosis and microvascular infarction. This explains the appearance of the corpus callosum lesions as there is predominantly microvascular supply at this location. Pathologically, retinal and brain biopsy shows small vessel vasculopathy resulting in arteriolar occlusion and microinfarction. Sensorineural hearing loss in Susac's syndrome is secondary to microinfarction of cochlear tissue at the apex of the cochlea.

One of the keys to making a diagnosis of Susac's syndrome-syndrome is the identification of branch retinal artery occlusions on fluorescein angiography. Such findings are not present in multiple sclerosis. Some authors recommend that in any unexplained encephalopathy involving the white matter, gray matter and leptomeninges, fundoscopy, and fluorescein angiography should be performed.

9.2.4 Imaging Findings

MRI is the mainstay in the imaging diagnosis of Susac's syndrome. The pathognomonic imaging finding is the presence of multiple 5-mm T2 hyperintense white matter lesions in the corpus callosum, which have a snowball appearance. These will involve the central fibers of the body and splenium as well as the roof of the corpus. The lesions spare the callososeptal interface and undersurface and periphery of the corpus callosum (▶ Fig. 9.5). Periventricular T2 hyperintensities are generally not present in Susac's syndrome. These imaging characteristics are key in

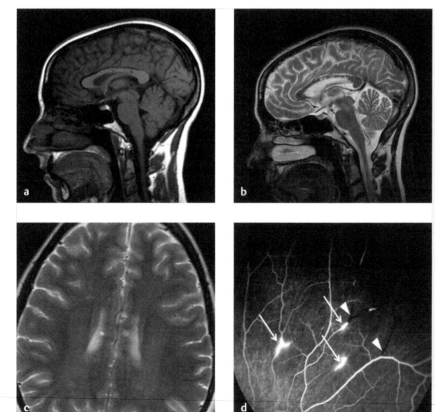

Fig. 9.4 Classic neuroimaging manifestations of Susac's disease. (**a**) Sagittal T1-weighted MRI demonstrates multiple T1 hypointense lesions in the corpus callosum which are also hyperinense on sagittal T2-weighted MRI as well (**b**). These lesions have the classic "snowball" pattern as they are more or less spherical in shape. (**c**) Axial T2-weighted MRI demonstrates the lesions in the axial plane (**d**). Fluorescein angiogram of the eye demonstrates multiple retinal artery branch occlusions (*arrows* and *arrowheads*).

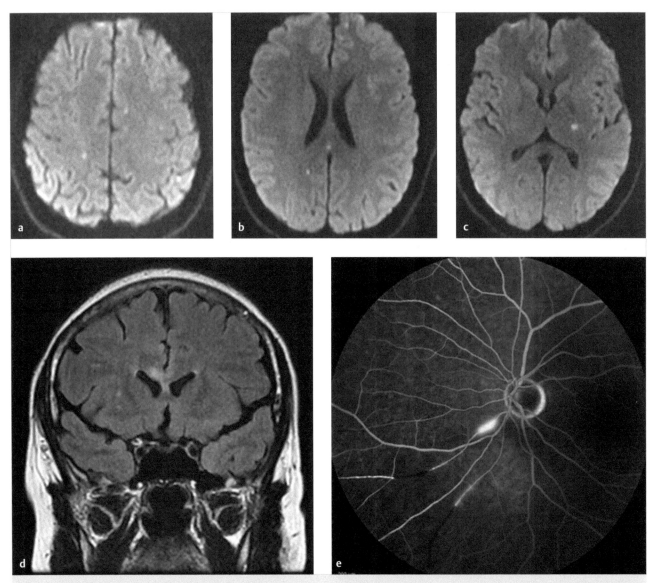

Fig. 9.5 A 57-year female with sudden headache, encephalopathy, tinnitus, and hearing loss but no visual symptoms. **(a-c)** Axial DWI show multiple punctate infarcts in the bihemispheric white matter including on lesion in the splenium of the corpus callosum. **(d)** Coronal T2/FLAIR MRI shows a T2 hyperintense lesion in the body of the corpus callosum. A possible diagnosis of Susac's was brought up and the patient underwent a fluorescein angiogram which showed multiple branch retinal artery occlusions **(e)**.

differentiating Susac's syndrome from multiple sclerosis; especially, since these two entities have overlapping clinical presentations and imaging findings. Another key differentiator between Susac and MS is the fact that over time, the T2 hyperintense lesions in Susac's syndrome become T1 hypointense; whereas in MS, T2 hyperintense lesions generally resolve and leave behind an atrophic corpus callosum. As in MS, sagittal views are extremely helpful in making the diagnosis (▶ Fig. 9.6).

Larger series' of Susac's syndrome patients have found that 70% of patients also have deep gray nuclei involvement (not seen in MS), 70% have parenchymal enhancement, and 33% have leptomeningeal enhancement (not seen in MS or ADEM). White matter lesions not only involve the corpus callosum, but also the cerebellum, middle cerebellar peduncles, and brainstem. Parenchymal enhancement can be focal or diffuse and occasionally have a miliary appearance. Many of the infarctions that occur in Susac's syndrome are below the resolution of current MRI techniques as evident by the fact that almost all biopsies performed of Susac's syndrome patients show small cortical and subcortical microinfarctions (▶ Fig. 9.5).

Vascular imaging in suspected Susac's syndrome can be helpful in distinguishing it from primary CNS vasculitis. Because Susac's syndrome typically affects pre-capillary arteriolar beds, there is rarely, if ever, involvement of arteries that are at the resolution of CTA, MRA, and digital subtraction angiography (DSA). This is in contrary to most large and medium vessel vasculitides, which demonstrate multifocal vascular narrowing.

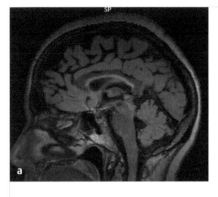
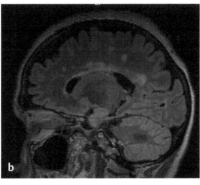
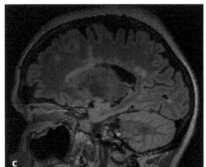
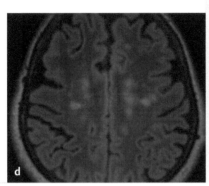

Fig. 9.6 Classic imaging manifestations of multiple sclerosis. (**a**) Sagittal T2/FLAIR MRI demonstrates T2 hyperintensity in the callososeptal interface, a classic imaging finding for multiple sclerosis. (**b-c**). Sagittal T2/FLAIR MRIs demonstrate classic "Dawson's Fingers." (**d**) Axial T2/FLAIR MRI shows multiple oval-shaped white matter hyperintensities consistent with demyelinating lesions.

9.2.5 What the Clinician Needs to Know

- Fluorescein angiography essential to diagnosis of Susac's syndrome and key to differentiating Susac's syndrome from MS, which has a similar presentation.
- The location of cortical, subcortical, and leptomeningeal disease as this can help guide biopsies when indicated.
- Key imaging differentiators of Susac's syndrome from MS-radiologist must relay the fact that central callosal lesions could be Susac's syndrome, especially in the absence of periventricular lesions such as Dawson's fingers.

9.2.6 High-yield Facts

- Susac's syndrome can be differentiated from MS by lack of involvement of the callososeptal interface and periphery of

the corpus callosum. In addition, Susac's syndrome is more likely to involve the gray matter than MS.
- Leptomeningeal enhancement occurs in up to 1/3 of cases and can help in differentiating Susac's syndrome from ADEM.
- There is often little correlation between extent/severity of imaging findings and clinical symptoms in Susac's syndrome.

Further Reading

[1] Susac JO. Susac's syndrome. AJNR Am J Neuroradiol. 2004; 25(3):351–352

[2] Demir MK. Case 142: Susac's syndrome. Radiology. 2009; 250(2):598–602

[3] Susac JO, Murtagh FR, Egan RA, et al. MRI findings in Susac's syndrome. Neurology. 2003; 61(12):1783–1787

9.3 Leukoaraiosis

9.3.1 Clinical Case

A 74-year-old male with memory loss, history of multiple cardiovascular risk factors (▶ Fig. 9.7).

9.3.2 Description of Imaging Findings and Diagnosis

Diffuse bilateral T2/FLAIR white matter hyperintensities, semiconfluent, consistent with leukoaraiosis.

9.3.3 Background

Leukoaraiosis is one of the most common imaging findings in the elderly population. This is a radiological term describing diffuse or patchy white matter changes seen on T2/FLAIR imaging. The pathogenesis of leukoaraiosis is poorly understood. There are data to suggest that it is secondary to atherosclerotic changes of deep brain arterioles. This hypothesis is supported by the fact that leukoaraiosis is commonly associated with diabetes, hypercholesterolemia, and hypertension. Other authors posit that leukoaraiosis could also be due to impaired cerebral lymphatic drainage through the recently described glymphatic system. In a recent longitudinal study employing weekly imaging on patients with leukoaraiosis, evidence was found for silent DWI-positive microinfarctions as the cause for this phenomenon.

Leukoaraiosis has been associated with a wide range of neurological complications. Case control studies of patients with and without leukoaraiosis have linked this entity to worse functional outcome after acute ischemic stroke and intracerebral hemorrhage. Patients with leukoaraiosis are also at increased risk of stroke recurrence when compared to non-leukoaraiosis counterparts. Leukoaraiosis has also been shown to be a strong risk factor for cognitive impairment.

9.3.4 Imaging Findings

On CT, leukoaraiosis is identified by non-enhancing periventricular white matter hypodensities, which are confluent or semiconfluent.

On MRI, leukoaraiosis is identified as non-enhancing T2/FLAIR white matter hyperintensities, which are confluent or semiconfluent. T1 can occasionally show these white matter lesions to be hypointense; however, they are usually isointense.

There is a commonly used scale for grading degree of leukoaraiosis called the Fazekas score. This score is commonly used in research studies and is generally not clinically applicable; however, it does help in conceptualizing the severity of leukoaraosis. In the Fazekas scoring system, the white matter is divided into periventricular and deep white matter and each region is given a grade depending on the extent of white matter changes. It is important to point out that deep white matter changes are usually secondary to chronic ischemic disease while periventricular white matter changes are due to subependymal gliosis, ependymitis granularis, and demyelination. A summary of deep white matter Fazekas score is as follows: Grade 0 = no white matter changes, Grade 1 = multiple punctate foci of T2/FLAIR hyperintensity without confluence, Grade 2 = beginning of confluent white matter T2/FLAIR changes, and Grade 3 = large confluent areas of T2/FLAIR white matter hyperintensity.

Ultimately, the role of the radiologist in the evaluation of leukoaraiosis is to distinguish it from more aggressive and reversible white matter processes. Leukoaraiosis is commonly mistaken for demyelinating diseases such as multiple sclerosis. The key distinguish feature is the fact that leukoaraiosis lesions are less likely to be oval shapes, less likely to run perpendicular to the ventricular system, and more likely to be confluent or semiconfluent. In addition, leukoaraiosis does not enhance or demonstrate restricted diffusion, something that is often present in demyelinating disease. CNS vasculitides are sometimes included in the differential of patients with leukoaraiosis type changes. Key distinguishing features of CNS vasculitis from leukoaraiosis include the lack of cortical and subcortical involvement in leukoaraiosis along with lack of leptomeningeal enhancement (▶ Fig. 9.8, ▶ Fig. 9.9).

One interesting facet of leukoaraiosis that is currently being explored is cerebrovascular reactivity in the affected cerebral white matter. Cerebrovascular reactivity can be studied using dynamic susceptibility contrast (DSC) perfusion techniques as well as by studying changes in blood oxygen level dependent (BOLD) signal in the setting of a change in arterial CO_2 levels. Studies of

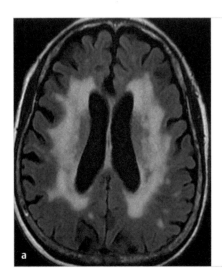
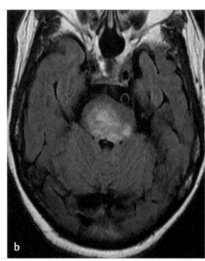

Fig. 9.7 Classic case of severe leukoaraiosis in a 74-year-old male with memory loss and the history of multiple cardiovascular risk factors. (a) Axial T2/FLAIR MRI shows bilateral large areas of confluent T2 white matter hyperintensity consistent with leukoaraosis. (b) Axial T2/FLAIR MRI at the level of the brainstem shows white matter hyperintensity of the pons as well, also consistent with chronic small vessel ischemic disease/leukoaraiosis.

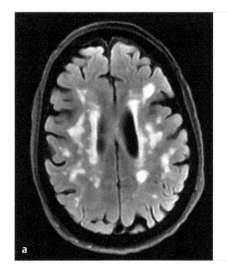
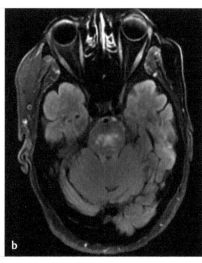

Fig. 9.8 A 74-year-old male with nonspecific tremor. (**a**) Axial T2/FLAIR MRI shows multiple foci of T2/FLAIR white matter hyperintensity in the periventricular, deep, and subcortical white matter. A number of these lesions have an oval shape. Differential diagnosis in this case included leukoaraiosis and demyelinating disease. (**b**) Axial T2/FLAIR MRI at the level of the pons shows patchy white matter hyperintensity. This appearance is most consistent with chronic small vessel ischemic disease. The combination of the pontine and supratentorial findings in addition to the patient's history of cardiovascular risk factors and lack of clinical evidence of demyelinating disease led to a diagnosis of leukoaraiosis. This would be consistent with a Fazekas Type 2 score.

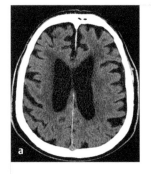
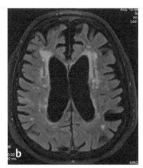
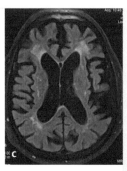

Fig. 9.9 White matter perfusion abnormalities in leukoaraiosis. (**a**) Non-contrast CT demonstrates diffusely hypodense white matter consistent with leukoaraiosis. (**b**) and (**c**). T2/FLAIR MRI demonstrates diffuse bilateral deep white matter T2 hyperintensities consistent with small vessel ischemic disease/leukoaraiosis. (**d**) and (**e**). CT perfusion mean transit time images demonstrate increase mean transit time in the deep and periventricular white matter bilaterally, a finding which has been associated with chronic small vessel ischemic disease.

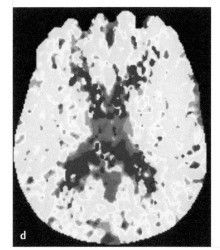
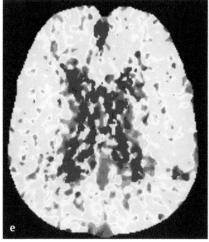

patients with leukoaraisis using both of these techniques have found that resting blood flow metrics are abnormal in these patients as CBV is abnormally low and time to peak (TTP) is abnormally high–indicating impaired blood flow. In addition, these patients have impaired cerebrovascular reactivity suggesting that these patients may have impaired responses to ischemic insults.

9.3.5 What the Clinician Needs to Know

- Extensive leukoaraiosis is a risk factor for dementia, ischemic stroke, and hemorrhage.
- Leukoaraiosis patients have worse prognosis following ischemic stroke and intracerebral hemorrhage, possibly due to impaired cerebrovascular reactivity.

- There is some overlap between imaging findings of leukoaraiosis and treatable white matter diseases such as MS and vasculitis. Relying on demographics, presentation, and imaging findings is invaluable in such circumstances.

9.3.6 High-yield Facts

- Leukoaraiosis involves the deep white matter and generally spares the subcortical white matter. It should not involve the gray matter, a key distinguishing feature from vasculitides.
- Leukoaraiosis does not have DWI restriction or enhancement.

- Perfusion imaging in leukoaraiosis patients shows decreased CVR (cerebral vascular reserve), CBV, and increased MTT and TTP, suggesting that the etiology of the disease is from microvascular ischemic changes.

Further Reading

[1] Inzitari D. Leukoaraiosis: an independent risk factor for stroke? Stroke. 2003; 34(8):2067–2071

[2] Sam K, Crawley AP, Poublanc J, et al. Vascular Dysfunction in Leukoaraiosis. AJNR Am J Neuroradiol. 2016; 37(12):2258–2264

[3] Conklin J, Silver FL, Mikulis DJ, Mandell DM. Are acute infarcts the cause of leukoaraiosis? Brain mapping for 16 consecutive weeks. Ann Neurol. 2014; 76(6):899–904

Chapter 10

Intracranial Hemorrhage

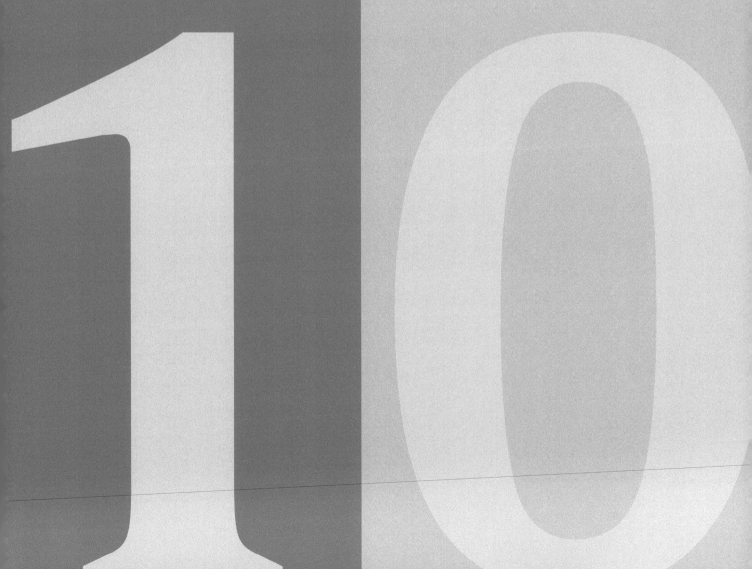

10 Intracranial Hemorrhage

10.1 Aneurysmal Subarachnoid Hemorrhage

10.1.1 Clinical Case

A 55-year-old male with sudden onset of worst headache of life.

10.1.2 Description of Imaging Findings and Diagnosis

Diffuse hyperdense blood in the subarachnoid space centered in the interhemispheric fissure. There is also a small amount of right-sided subdural hemorrhage. Severe hydrocephalus. Findings most consistent with a ruptured anterior communicating artery aneurysm (▶ Fig. 10.1).

10.1.3 Background

Aneurysmal subarachnoid hemorrhage (SAH) is the most common form of nontraumatic SAH affecting up to 20 individuals per 100,000 persons/year. Rupture of a cerebral aneurysm results in the extravasation of blood into the subarachnoid space, which triggers a cascade of events that can result in severe disability or death. Failure to diagnose and treat an aneurysmal SAH can result

in further impairment due to aneurysm rebleeding and delayed cerebral ischemia from cerebral vasospasm. While lumbar puncture is the gold standard for the diagnosis of SAH, CT has emerged as the diagnostic modality of choice with sensitivity and specificity of over 99% in the first days after the SAH.

It is important for neuroradiologists to understand some basic tenants of the pathophysiology of aneurysmal SAH. First, in general, once an aneurysm ruptures, the rupture point soon thromboses resulting in temporary cessation of bleeding. For this reason, active extravasation is rarely identified on cross-sectional imaging. However, rebleeding of an unsecured aneurysm is relatively common as the rate ranges from 1–2% per day for the first month following the initial insult. Rebleeding has a 60% mortality and severe disability rate; hence, the importance of identifying the aneurysm. Hydrocephalus is a relatively common complication of aneurysmal SAH and often presents with slowly progressive reduction in the level of consciousness, downward deviation of the eyes, and small pupils from pressure on the tectal area. Early identification of hydrocephalus is important so that EVD placement can be considered. Acute hydrocephalus typically occurs in the first 3 days following aneurysm rupture. Symptomatic and delayed cerebral infarction are also relatively common (10–20% of cases). These are important causes of SAH-associated morbidity and typically occur from 5–14 days following the initial insult. The neuroradiologist

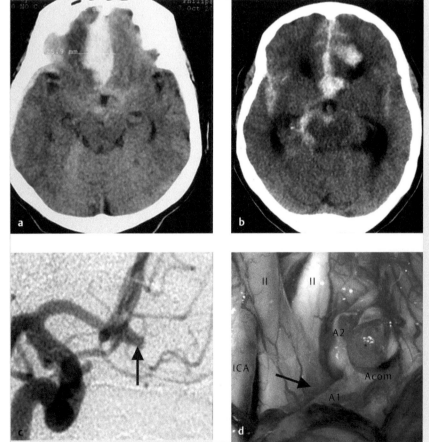

Fig. 10.1 A 62-year-old male with ruptured anterior communicating artery aneurysm. (a) Non-contrast CT shows dense intraparenchymal hemorrhage in the right gyrus rectus along with dense SAH in the interhemispheric fissure. There is also a thin subdural hematoma overlying the right cerebral hemisphere. Severe hydrocephalus is present with marked dilatation of the bilateral temporal horns. (b) Non-contrast CT shows blood extending to the interpeduncular cistern, ambient cistern, and bilateral sylvian fissures. (c) Cerebral angiogram shows a small aneurysm of the anterior communicating artery complex (arrow). (d) Surgical microscopic image shows the aneurysm (*). Note the proximity of the aneurysm to the optic nerve (II) and optic chiasm (arrow).

plays an essential role in the identification and prediction of these pathophysiologic processes.

10.1.4 Imaging Findings

The diagnosis of aneurysmal SAH on imaging is straight forward.

Non-contrast CT is the imaging modality of choice as it easily identifies hemorrhage and allows for quick identification of hydrocephalus. SAH is identified as hyperdense blood products, usually centered in the suprasellar cistern with extension into the interhemispheric and sylvian fissures. Sensitivity of CT for the identification of SAH decreases over time from about 99% in the first 24 hours to 30–50% after 1 week. In cases where CT is equivocal, MRI with FLAIR (fluid attenuation inversion recovery) or T2* sequences is helpful. Potential mimics of SAH include iodinated contrast, diffuse basal meningitis (i.e., tuberculosis), and pus.

The modified Fisher scale is the most commonly used scale in grading SAH and is described in ▶ Table 10.1. It serves as a good template for describing imaging findings in aneurysmal SAH and is a useful tool in predicting future risk of vasospasm. Key points are the following: (1) thin SAH is < 1-mm thick and thick SAH is > 1-mm thick, (2) presence of IVH is key, and (3) the radiologist must seek out the presence of areas of focal SAH. Risk of vasospasm ranges from 24% for a mFisher of 1 to 40% for a mFisher of 4. Another key point is that the Fisher score does not account for degree of hydrocephalus. Thus, the neuroradiologist must be attuned to imaging findings of hydrocephalus including

(1) temporal horn expansion, (2) convexity of the third ventricular walls, (3) rounding of the frontal horns, (4) sulcal effacement, and (5) ventricular enlargement out of proportion to sulcal dilatation.

Aneurysm detection is typically performed with CTA in most centers. However, given the fact that most ruptured aneurysms are treated endovascularly, some centers have advocated for skipping the initial CTA and going directly to diagnostic cerebral angiography. While it may be more cost effective to go straight to digital subtraction angiography (DSA), there is some benefit in doing an initial CTA as it can triage patients who are not typically endovascular candidates to surgery and allow them the possibility of skipping the DSA. DSA with 3DRA is the gold standard in aneurysm detection and characterization. CTA has a sensitivity of 100% for identifying ruptured aneurysms ≥ 4 mm in size but just 92% for aneurysms < 4 mm. Thus, a negative CTA in the setting of diffuse SAH should prompt a diagnostic cerebral angiogram. 3D and MPR reconstructions are often essential in identifying smaller aneurysms on CTA. In cases of aneurysm multiplicity, one can refer to aneurysm size, morphology, and wall-imaging characteristics to identify the culprit lesion. In general, the ruptured aneurysm is the larger and more irregular lesion. MRI vessel wall imaging (VWI), described in a previous chapter may also be helpful as some studies have suggested that ruptured aneurysms are more likely to demonstrate circumferential wall enhancement than unruptured lesions.

It is important to point out that non-contrast CT can be very helpful in identifying the bleeding site, particularly in patients with multiple aneurysms. The location of the thickest/highest density blood is often the site of the aneurysm. If there is dense thick blood in the interhemispheric fissure, then an Acom aneurysm can be considered, sylvian fissure indicates MCA, interpeduncular cistern indicates basilar tip, and asymmetric blood in the suprasellar cistern suggests an ICA/Pcom etiology (▶ Fig. 10.2).

Serial imaging is often performed in *aSAH* patients during their hospitalization. Over time, one should expect reduction in blood volume and density and improvement in hydrocephalus. Around days 5–14, screening for cerebral vasospasm is often performed. Vasospasm is identified by narrowing of intracranial arteries on CTA, MRA, or DSA. The narrowing is often most

Table 10.1 Fisher and Modified Fisher Scales

Score	Fisher Scale	Modified Fisher Scale
1	Focal Thin SAH	Focal or Diffuse Thin SAH, No IVH
2	Diffuse Thin SAH	Focal or Diffuse Thin SAH, With IVH
3	Thick SAH	Thick SAH, No IVH
4	Focal or Diffuse Thin SAH with Significant ICH or IVH	Thick SAH with IVH

Abbreviations: SAH, Subarachnoid hemorrhage; IVH, Intraventricular Hemorrhage.

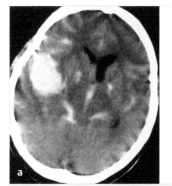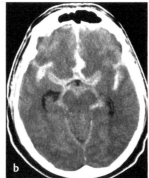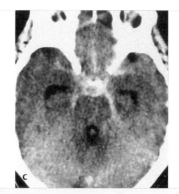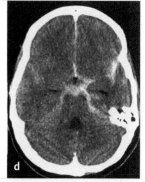

Fig. 10.2 Example of typical blood distribution patterns by aneurysm location. (**a**) Ruptured MCA aneurysm with dense hemorrhage in the right sylvian fissure and associated intraparenchymal hematoma. (**b**) Ruptured anterior communicating/anterior cerebral artery (ACA) aneurysm with densest blood in the interhemispheric fissure. (**c**) Ruptured basilar artery aneurysm with dense blood in the suprasellar cistern but a focal filling defect indicative of the aneurysm itself. (**d**) Ruptured ICA terminus aneurysm on the left with slight asymmetry of subarachnoid blood products on the left side of the suprasellar cistern.

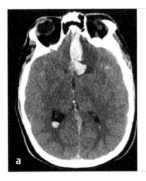
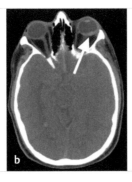
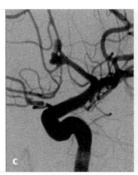

Fig. 10.3 Example of Terson's syndrome. (a) Non-contrast CT shows dense hemorrhage and edema in the left gyrus rectus and inter-hemispheric fissure. There is also marked vasogenic edema in the inferior left frontal lobe and blood laying in the dependent lateral ventricles. (b) Close inspection of the left eye demonstrates layering blood in the left globe (*arrow*). (c) Cerebral angiogram shows a ruptured anterior communicating artery aneurysm with a slow flow pseudoaneurysm.

severe at the location of the densest blood. Perfusion imaging, particularly CT perfusion, is very helpful in determining how flow limiting the vasospasm is. Delayed cerebral ischemia from vasospasm is associated with high rates of infarction and poor neurological outcome. It is important to point out that about 20% of patients without cerebral vasospasm will develop DCI suggesting that factors other than vasospasm play a role. CTP perfusion studies of aSAH patients have found that patients with perfusion changes on CTP have a 23 times higher odds of DCI than patients with normal CTP. In addition, CTP performed within 4–14 days after aSAH predicts DCI. The best parameters to study in such cases are CBF and MTT.

One common imaging finding that is often not picked up on during the initial evaluation of SAH patients is the presence of blood in the globes (i.e., Terson's syndrome). This finding is present in 20–50% of SAH patients and can be identified as layering blood in the posterior portion of the globe. Terson's syndrome is a common cause of long-term vision loss in SAH and can be treated with vitrectomy (▶ Fig. 10.3).

10.1.5 What the Clinician Needs to Know

- Extent and distribution of subarachnoid blood with focus on parameters identified in Fisher scale.
- The presence or absence of hydrocephalus and intraventricular blood.

- Aneurysm location.
- The presence or absence or risk factors for vasospasm and delayed cerebral ischemia. Discussion of role of perfusion imaging in prognosticating DCI can help guide critical care physicians in how aggressive they need to be in medical management. In setting of suspected vasospasm, CTP can help identify severity of perfusion deficit.

10.1.6 High-yield Facts

- Sensitivity of CTA is 92% for aneurysms < 4 mm in size. A negative CTA in the setting of a suspected aneurysmal SAH should prompt an immediate DSA.
- Cerebral vasospasm is most common on days 5–14 post-SAH. CTA and CTP are useful screening tools in evaluating both anatomic and functional effects of vasospasm.
- In setting of multiple aneurysms, factors that can help identify the culprit lesion include aneurysm wall enhancement on MRI, aneurysm morphology, aneurysm size, and location of the densest amount of blood products.

Further Reading

[1] de Oliveira Manoel AL, Mansur A, Murphy A, et al. Aneurysmal subarachnoid haemorrhage from a neuroimaging perspective. Crit Care. 2014; 18(6):557
[2] Dupont SA, Wijdicks EFM, Lanzino G, Rabinstein AA. Aneurysmal subarachnoid hemorrhage: an overview for the practicing neurologist. Semin Neurol. 2010; 30(5):545–554

10.2 Non-Aneurysmal Perimesencephalic Hemorrhage

10.2.1 Clinical Case

A 43-year-old male with post-coital severe headache. No loss of consciousness (▶ Fig. 10.4).

10.2.2 Description of Imaging Findings and Diagnosis

Diagnosis

Focal SAH isolated to the perimesencephalic cistern in the setting of a negative CTA and cerebral angiogram. Consistent with non-aneurysmal perimesencephalic hemorrhage.

10.2.3 Background

Non-aneurysmal perimesencephalic subarachnoid hemorrhage (pSAH) was first described by van Gijn in 1985 as an SAH in which blood was limited primarily to the perimesencephalic cisterns with no evidence of aneurysm on angiography. Definition of pSAH is somewhat variable across studies; however, in general, most authors seem to agree that for an SAH to be considered a pSAH it has to meet the following imaging criteria: (1) center of hemorrhage located in front of the brainstem, (2) no blood in the interhemispheric or lateral Sylvian fissures (except for minute amounts), (3) minimal intraventricular hemorrhage, and (4) no intraparenchymal hemorrhage. In addition

to imaging findings, patients need to have minimal symptoms beyond a severe headache. Non-aneurysmal pSAH patients are typically alert, orientated, and have a Glasgow Coma Scale of 15. These relatively minor symptoms are the reason why many authors believe that non-aneurysmal pSAH is the result of a venous hemorrhage rather than an arterial bleed. The differential diagnosis of a pSAH is fairly broad. The prevalence of a saccular aneurysm in the setting of a pSAH ranges from 1–9% depending on the study, with most aneurysms being located in the posterior fossa. Other potential etiologies include arterial dissection/dissecting aneurysm, posterior fossa or spinal vascular malformation, and hypervascular tumors like hemangioblastomas. In most cases, the hemorrhage is idiopathic with no structural lesion to account for the hemorrhage.

Many authors have claimed that the etiology of idiopathic pSAHs is venous in nature. Many patients with pSAH report performing some variant of a Valsalva maneuver at the time of the initial ictus. It is thought that the Valsalva maneuver can result in intracranial venous engorgement and rupture due to the fact that Valsalva increases intrathoracic pressure, which blocks internal jugular venous return thus resulting in increased intracranial venous pressure. A number of studies have found that patients with non-aneurysmal pSAH have variant venous drainage patterns as well, further lending support to the venous hypothesis. Patients with pSAH have been found to have more primitive drainage patterns of the basal vein of Rosenthal including drainage directly into the dural sinuses (cavernous sinus via the uncal vein, the superior petrosal sinus via the tentorial sinus or the pontomesencephalic vein) rather than into the Galenic system as classically described. The direct connection of the perimesencephalic and basal veins with the dural

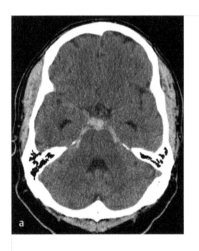
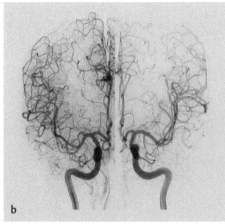
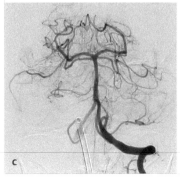
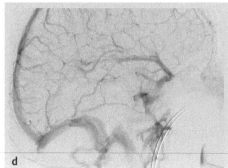

Fig. 10.4 Typical non-aneurysmal SAH. (a) Non-contrast CT demonstrates blood in the prepontine cistern with a small amount of blood extending to the ambient cisterns. There is no hydrocephalus or intraventricular hemorrhage. (b) and (c). Bilateral ICA and vertebral artery cerebral angiography demonstrates no intracranial aneurysm or AVM. (d) Interestingly, in the venous phase, the basal vein of Rosenthal did not drain into the vein of Galen. This would be consistent with a primitive venous drainage pattern and is associated with non-aneurysmal perimesencephalic hemorrhage.

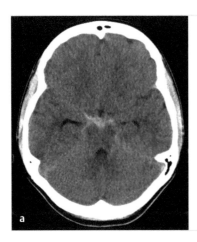
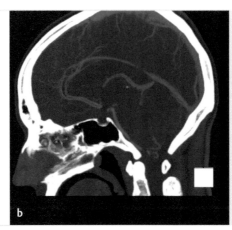

Fig. 10.5 Non-aneurysmal perimesenephalic hemorrhage with vein of Galen stenosis. (a) Non-contrast CT shows typical perimesencephalic hemorrhage without hydrocephalus or extension to the suprasellar cistern. (b) CTA demonstrates a focal narrowing at the entry of the vein of Galen into the straight sinus. Some authors suspect that this is associated with non-aneurysmal perimesencephalic hemorrhage. However, this is controversial as there is a dural ring surrounding the vein of Galen as it enters the straight sinus; thus, this finding is present in a substantial proportion of the population.

sinuses may predispose to sudden increases in venous pressure and venous rupture during Valsalva. Other reported venous culprits for pSAH include the vein of Galen stenosis and straight sinus stenosis (▶ Fig. 10.5).

10.2.4 Imaging Findings

The ideal initial imaging strategy for patients with pSAH has been a point of debate for several years. With improvements in CTA techniques, the diagnostic accuracy and negative predictive value of CTA is clearly improving. The negative predictive value of CTA in the setting of pSAH is roughly 98%. The diagnostic yield of DSA after a negative CTA is approximately 1–10%. It is important to point out that even though CTA may have a high sensitivity for intracranial aneurysms, CTA is not effective in excluding other causes of pSAH such as tiny vascular malformations, vasculitis, dissections, and blister aneurysms. Given the excellent safety profile of diagnostic cerebral angiography and the potentially devastating effect of missing a treatable vascular lesion, it is reasonable (and in most cases, preferred) to perform cerebral angiography, even in the setting of a CTA-negative pSAH, although this is controversial.

The previously held dogma for diagnostic evaluation of pSAH is two negative cerebral angiograms performed within a month or so of each other. However, over the past several years, there have been several studies which have found that the diagnostic yield of a second short-term or long-term repeat cerebral angiographic evaluation in the setting of a strictly pSAH is less than 2%. Based on such data, most practitioners appear to be comfortable with the idea that a single negative DSA with 3DRA in the setting of a pSAH is sufficient in excluding a vascular lesion as the source of the bleed. The diagnostic yield of a long-term follow-up CTA or MRA following an initially negative cerebral angiogram is also very low and generally not performed.

Many centers still routinely perform brain MRI in pSAH patients with negative angiographic imaging in order to exclude other causes of pSAH such as an angiographically occult vascular malformation, tiny hypervascular tumor, dissection, etc. However, a number of studies have demonstrated that the diagnostic yield of a follow-up MRI is essentially nil. Another dogma of pSAH evaluation is MR imaging of the cervical spine to rule out a cervical cord tumor or vascular lesion, which could result

in a pSAH distribution. While there have been case reports of spinal dural fistulae resulting in a pSAH, this is extremely rare. In general, large case series on spinal axis imaging for pSAH have found that the diagnostic yield is essentially nil. The largest study to date included 51 patients with angiographically negative pSAH and found no cases in which spinal axis imaging demonstrated a source of hemorrhage.

Over the past several years, there has been growing interest in the role of VWI in the characterization of cerebrovascular diseases. While the most common assumption is that pSAH is due to venous pathology, others have suggested that microdissections or microaneurysms related to tiny perforators are the cause of bleeding. High-resolution VWI allows for excellent spatial resolution (0.4 mm) and can delineate such pathologies. However, while no large studies have been performed to evaluate the diagnostic yield of VWI in the evaluation of pSAH, one recently published study of seven patients with angiogram negative pSAH found that the diagnostic yield was nil.

10.2.5 What the Clinician Needs to Know

- The extent of subarachnoid blood and whether there is enough blood for the clinician to suspect aneurysmal SAH.
- The presence or absence of hydrocephalus and intraventricular blood as hydrocephalus would exclude a non-aneurysmal pSAH and require a full diagnostic work-up.

10.2.6 High-yield Facts

- DSA is relatively low yield in setting of pSAH, however, is recommended by some and performed at some institutions.
- Diagnostic yield of brain and spine MRI is very low and probably should not be routinely performed.
- For an SAH to be considered a pSAH it has to meet the following criteria: (1) center of hemorrhage located in front of the brainstem, (2) no blood in the interhemispheric or lateral Sylvian fissures (except for minute amounts), (3) minimal intraventricular hemorrhage, (4) no intraparenchymal hemorrhage, and (5) no hydrocephalus.

Further Reading

[1] Brinjikji W, Kallmes DF, White JB, Lanzino G, Morris JM, Cloft HJ. Inter- and intraobserver agreement in CT characterization of nonaneurysmal perimesencephalic subarachnoid hemorrhage. AJNR Am J Neuroradiol. 2010; 31(6): 1103–1105

[2] Coutinho JM, Sacho RH, Schaafsma JD, et al. High-Resolution Vessel Wall Magnetic Resonance Imaging in Angiogram-Negative Non-Perimesencephalic Subarachnoid Hemorrhage. Clin Neuroradiol. 2015

[3] Agid R, Andersson T, Almqvist H, et al. Negative CT angiography findings in patients with spontaneous subarachnoid hemorrhage: When is digital subtraction angiography still needed? AJNR Am J Neuroradiol. 2010; 31(4): 696–705

10.3 Sulcal Subarachnoid Hemorrhage

10.3.1 Clinical Case

A 65-year-old male with seizure and a known history of mild cognitive impairment (▶ Fig. 10.6).

10.3.2 Description of Imaging Findings and Diagnosis

Focal sulcal SAH overlying the right frontal lobe. MRI demonstrates multiple T2* hypointensities consistent with microhemorrhages. Findings consistent with amyloid angiopathy.

10.3.3 Background

Sulcal, convexal, or atypical SAH is defined as a hemorrhage isolated to the cerebral sulci without associated intraventricular or basal cistern blood products. Hemorrhage can be identified on CT or on hemosiderin sensitive sequences such as SWI and GRE on MRI. Approximately 5% of all spontaneous SAH are thought to be due to sulcal subarachnoid hemorrhage (sSAH). The differential diagnosis of sulcal sSAH is broad and includes remote aneurysmal SAH, trauma, reversible cerebral vasoconstriction syndrome, cerebral amyloid angiopathy, posterior reversible encephalopathy syndrome, cerebral venous thrombosis, septic emboli, coagulopathy, moyamoya disease, superficial vascular malformation (including cavernoma or AVM), dural AVF, tumor,

and vasculitis. The largest series to date on sSAH included 88 patients and the authors found that reversible cerebral vasoconstriction syndrome and cerebral amyloid angiopathy each comprised approximately 30% of causes of sSAH. In approximately 20% of cases however, the cause was indeterminate.

There are two main clinical presentations for sSAH. Younger patients are more likely to have reversible cerebral vasoconstriction syndrome and often present with a thunderclap headache which can sometimes be accompanied by neurological deficits or stroke. Meanwhile, older patients, who are more likely to have cerebral amyloid angiopathy, can present with transient motor or neurological symptoms presumably due to cortical irritation by blood in the subarachnoid space. Patients with sSAH can also present with altered mental status, seizures, confusion, or lethargy.

10.3.4 Imaging Findings

Identification and definition of sSAH is relatively straight forward, the challenge presents itself in determining the cause of the sSAH. On CT, curvilinear hyperdensity within the surface sulci of the brain is the finding. On MRI, it is defined by curvilinear T2* artifact or FLAIR hyperintensity along the surface sulci. Any patient with a sSAH should undergo noninvasive vascular imaging including CTA or MRA. This is needed to identify an underlying vascular lesion such as a tiny aneurysm, superficial vascular malformation, vasoconstriction, or vasculitis. The diagnostic yield of vascular imaging in patients with sSAH is high at around 66%. DSA is generally not indicated in the evaluation of sSAH. DSA should only be considered after all

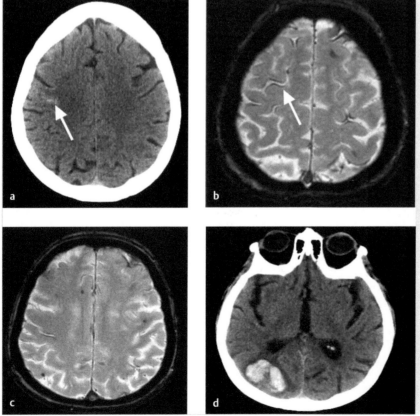

Fig. 10.6 A 71-year-old male with amyloid angiopathy first presenting with sulcal SAH. (a) Non-contrast CT demonstrates subtle SAH overlying the right frontal lobe (*arrow*). (b) (*arrow*) and (c). Over the ensuing 3 years, the patient was noted to have gradual cognitive decline. T2*-weighted MRI demonstrates multiple foci of chronic sulcal hemosiderin deposition overlying the bilateral frontal and parietal lobes. In addition, there are multiple foci of microhemorrhage at the gray white junctions bilaterally. Findings were consistent with amyloid angiopathy. (d) The following year, the patient presented with a spontaneous right temporo-occipital intraparenchymal hematoma. This lobar hemorrhage is typical of amyloid angiopathy.

other noninvasive imaging methods have been exhausted including CTA, MRA, and brain MRI. When sending a patient to cerebral angiography with sSAH, the clinician should have a high diagnostic suspicion for a vascular cause such as vasculitis, mycotic aneurysm, or RCVS (▶ Fig. 10.7, ▶ Fig. 10.8). Studies on the role of diagnostic angiography after a negative CTA or MRA have found that the yield is very low (< 5%).

Brain MRI is instrumental in the evaluation of sSAH as it can be helpful in identifying nonvascular causes of sSAH as well as determining if there is evidence of chronic sSAH or infarct associated with the original ictus. Brain MRI imaging with susceptibility weighted sequences is essential in the diagnosis and characterization of cerebral amyloid angiopathy and can also be helpful in identifying thrombosed mycotic aneurysms. Brain MRI imaging is also essential to the diagnosis of angiographically negative vascular pathologies such as cavernous malformations, posterior reversible encephalopathy syndrome, and cerebral venous thrombosis. In cases where no clear etiology is present, repeat brain MRI can be considered.

Advanced VWI has emerged as a useful tool in differentiating various vascular pathologies that can present with sSAH. Both RCVS and vasculitis can present with sSAH, and at times can have a similar presentation. In cases where CSF testing and serum biomarkers are negative or indeterminate, advanced VWI can help in distinguishing between vasculitis and RCVS, both of which demonstrate multifocal vascular narrowing on angiographic imaging. In vasculitis, there is typically circumferential enhancement of the vessel wall whereas in RCVS there is no wall enhancement.

10.3.5 What the Clinician Needs to Know

- Important to provide clinician with differential diagnosis for sSAH as well as which imaging modalities/sequences can be considered to narrow the differential.
- Vascular imaging and T2*-weighted imaging have a very high diagnostic yield in these cases. Vascular imaging can identify

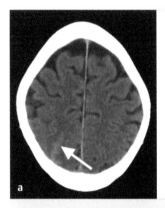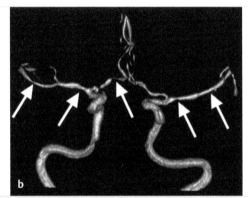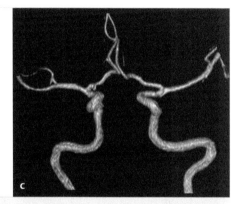

Fig. 10.7 Sulcal subarachnoid hemorrhage (sSAH) from reversible cerebral vasoconstriction syndrome. (a) Non-contrast CT shows subtle sulcal SAH overlying the right parietal lobe (*arrow*). (b) MIP image from MRA demonstrates multifocal narrowing of the proximal cerebral vasculature including the bilateral MCAs and ACAs (*arrow*). (c) After 6 weeks of verapamil treatment, there is reversal of the vascular narrowing. Findings were consistent with reversible cerebral vasoconstriction syndrome.

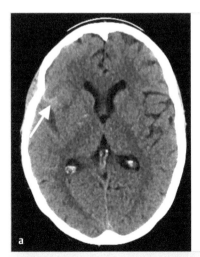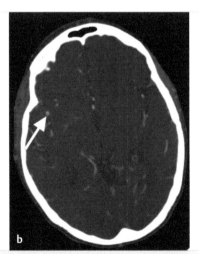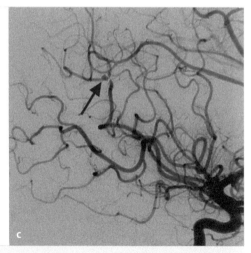

Fig. 10.8 Sulcal subarachnoid hemorrhage from mycotic aneurysm. (a) Non-contrast CT demonstrates focal sulcal subarachnoid hemorrhage overlying the right frontal lobe (*arrow*). (b) At the site of hemorrhage on the CTA, there is a focal aneurysmal dilatation of an MCA branch, concerning for mycotic aneurysm in this 28-year-old IV drug user (*arrow*). (c) Cerebral angiography was performed which demonstrated a mycotic aneurysm of a frontal MCA branch on a right ICA cerebral angiogram oblique projection (*arrow*).

RCVS while T2*-weighted imaging can help identify amyloid angiopathy. These are the two most common causes of sSAH.

10.3.6 High-yield Facts

- The differential diagnosis of sSAH is broad and includes trauma, reversible cerebral vasoconstriction syndrome, cerebral amyloid angiopathy, posterior reversible encephalopathy syndrome, cerebral venous thrombosis, septic embolic, coagulopathy, moyamoya disease, superficial vascular malformation, tumor, and vasculitis.

- Amyloid angiopathy is most common cause in the elderly and RCVS in the young.
- Clinical symptoms at presentation are a major component in making the diagnosis.

Further Reading

[1] Graff-Radford J, Fugate JE, Klaas J, Flemming KD, Brown RD, Rabinstein AA. Distinguishing clinical and radiological features of nontraumatic convexal subarachnoid hemorrhage. Eur J Neurol. 2016; 23(5):839–846
[2] Marder CP, Narla V, Fink JR, Tozer Fink KR. Subarachnoid hemorrhage: beyond aneurysms. AJR Am J Roentgenol. 2014; 202(1):25–37

10.4 Isolated Intraventricular Hemorrhage

10.4.1 Clinical Case

A 43-year-old female with headache and drowsiness (▶ Fig. 10.9).

10.4.2 Description of Imaging Findings and Diagnosis

Dense intraventricular blood in the left lateral ventricle. CTA demonstrates a focal aneurysm projecting into the left lateral ventricle. Cerebral angiography confirmed the presence of the aneurysm supplied by the left posterior choroidal artery as well as bilateral ICA occlusions from moyamoya disease (▶ Fig. 10.10).

10.4.3 Background

Primarily intraventricular hemorrhage is defined as hemorrhage isolated to the ventricular system without associated intraparenchymal hemorrhage, or basilar cistern subarachnoid hemorrhage. This entity is very rare and comprises approximately 1% of patients with intracerebral hemorrhage. By far, the most common etiology for primary intraventricular hemorrhage is hypertension with most series reporting that approximately 50–80% of patients with primary intraventricular hemorrhage have severe hypertension. Other series suggest that vascular malformations comprise a sizeable minority of patients with primary intraventricular hemorrhage with about 10–30% of cases being related to the presence of a vascular malformation. Coagulopathy is found in about 10% of intraventricular hemorrhage patients. In approximately one-fifth of cases, the cause of intraventricular hemorrhage remains unknown.

The most common presentation of patients with primary intraventricular hemorrhage is altered mental status and headache. About 25% of patients present with nausea and vomiting and about 10% of patients present with seizure. Hydrocephalus is found in approximately 50% of patients and approximately 50% of patients require EVD placement.

10.4.4 Imaging Findings

Identification of intraventricular hemorrhage is straightforward. Perhaps, the biggest diagnostic dilemma in these cases is whether the hemorrhage is primarily intraventricular or if it is

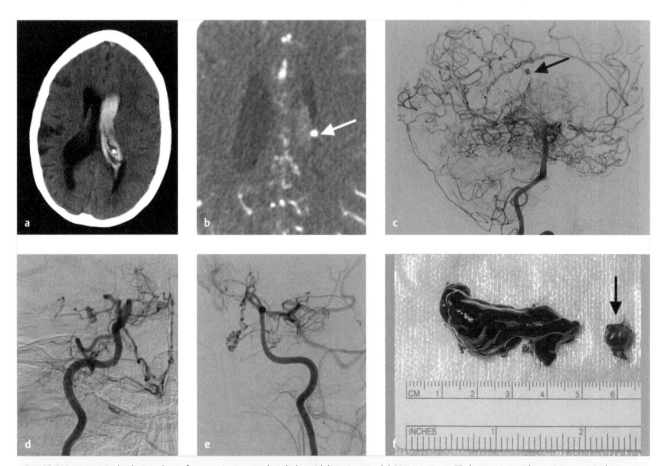

Fig. 10.9 Intraventricular hemorrhage from moyamoya-related choroidal aneurysm. (**a**) Non-contrast CT demonstrates dense intraventricular hemorrhage isolated to the left lateral ventricle. (**b**) CTA demonstrates a focal aneurysm of a subependymal vessel in the left lateral ventricle (*arrow*). (**c**) Cerebral angiography confirms the aneurysm, which arises from the posterior choroidal artery (*arrow*). There are extensive splenial collateral and leptomeningeal collaterals as well, which are typical of moyamoya disease. (**d**) Right internal carotid artery and (**e**) left internal carotid artery cerebral angiograms demonstrate occlusion of the supraclinoid ICAs bilaterally, consistent with moyamoya. (**f**) Operative specimen including the evacuated hematoma and the resected aneurysm (*arrow*).

intraparenchymal or subependymal bleed with intraventricular extension. This differentiation is important because it can guide the diagnostic work-up in the patient. For example, if there is hemorrhage in the caudate nucleus that dissects into the ventricular system and the patient is known to have a history of hypertension, one may be satisfied with a negative CTA that the hemorrhage was related to hypertension (▶ Fig. 10.10). However, if the hemorrhage is isolated to the ventricular system, one must be more discerning and rule out a whole host of entities, including vascular lesions and metastatic disease. Key information that must be relayed to the primary team includes extent of hemorrhage, location of hemorrhage, where the densest amount of clot is and the severity of hydrocephalus. If a

vascular malformation is identified, identification of a false aneurysm pointing into the ventricle from a subependymal or a choroidal feeder has to be sought for.

Many authors recommend routine CTA or MRA in patients with intraventricular hemorrhage in order to exclude a vascular lesion. MRI with contrast is a mainstay in work-up of patients with primary intraventricular hemorrhage-particularly to rule out a neoplasm. Repeat MRI should be performed if the initial one is negative. As already mentioned, approximately 20% of patients with a primary intraventricular hemorrhage will have a vascular lesion that is responsible for the hemorrhage (i.e., microaneurysm, choroidal arteriovenous malformation, etc.) (▶ Fig. 10.11). Close attention should be paid to any abnormal intraventricular

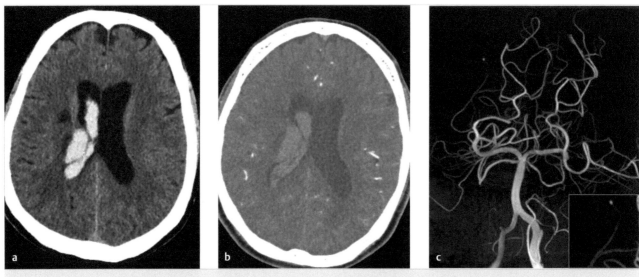

Fig. 10.10 Intraparenchymal hematoma with intraventricular extension secondary to Bouchard aneurysm. (a) Non-contrast CT demonstrates hemorrhage in the posterior body of the caudate with extension into the right lateral ventricle. (b) CTA demonstrates no vascular abnormality to account for the hemorrhage. The patient was very hypertensive at presentation. (c) Because the patient was only 54 years old, a cerebral angiogram was performed to rule out vascular malformation. This demonstrates a tiny Bouchard aneurysm.

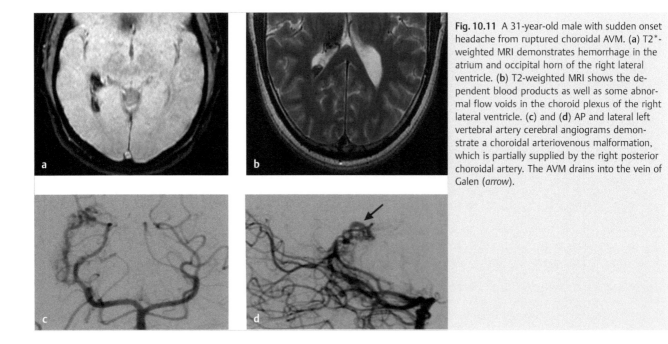

Fig. 10.11 A 31-year-old male with sudden onset headache from ruptured choroidal AVM. (a) T2*-weighted MRI demonstrates hemorrhage in the atrium and occipital horn of the right lateral ventricle. (b) T2-weighted MRI shows the dependent blood products as well as some abnormal flow voids in the choroid plexus of the right lateral ventricle. (c) and (d) AP and lateral left vertebral artery cerebral angiograms demonstrate a choroidal arteriovenous malformation, which is partially supplied by the right posterior choroidal artery. The AVM drains into the vein of Galen (arrow).

vascular flow voids or subependymal enhancement which can clue one in on the presence of a vascular lesion. DSA can be considered in cases in which CTA or MRA is equivocal and where no offending lesion is identified on MRI. In cases in which the initial CTA, MRA, and MRI is negative, the yield of DSA is low (~5%) but not negligible.

10.4.5 What the Clinician Needs to Know

- The presence or absence of any intraparenchymal hemorrhage which could suggest that the hemorrhage was an intraparenchymal hemorrhage which extended into the ventricular system.
- The severity of hydrocephalus and extent/location of hemorrhage; particularly, the area of densest hemorrhage.
- In cases where no etiology is identified on CTA/MRA and MRI, DSA plays a role in.

10.4.6 High-yield Facts

- Most common causes of primary intraventricular hemorrhage include hypertension, vascular lesion (AVM, microaneuyrsm, etc.), coagulopathy, and neoplasm. In 20% of cases, cause is unknown.
- All intraventricular hemorrhage patients should undergo vascular imaging and MRI. Repeat MRI and DSA should be considered in cases where etiology is not identified.

Further Reading

[1] Weinstein R, Ess K, Sirdar B, Song S, Cutting S. Primary Intraventricular Hemorrhage: Clinical Characteristics and Outcomes. J Stroke Cerebrovasc Dis. 2017; 26(5):995–999

[2] Marder CP, Narla V, Fink JR, Tozer Fink KR. Subarachnoid hemorrhage: beyond aneurysms. AJR Am J Roentgenol. 2014; 202(1):25–37

10.5 Spontaneous Intraparenchymal Hemorrhage

10.5.1 Clinical Case

A 67-year-old male with headache, drowsiness, no history of trauma. BP 250/120 (▶ Fig. 10.12).

10.5.2 Description of Imaging Findings and Diagnosis

Intraparenchymal hemorrhage in the ventrolateral left thalamus and internal capsule with intraventricular extension; hypertensive etiology suspected.

10.5.3 Background

Primary intraparenchymal hemorrhage is the second most common cause of stroke and is associated with high rates of morbidity and mortality. The pathogenesis of ICH is generally due to rupture of tiny blood vessels, which are deeply embedded in the brain parenchyma. Common clinical presentation includes focal neurological deficits, severe headache, hypertension, vomiting, and decreased level of consciousness.

In general, the prognosis of primary ICH is very poor with a majority of patients suffering permanent morbidity and mortality. There has been a lot of interest in determining the prognosis of ICH as well as the risk of hematoma expansion. The ICH score is probably the most widespread scoring system used for determining ICH prognosis. It factors in variables including Glasgow Coma Scale, ICH volume, presence of intraventricular hemorrhage, location of hemorrhage, and age (▶ Table 10.2). Regarding management, medical management in the acute setting is a key factor for preventing or abating morbidity and mortality. Regarding surgical treatment; patients with cerebellar hemorrhage > 3 cm in diameter or those with brainstem compression or hydrocephalus are often treated with surgical decompression and hematoma evaluation. Brainstem hemorrhages are usually managed conservatively. The beneficial effects of surgical management of supratentorial ICH is controversial and is usually reserved for patients with neurological deterioration, significant midline shift or medically intractable intracranial pressure.

10.5.4 Imaging Findings

When evaluating a patient with an intraparenchymal hemorrhage, it helps to have a standard checklist. Important imaging findings that need to be reported include: (1) hematoma volume (cm³), (2) the location of hemorrhage (supratentorial, brainstem, and cerebellum), (3) the presence of intraventricular extension of the hematoma, (4) the presence of hydrocephalus, (5) extension to other extra-axial spaces (i.e., subdural, subarachnoid, etc.), (6) mass effect including midline shift, downward, or upward herniation, (7) risk factors for hemataoma expansion, and (8) the presence of any imaging findings that would suggest a secondary

Table 10.2 ICH Score

Component	ICH Score Points
GCS Score	
3–4	2
5–12	1
13–15	0
ICH Volume (cm³)	
≥ 30	1
< 30	0
IVH	
Yes	1
No	0
Infratentorial origin of ICH	
Yes	1
No	0
Age	
≥ 80	1
< 80	0

Abbreviations: ICH, Intracerebral hemorrhage; GCS, Glasgow coma scale, IVH, Intraventricular haemorrhage.

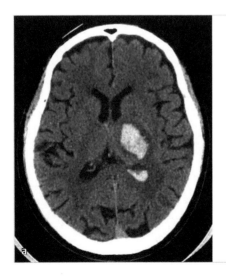 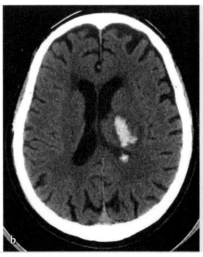

Fig. 10.12 Classic deep hemorrhage secondary to hypertension in an elderly male. (a) and (b). Non-contrast CT demonstrates intraparenchymal hemorrhage in the ventrolateral left thalamus and internal capsule with intraventricular extension.

source such as a tumor, aneurysm, arteriovenous malformation, amyloid angiopathy, venous thrombosis, etc.

Regarding hematoma location, a deep location (i.e., basal ganglia, pons, and thalamus) is strongly suggestive of a hypertensive cause. Often, these patients will have other stigmata of chronic hypertension such as T2 hyperintensities in these deep structures as well as deep structure microhemorrhages. Lobar hemorrhages have a broader differential including amyloid angiopathy, distal aneurysms, hypertension, vasospastic diseases, tumors, coagulopathies, vasculitis, and venous thrombosis.

Regarding hematoma volume, the most commonly used formula/technique is the abc/2 method. "a" is the largest cross-sectional diameter of the hematoma, "b" is the diameter of the hematoma measured at a right angle to "a" and "c" is the height, measured either on the coronal images or by determining the number of slices, which contain the hematoma. More accurate and reproducible methods for the evaluation of hematoma volume will likely come to the forefront with the rise of artificial intelligence.

One of the key roles of imaging in evaluating intraparenchymal hematomas is determining the risk of hematoma expansion. The CTA "spot sign" has emerged as one of the most consistent imaging findings to be associated with hematoma expansion. The presence of a focal area of vascular enhancement within the hematoma, aka a spot, is strongly associated with hematoma expansion. In fact, > 90% of hematomas with a spot sign will expand whereas > 90% of hematomas without a spot sign will remain stable. Another imaging finding that has been associated with hematoma expansion is the CT swirl sign. The CT swirl sign is defined as a swirling pattern of mixed attenuation (low and high) with a hematoma on non-contrast CT. The mixed attenuation is a result of both clotted (bright) and non-clotted flowing blood (dark). One advantage of this sign is the lack of need for a CTA; however, it has yet to be validated as extensively as the CTA spot sign. Examples of patients with both the CTA spot and CT swirl sign is provided in ▸ Fig. 10.13 and ▸ Fig. 10.14.

CTA has become a standard part of the workup for intraparenchymal hemorrhage. Its value lies in its ability to determine whether a hematoma is at risk of expansion (i.e., spot sign), as well as excluding vascular pathologies as the source of hemorrhage. Lesions such as lenticulostriate/bouchard aneurysms (▸ Fig. 10.14), saccular aneurysms (▸ Fig. 10.15), arteriovenous malformations, venous thrombosis, reversible cerebral vasoconstriction, vasculitis, and developmental venous anomalies can all present with isolated intraparenchymal hemorrhage. Identification of structural causes for an isolated intraparenchymal hemorrhage is essential to allow for further treatment. Because the initial hematoma can compress the culprit lesion, repeat CTA in 3 months is generally recommended. DSA can be considered in select cases where no clear etiology is identified on clinical history or cross-sectional imaging.

Aside from vascular causes, isolated intraparenchymal hemorrhage can be due to underlying mass lesions such as primary tumors and metastases. For these reasons, most centers do perform brain MRI with contrast in the work-up for intraparenchymal hemorrhage. Because subacute hematoma is T1 bright, it can mask the presence of any underlying enhancement. For this reason, even when the initial MRI is negative, MRI is often repeated a few months later. In elderly patient, the most common cause of lobar hemorrhage is amyloid angiopathy. This is discussed in a previous chapter, but the presence of multiple microhemorrhages in a patient with an isolated lobar hemorrhage is more or less diagnostic of amyloid angiopathy (▸ Fig. 10.16).

10.5.5 What the Clinician Needs to Know

- Imaging findings indicating a high risk for hematoma expansion.
- The severity of hydrocephalus and mass effect and extent/location of hemorrhage-particularly the area of densest hemorrhage.

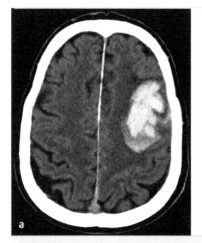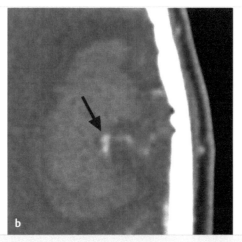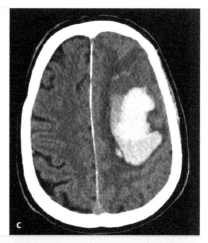

Fig. 10.13 Example of expanding hematoma with CTA spot sign. (a) Non-contrast CT shows a mixed density hematoma measuring 5 cm in maximum diameter. There is also a suggestion of a CT swirl sign. (b) CTA shows a focal area of enhancement, aka the CTA spot sign, in the middle of the hematoma (arrow). (c) Follow-up CT performed for increasing drowsiness shows expansion of the hematoma.

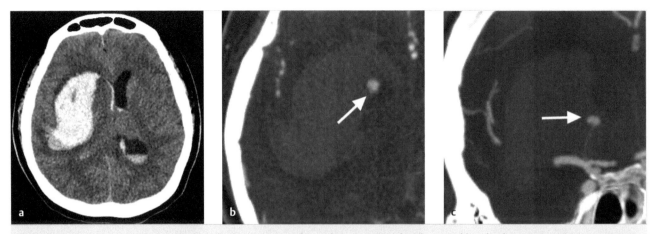

Fig. 10.14 Deep hemorrhage with intraventricular extension secondary to hypertension induced ruptured bouchard aneurysm. (a) Non-contrast CT shows a large intraparenchymal hematoma in the right basal ganglia and deep white matter with rightward shift and intraventricular hemorrhage. (b) CTA shows a focal area of enhancement in the hematoma, a spot sign (*arrow*). (c) Coronal CTA shows that the spot sign is in fact a bouchard aneurysm at the end of a lateral lenticulostriate vessel (*arrow*).

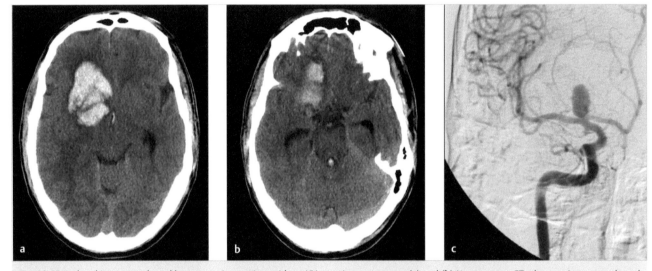

Fig. 10.15 Isolated intraparenchymal hematoma in a patient with an ICA terminus aneurysm. (a) and (b) Non-contrast CTs show an intraparenchymal hematoma in the right basal ganglia and frontal lobe. (c) DSA shows a large, superiorly projecting ICA terminus aneurysm, which was the cause of the hemorrhage.

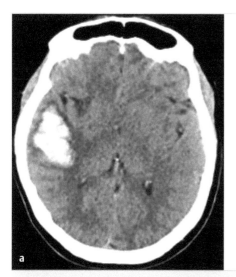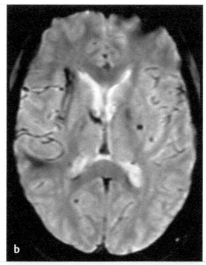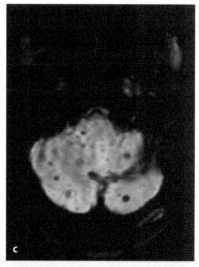

Fig. 10.16 Lobar hemorrhage from amyloid angiopathy in an 84-year-old patient. (**a**) Non-contrast CT shows a lobar hemorrhage in the right temporal lobe. (**b**) and (**c**). T2*MRI shows multiple punctate microhemorrhages in the bilateral cerebral and cerebellar hemispheres. This imaging finding is classic for amyloid angiopathy.

- Secondary causes for parenchymal hemorrhage.
- In cases where no etiology is identified on CTA/MRA and MRI, DSA plays a role in diagnosis and should be considered.

10.5.6 High-yield Facts

- Most common cause of deep hemorrhage is hypertension and most common cause of lobar hemorrhage in elderly patients is amyloid angiopathy.

- CTA spot sign has a > 90% positive predictive value (PPV) and negative predictive value (NPV) for hematoma expansion.

Further Reading

[1] Demchuk AM, Dowlatshahi D, Rodriguez-Luna D, et al. PREDICT/Sunnybrook ICH CTA study group. Prediction of haematoma growth and outcome in patients with intracerebral haemorrhage using the CT-angiography spot sign (PREDICT): a prospective observational study. Lancet Neurol. 2012; 11(4): 307–314

[2] Koculym A, Huynh TJ, Jakubovic R, Zhang L, Aviv RI. CT perfusion spot sign improves sensitivity for prediction of outcome compared with CTA and post-contrast CT. AJNR Am J Neuroradiol. 2013; 34(5):965–970, S1

Chapter 11

Spinal Vascular Disease

11 Spinal Vascular Disease

11.1 Spinal Cord Infarction

11.1.1 Clinical Case

A 67-year-old male with sudden onset paraplegia following a motor vehicle accident (▶ Fig. 11.1).

11.1.2 Description of Imaging Findings and Diagnosis

Diagnosis

T2 hyperintensity in the anterior spinal cord with associated restricted diffusion. There is a small disc protrusion at the level of the signal abnormality. Findings consistent with cord infarct, possibly related to fibrocartilaginous embolism.

11.1.3 Background

Given the dense anastomotic network, spinal cord infarcts are rare and account for 8% of myelopathies. Spinal cord infarction presents with abrupt onset of pain in 60–70% of cases. Pain is generally located at the dermatomal level of the cord along with weakness and/or sensory loss, with the possible loss of sphincter tone. In spinal cord arterial infarcts, the constellation of presenting symptoms is determined by the level and artery affected. Anterior spinal artery infarcts are the most common and can be seen in the setting of aortic or spinal procedures. Anterior spinal artery infarcts can cause respiratory compromise and tetraparesis if in the upper cervical segments, and paraplegia in the thoraco-lumbar segments due to corticospinal tract involvement and loss of pain and temperature due to spinothalamic involvement. Posterior spinal artery infarcts are rare and affect the dorsal column and therefore present with isolated loss of vibration and proprioception. Combined anterior and posterior spinal artery infarcts can also be seen from mechanical hyperflexion or hyperextension injuries.

Spinal sulcal artery infarcts presents with a sulcocommisural syndrome also known as Brown Sequard syndrome due to "hemi-cord" involvement. This includes ipsilateral weakness, loss of vibratory sense, and proprioception and contralateral loss of pain and temperature due to the spinothalamic tracts decussation. Central spinal artery infarcts are most likely due to prolonged hypoperfusion from hypotension or cardiac arrest and present with bilateral loss of pain and temperature without any weakness or proprioceptive loss. A complete transverse infarct would lead to bilateral loss of sensation and weakness and more likely due to embolic etiology. Examples of different territories of spinal cord infarcts is provided in ▶ Fig. 11.2.

There are numerous etiologies implicated in spinal cord infarctions including aortic disease, iatrogenic causes, vertebral dissection, emboli (large artery or cardiac), hypercoagulable states (i.e., sickle cell disease, antiphospholipid syndrome, malignancy, etc.), decompression sickness, vasculitis, systemic hypotension or global hypoperfusion from cardiac arrest, radicular artery compression, discocartilagnious emboli, and trauma. However, approximately one-third of spinal cord infarcts do not have an identifiable etiology and therefor deemed to be idiopathic or cryptogenic. Treatments include blood pressure augmentation and sometimes, lumbar drain placement.

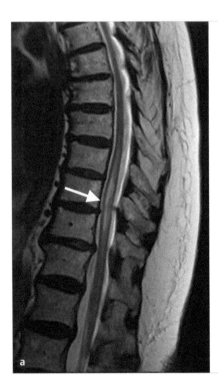
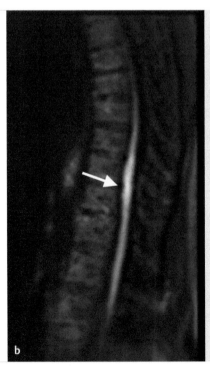

Fig. 11.1 Spinal cord infarct with restricted diffusion possibly related to fibrocartilaginous embolism. (a) Sagittal T2-weighted MRI demonstrates high T2 cord signal from T8-T10 (*arrow*). There was no fracture or epidural hematoma seen in this patient who had suffered light trauma. Note the small disc protrusions at the T9-T10 and T10-T11 levels. (b) Sagittal diffusion weighted imaging (DWI) MRI of the spine demonstrates restricted diffusion at the level of the T2 hyperintensity (*arrow*) which was confirmed on the apparent diffusion coefficient (ADC) map (not shown).

11.1.4 Imaging Findings

MRI is the preferred imaging modality for diagnosis of a spinal cord infarction; however, it is not very sensitive in detecting acute spinal cord infarction. Urgent MRI is vital in excluding other diagnosis on the differential with the most urgent being spinal cord compression. MRI can also be useful in differentiating spinal cord infarction from other vascular myelopathies (i.e., vascular malformations) or autoimmune myelopathies. Lumbar puncture is generally recommended to rule out an inflammatory etiology.

The ideal protocol for the assessment of spinal cord ischemia is sagittal spin-echo T2 or T2- STIR, sagittal spin echo T1, axial gradient echo T2 in the cervical spine and axial spin-echo T2 of the thoracic and lumbar spine. Diffusion-weighted imaging (DWI) should be performed in both the axial and sagittal planes in order to give the radiologist two shots at identifying the infarct. DWI is rife with technical challenges; however, due to motion artifact from physiological spinal cord movement, susceptibility artifacts and low signal-to-noise ratio due to the small pixel size required for appropriate imaging of the spinal cord. Contrast is not necessary but is helpful in excluding inflammatory, infectious, and neoplastic etiologies. The sensitivity of DWI in detecting acute spinal cord infarcts varies across studies, but more recent studies have suggested it is on the order of 90%. There is typically no role for spinal vascular imaging in the setting of spinal cord infarction. However, CTA of the neck, chest, abdomen, and pelvis can be helpful in identifying potential culprits such as atheroma, dissection or aneurysm (▶ Fig. 11.3).

In the acute phase, spinal cord infarction presents with restricted diffusion and T2 hyperintensity (▶ Fig. 11.1). Enhancement can occur in the subacute phase (▶ Fig. 11.4). Infarction in the anterior spinal artery territory includes the anterior horns with or without adjacent white matter changes. Isolated gray matter changes are due to the fact that the gray matter is more vulnerable to ischemia. This gives a characteristic "owl eyes" appearance. Posterior spinal cord infarcts affect the posterior columns and/or surrounding white matter and can be unilateral or bilateral.

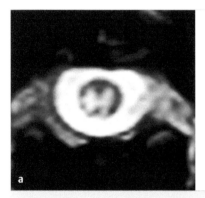 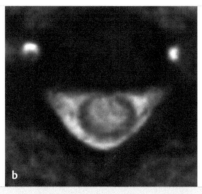 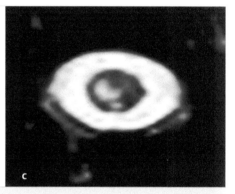

Fig. 11.2 Various patterns of spinal cord infarction on axial T2 MRI. (**a**) Sulcocommisural artery infarct affecting entirety of grey matter with sparing of white matter tracts. (**b**) Anterior spinal artery infarct affecting both grey and white matter. (**c**) Hemicord infarct resulting from occlusion of a sulcocommisural artery branch. This resulted in a Brown-Sequard syndrome.

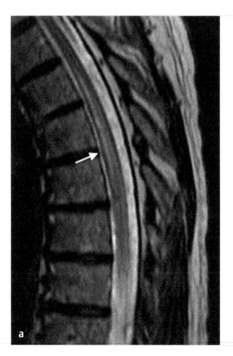 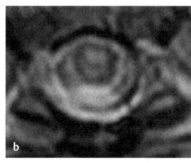 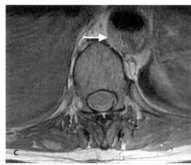

Fig. 11.3 Spinal cord infarct secondary to aortic dissection. (**a**) Sagittal T2-weighted MRI demonstrates high cord signal in the anterior portion of the cord extending 4 levels (*arrow*). (**b**) Axial T2-weighted MRI demonstrates high T2 signal affecting the nearly the entirety of the cross-section of the spinal cord. (**c**) Larger field of view axial T2-weighted MRI demonstrates a large intramural hematoma of the descending thoracic aorta consistent with dissection (*arrow*). This was the cause of the patient's infarct.

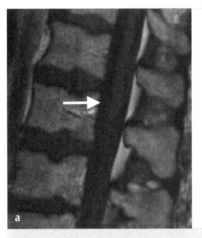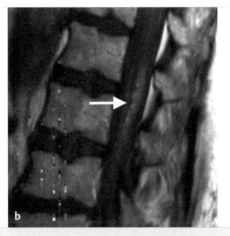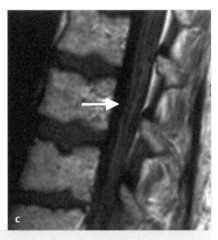

Fig. 11.4 Time onset of enhancement in cord infarct. Sagittal post-contrast T1-weighted MRIs at days 1 (**a**), 9 (**b**), and 19 (**c**) post-symptom onset. Note the absence of enhancement at day 1 (*arrow*) (**a**), marked enhancement at day 9 (*arrow*) (**b**), and faint enhancement at 19 (*arrow*) (**c**).

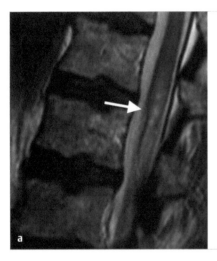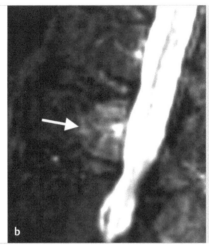

Fig. 11.5 Conus infarct with vertebral body infarct. (**a**) Sagittal T2-weighted MRI demonstrates high signal in the conus medullaris (*arrow*). (**b**) Sagittal T2 STIR MRI demonstrates high marrow signal of the posterior aspect of the L1 vertebral body. The presence of the high conus signal along with the high vertebral body is diagnostic of a segmental artery infarction result in both cord and vertebral body infarcts (*arrow*).

Myelomalacia can be seen in the infarct territory in the chronic phase. Vertebral body infarct has been reported in the setting of spinal cord infarct as well and presents with high T2 signal and enhancement of the body and adjacent disc (▶ Fig. 11.5). Hemorrhagic transformation is rare.

Distinguishing spinal cord infarction from other causes of myelopathy is essential. The most common mimicker is demyelinating disease. In demyelinating disease the lesions typically are smaller than cord infarct and involve the lateral and posterior aspects of the cord. Venous ischemia from congestive myelopathy (i.e., dural fistula) will result in cord expansion and diffuse T2 cord signal usually involving the conus and extending superiorly.

11.1.5 What the Clinician Needs to Know

- Any imaging findings that can help point to an etiology for the cord infarct (i.e., dissection, aortic aneurysm, atheroma, etc.).
- Distinguishing characteristics of spinal cord infarct from potentially reversible causes of myelopathy.

- The presence of any mechanical injury which could have caused the infarct (i.e., cervical canal stenosis, compression of radicular artery by disc material, etc.).

11.1.6 High-yield Facts

- DWI is essential to the diagnosis of spinal cord infarction.
- The distribution of spinal cord infarct is highly dependent on the type of artery affected. Owl eye appearance is seen in anterior spinal artery infarct.
- Spinal cord infarcts can enhance in subacute phase.

Further Reading

[1] Nogueira RG, Ferreira R, Grant PE, et al. Restricted diffusion in spinal cord infarction demonstrated by magnetic resonance line scan diffusion imaging. Stroke. 2012; 43(2):532–535

[2] Vargas MI, Gariani J, Sztajzel R, et al. Spinal cord ischemia: practical imaging tips, pearls, and pitfalls. AJNR Am J Neuroradiol. 2015; 36(5):825–830

11.2 Spinal Dural Arteriovenous Fistula (MRI Findings)

11.2.1 Clinical Case

A 68-year-old right-handed white female who presents right lower extremity weakness with difficulty of getting off low chairs and difficulty going up stairs. Provided MRI interpreted as negative for cord or nerve root compression.

11.2.2 Description of Imaging Findings and Diagnosis

T2 hyperintensity of the conus with associated flow voids running up the dorsal aspect of the cord. Findings most consistent with spinal dural fistula or other spinal vascular malformation (▶ Fig. 11.6).

11.2.3 Background

Spinal dural arteriovenous fistulas (SDAVF) are spinal vascular lesions that classically present with vague symptoms such as leg dysesthesias and exertional leg weakness, but slowly progress to severe myelopathy with paraplegia and sphincter dysfunction. The slow and insidious onset of symptoms is generally considered to be the reason why so many of these lesions are diagnosed late or misdiagnosed. SDAVFs have been reported to be misdiagnosed and even treated as peripheral neuropathy, radiculopathies, multiple sclerosis, intramedullary tumors, neuromyelitis optica, and transverse myelitis. Furthermore, because of the demographic characteristics of patients affected by these lesions (typically, older men), they are often misdiagnosed as central spinal canal stenosis secondary to degenerative changes. The consequences of misdiagnosis are severe as each month in delay of diagnosis results in added morbidity which is often irreversible. With or without initial misdiagnosis, diagnostic delays are common and can be quite long. In fact, the estimated time from clinical symptom onset to diagnosis ranges from 11 to 27 months depending on the series.

It has been proposed that SDAVFs result from loss of normal physiologic control of the glomeruli of Manelfe, a structure located between two layers of dura mater that is composed of two or more arterioles converging with a vascular ball (glomerulus) and being drained by a single intradural vein. However, the means by which the glomeruli of Manelfe lose their ability to be physiologically controlled is still unknown. Following formation of the fistula between the radiculomeningeal artery and radicular vein, venous congestion along the longitudinal venous network draining the spinal cord can occur. Congestion is generally most marked in the conus due to its dependent location resulting in the classic sensorimotor deficits and bowel and bladder symptoms. Progression of the lesion results in increased venous congestion and, in turn, chronic hypoxia and progressive myelopathy with the worsening of symptoms. The onset of symptoms is often insidious and can take place years after the fistula develops. In general, when left untreated, symptomatic SDAVFs progress to severe irreversible myelopathy with paraparesis and sphincter dysfunction. While the natural history of asymptomatic, incidentally discovered SDAVFs is unknown, it is believed that they will progress to become symptomatic with progressive loss of radicular venous outlets and thus formation of venous congestion.

11.2.4 Imaging Findings

MRI is essential to diagnosis of SDAVFs. These lesions have a characteristic appearance which includes T2 signal intensity of the conus extending superiorly across multiple segments (95% of cases), serpiginous enlarged intradural vessels seen as flow voids on T2-weighted imaging that are more pronounced along the dorsal compared to the ventral aspect of the cord (96% of cases) and

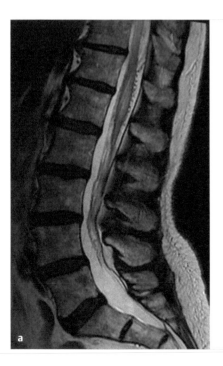 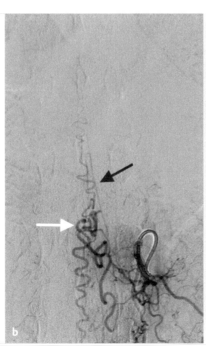

Fig. 11.6 SDAVF missed on initial MRI. **(a)** Sagittal T2-weighted MRI of the lumbar spine performed for evaluation of lower extremity weakness demonstrates no disc disease or cord compression. No note was made of the high signal of the conus medullaris nor the prominent flow voids running up along the conus and down the cauda equina. Repeat interpretation of the MRI at a tertiary referral center prompted a spinal angiogram **(b)** which demonstrated the fistula and a dilated coronal venous plexus (*white arrow*) supplied by the left T12 intercostal artery. The presence of both posterior and anterior spinal arteries at this level precluded embolization (*black arrow*).

sometimes, gadolinium enhancement of the cord itself (80% of cases). Of note, cord enhancement is often patchy (▶ Fig. 11.7). High conus signal is unrelated to the level of the fistula due to the fact that the pathophysiology of the lesion is due to venous congestion, which affects the inferior aspect of the cord first.

Despite the characteristic imaging findings, up to 50% of these lesions are missed on initial imaging evaluation (▶ Fig. 11.7). Because most of these patients will only receive imaging of the lumbar spine without contrast during the initial evaluation of their symptoms, oftentimes the only sign of a SDAVF will be a slightly increased signal in the conus with flow voids. These "edge of the film" findings are commonly missed, highlighting the importance for the radiologist to specifically

examine the conus in every lumbar spine MRI. In cases of patients with unexplained myelopathy, a spinal MRA should be considered as a SDAVF is present in up to 30% of these patients. Spinal contrast-enhanced, time resolved MRA has a high sensitivity for the detection of SDAVFs. In cases where there is a high clinical suspicion, conventional spinal angiography should be performed as it is both safe, and the gold standard for detection of SDAVFs. In cases where an artery cannot be accessed or assessed on the first attempt, there should be a low threshold for repeat angiography at a later date in order to ensure that all vessels are fully evaluated.

Of note, there are some imaging findings which can help in the localization of the fistula. One finding which has been

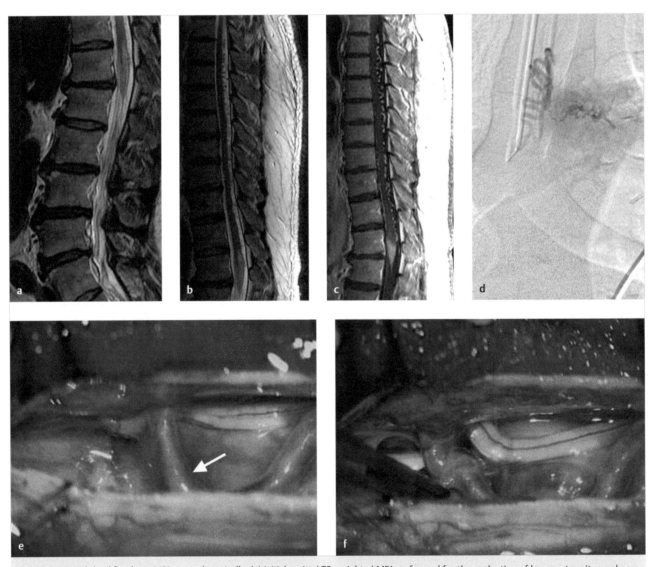

Fig. 11.7 Missed dural fistula on MRI, treated surgically. **(a)** Initial sagittal T2-weighted MRI performed for the evaluation of lower extremity weakness demonstrates high cord signal of the conus, an edge of the film finding. This was interpreted as negative, aside from a few degenerative disc findings. The patient's myelopathy progressed, prompting a thoracic spine MRI. **(b)** Sagittal T2-weighted MRI of the thoracic spine demonstrated high conus signal (again) and prominent flow voids running up the cord for ten levels. **(c)** Sagittal T1 post-contrast MRI demonstrates marked enhancement of the conus and enhancement of the previously mentioned flow voids. These findings are consistent with engorgement of the coronal venous plexus from venous congestive myelopathy. **(d)** Spinal angiogram at the T8 level demonstrates the dural fistula with the marked dilatation and tortuosity of the intradural veins. **(e)** The patient was brought to surgery. Following laminectomy and durotomy at the T8 level, a prominent dilated vein, which was draining the fistula was identified (*arrow*) and **(f)** ligated.

recently described is the presence of a curvilinear vein extending from the sacrum to the conus. This is considered to be an enlarged vein of the filum terminale and is an indicator of a low-lying fistula (i.e., L3 and lower). This can help in guiding where to center a spinal MRA as well as guide the angiographer in knowing where to start the spinal angiogram (▶ Fig. 11.8).

There are many tips and tricks to interpretation of spinal MRAs in localizing a fistula. One key thing to keep in mind is that this needs practice. One piece of advice is as follows: familiarize yourself with dural fistulas and how they look on conventional angiography. Trace out the feeding artery as it arises from the aorta and segmental artery and identify the draining radicular vein and dilated coronal venous plexus. When interpreting spinal MRAs, it helps to look at the images in axial, sagittal, and coronal planes. The coronal plane will be the most likely to demonstrate a similar finding to what is seen on angiography (▶ Fig. 11.9). In general, what one is looking for is a prominent artery/vein coursing under the pedicle and along the expected course of the nerve root. It is important to distinguish between feeding arteries/arteriovenous fistula sites and prominent veins which may be draining the fistula. In order to do this, it helps to follow the course of the prominent foraminal vessel and determine if it connects with the aorta (in which case, this is likely the site of the fistula) or the vena cava (in which case it is a prominent draining vein).

11.2.5 What the Clinician Needs to Know

- The extent of T2 changes and presence of irreversible findings such as myelomalacia and cord atrophy
- Any potential imaging findings which can help identify the level of the fistula
- The role of noninvasive angiography in the assessment of unexplained causes of myelopathy
- IV steroids are contraindicated in SDAVF patients as they can exacerbate the congestive myelopathy

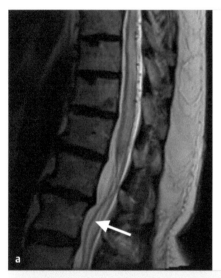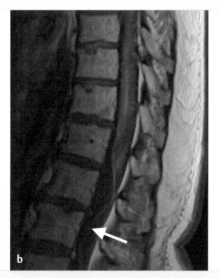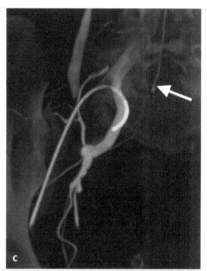

Fig. 11.8 Dilated vein of the Filum terminale indicating lower level fistula. (**a**) Sagittal T2-weighted MRI demonstrated markedly elevated conus and lower cord signal with multiple flow voids. There was also a prominent flow void extending below the conus, which was relatively straight compared to the flow voids coursing along the cord (*arrow*). (**b**) Sagittal T1 post-contrast MRI demonstrates patchy cord enhancement and enhancement of the flow voids coursing along the cord. The already mentioned straight flow void below the conus was enhancing suggesting this to be a vascular structure (*arrow*). Indeed, this was a dilated vein of the filum terminale. This prompted a spinal angiogram focused on the sacral or lower lumbar level. (**c**) The first vessel catheterized was the right internal iliac artery. Indeed, there was a fistula at this level with lateral sacral artery directly fistulizing with the vein of the filum terminale (*arrow*). This was treated endovascularly.

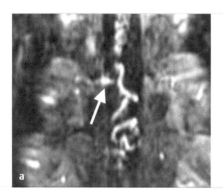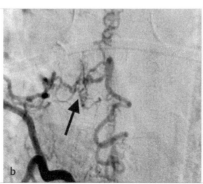

Fig. 11.9 Spinal MRA of spinal dural fistula. (**a**) Coronal reconstruction of a gadolinium bolus spinal MRA of a patient with a fistula supplied by the right T8 intercostal artery. The prominent artery coursing under the pedicle is the arterial feeder (*arrow*). The draining radicular vein is clearly seen as is its connection with the coronal venous plexus. (**b**) Conventional spinal angiogram demonstrates the exact same findings with the prominent radicular artery (*arrow*) and draining vein.

11.2.6 High-yield Facts

- SDAVFs almost always result in T2 changes of the conus, irrespective of the level involved.
- Typical imaging findings include T2 conus signal, vascular flow voids, and cord enhancement.
- The presence of a curvilinear vein extending from sacrum to conus suggests a low-lying fistula.

Further Reading

[1] Krings T, Geibprasert S. Spinal dural arteriovenous fistulas. AJNR Am J Neuroradiol. 2009; 30(4):639–648

[2] Morris JM. Imaging of dural arteriovenous fistula. Radiol Clin North Am. 2012; 50(4):823–839

[3] Brinjikji W, Nasr DM, Morris JM, et al. Clinical Outcomes of Patients with Delayed Diagnosis of Spinal Dural Arteriovenous Fistulas. AJNR Am J Neuroradiol. 2015; 36:1905–1911

11.3 Imaging Appearance of Other Spinal Vascular Malformations

11.3.1 Clinical Case

A 19-year-old female with acute onset lower extremity weakness.

11.3.2 Description of Imaging Findings and Diagnosis

Multiple intramedullary and perimedullary flow voids in the lower thoracic cord with associated cord edema and areas of hemorrhage. Spinal angiography confirms the presence of an intramedullary spinal AVM.

11.3.3 Background

Spinal arteriovenous malformations are a rare but treatable cause of myelopathy. The clinical presentation and ideal treatment of these lesions vary widely, primarily due to differences in anatomic and angioarchitectural features. While the Type I dural arteriovenous fistula is by far the most common spinal vascular malformation, several other types of spinal vascular malformation exist, each with their own unique clinical presentation, treatment strategies, and imaging features.

11.3.4 Imaging Findings

Given the often unspecific clinical symptomatology, responsibility for initial detection of the lesion often falls on the neuroradiologist. Characteristics of spinal vascular malformations, which should be noted include angioarchitecture (described here), location/level, arterial feeders, and effect of the lesion on the cord. Understanding the angioarchitectural characteristics of these lesions is essential and can in most instances only be

achieved by conventional angiography. However, spinal MRA may be used to guide the conventional angiography. A brief overview of the various spinal vascular malformations is provided here.

Intramedullary Spinal AVMs

Intramedullary AVMs have a similar angioarchitecture to cerebral parenchymal arteriovenous malformations in that they consist of a nidus that is embedded within the parenchyma (▶ Fig. 11.10). These lesions generally have multiple arterial feeders and drain into the coronal venous plexus. Arterial feeders can either be direct or indirect. Direct arterial feeders are the angiographically larger branches entering the AVM. These arteries typically are only supplying the AVM and provide little to no supply to the cord itself. In contrast, indirect feeders are smaller caliber vessels which also feed normal territories. These generally form as a result of a sump effect and local collateral circulation recruitment that is enabled through the physiological rich anastomotic network between spinal arteries. About one-third of these lesions have associated aneurysms. On MRI, the effect of these lesions on the cord is usually isolated to the level of the lesion although venous congestion may be present leading to edema distant from the nidus proper. Contrary to high-flow perimedullary fistulas, intramedullary AVMs are typically sporadic, non-hereditary lesions.

Cobb Syndrome

Cobb syndrome, also referred to as juvenile AVMs, or metameric AVMs are complex vascular malformations that involve the spinal cord, vertebral body, epidural space, paraspinal soft tissue, and skin and subcutaneous tissues within one or more of the 31 spinal segments. These lesions typically have both intradural and extradural components. The intradural lesion is most commonly an intramedullary nidus-type spinal AVM. In addition, these patients can get nerve root AVMs, which are

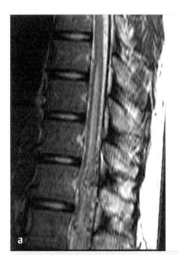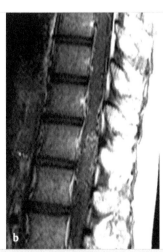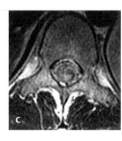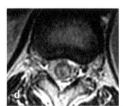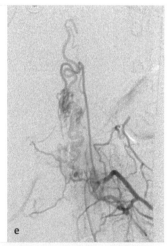

Fig. 11.10 18/F with acute onset lower extremity weakness secondary to intramedullary hemorrhage and edema from an intramedullary AVM. (a) Sagittal T2-weighted MRI demonstrates multiple vascular flow voids and long segment cord edema extending from T6-T10. (b) Sagittal T1 post-contrast MRI demonstrates enhancement of the intramedullary flow voids suggesting the presence of a spinal AVM. (c) and (d) are axial T2-weighted MRIs through the affected cord segments which demonstrate perimedullary flow voids as well as areas of T2 hypointensity in the cord, concerning for intramedullary hemorrhage. (e) Spinal angiogram demonstrates the AVM supplied by a radiculopial artery.

frequently missed on imaging, and AVMs within the vertebrae and/or the muscles. Arterial supply is typically from a segmental artery and venous drainage is both intradural, epidural, and extraspinal. Associated aneurysms are seen in about 50% of cases. The effect of these lesions is often isolated to the metamere of the AVM. MRI will show vascular flow voids involving an entire metamere (vertebral body, dura, cord, muscle, fat) (▶ Fig. 11.11).

Perimedullary AVFs

Perimedullary AVFs consist of a direct fistulous connection between an anterior or posterior spinal artery and a pial vein. These lesions form more often on the ventral surface of the spinal cord and typically have a midline location. There are three typical angioarchitectural features of these lesions:

(1) single feeder lesions with slow blood flow and mild venous hypertension, (2) high-flow lesions with multiple feeding arteries, and (3) giant fistulas with a markedly distended venous network. The giant fistulas can have multiple large venous varices, which can result in compressive symptoms. Similar to dural fistulas, these lesions cause symptoms from congestive myelopathy and T2 changes often extend from the conus on up. High-flow lesions are associated with Hereditary Hemorrhagic Telangiectasia and *RASA* mutations (▶ Fig. 11.12).

Filum Terminale AVFs

Filum terminale AVFs are essentially perimedullary AVFs, which are located along the filum terminale. These lesions are

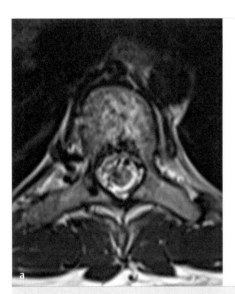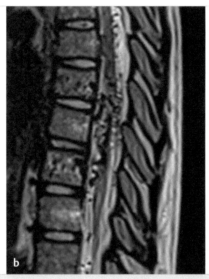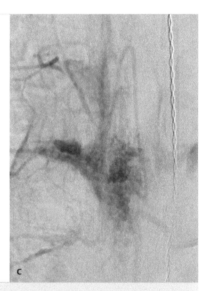

Fig. 11.11 A 17-year-old female with Cobb syndrome presenting with progressive myelopathy. (a) Axial T2-weighted MRI demonstrates prominent vascular flow voids in the vertebral body, paravertebral soft tissue, spinal canal, and in the cord itself. In addition, there is moderate T2 hyperintensity of the cord. (b) Findings are confirmed on the sagittal T2-weighted MRI, which demonstrates the flow voids involving the osseous, intradural, and intramedullary tissues in a segmental distribution, consistent with a Cobb syndrome. (c) AP projection of a spinal angiogram at T12 demonstrates the spinal vascular malformation supplied by an enlarged anterior spinal artery as well as dural and extradural branches of the right T12 intercostal artery.

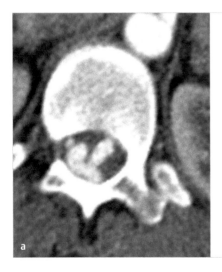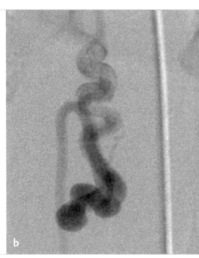

Fig. 11.12 Incidential perimedullary AV fistula in a patient with HHT. (a) CT chest with IV contrast was performed to evaluate for the presence of pulmonary AVMs (not shown). Incidentally discovered were large tortuous vessels in the thecal sac. (b) Spinal angiogram was performed which demonstrated a dilated posterior spinal artery with anastomosed with a spinal vein forming a single-hole perimedullary AV fistula. There is a dilated venous pouch which could produce mass effect if thrombosed.

typically located along the ventral aspect of the filum and have a midline location. The filum terminale's arterial supply is essentially a continuation of the anterior spinal artery. Because the filum terminale is non-neural structure derived from mesoderm, it can also be supplied by dural branches of the lateral sacral and median sacral arteries. Tell-tale signs of a filum terminale fistula include (1) prominent flow voids along the filum terminale on T2-weighted MRI, (2) a large prominent vein of the filum terminale/infra-conal straight flow void, and (3) hypertrophied anterior spinal artery on angiography, which continues well below the conus and continues along the filum terminale (▶ Fig. 11.13).

Spinal Epidural AVFs

Spinal epidural AVFs (SEDAVFs) consist of a fistulous connection between a segmental artery and an epidural vein. These lesions typically have multiple feeding arteries due to the rich vascular supply of the ventral epidural space. The feeding arteries typically drain into a shunted ventral epidural venous pouch which is often clearly visible on spinal MRA. These lesions are divided into three types based on pattern of venous drainage. Type 1 lesions have drainage into the perimedullary venous plexus (and are thus indistinguishable from a spinal dural AVF on MRI

without spinal MRA), type 2 lesions have only epidural venous drainage with thecal sac compression due to engorgement of the epidural venous plexus (and thus cause compressive myelopathy), and type 3 lesions have epidural venous drainage without compression. Cervical SEDAVFs generally demonstrate only paravertebral/extradural drainage while lumbosacral SEDAVFs generally demonstrate intradural venous drainage (60%). Interestingly, about 20% of lumbosacral SEDAVF patients have an associated neural tube defect (i.e., tethered cord, myelomeningocele, filum terminale lipoma, etc.). In approximately 10% of cases, SEDAVFs are located at the site of a prior discectomy (▶ Fig. 11.14).

Conus Medullaris AVMs

Conus medularis AVMs are essentially mixed intramedullary and perimedullary AVMs of the conus and are characterized by multiple feeding arteries, multiple niduses and complex venous drainage. These lesions typically have multiple direct AV shunts from the anterior and posterior spinal arteries as well as nidal-type arteriovenous connections that are usually extramedullary. These lesions are always located in the conus medullarus and cauda equina and can extend along the entire filum terminale (▶ Fig. 11.15).

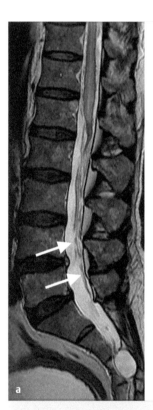 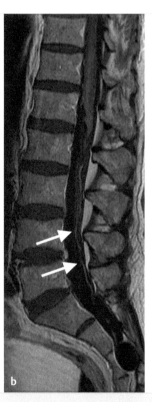 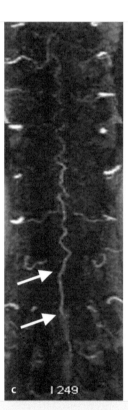 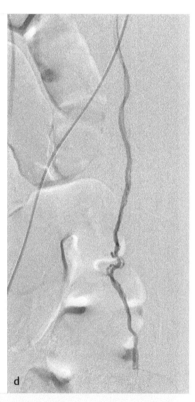

Fig. 11.13 Filum terminale AVF in a 60-year-old male patient presentation with myelopathy. (**a**) Sagittal T2-weighted MRI demonstrates marked edema in the conus and lower cord with subtle vascular flow voids coursing along the conus (*arrows*). (**b**) Sagittal T1 post-contrast MRI demonstrates patchy cord enhancement as well as mild enhancement of the flow voids of the coronal venous plexus. Note the enhancing curvilinear vascular structure coursing along the conus, this is a dilated vein of the filum terminale (*arrows*). (**c**) Coronal gadolinium bolus MRA demonstrates the filum terminale fistula supplied by the anterior spinal artery which extends down to the filum terminale (*arrows*). (**d**) This finding was confirmed on the conventional spinal angiogram.

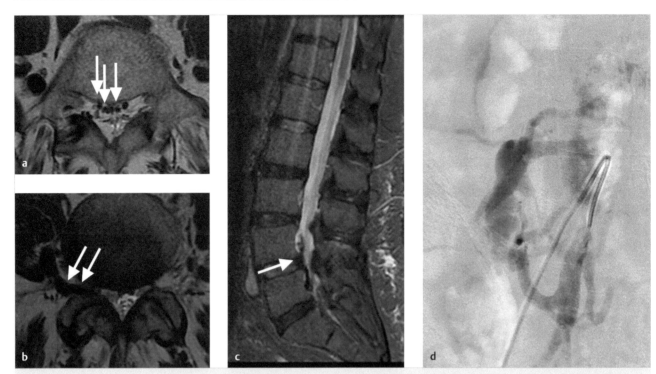

Fig. 11.14 Extradural fistula in a patient presenting with a right L4 radiculopathy. (**a**) Axial T2-weighted MRI demonstrates multiple vascular flow voids in the ventral epidural space at L5 (*arrows*). (**b**) Axial T2-weighted MRI demonstrates a large vascular flow void in the right L4 neural foramen (*arrows*). (**c**) Sagittal T2-weighted MRI demonstrates a T2 hypointense flow void in the ventral epidural space at L4/L5 (*arrow*). (**d**) Selective angiography of the right internal iliac artery shows a paraspinal and extradural fistula with no evidence of intradural venous drainage.

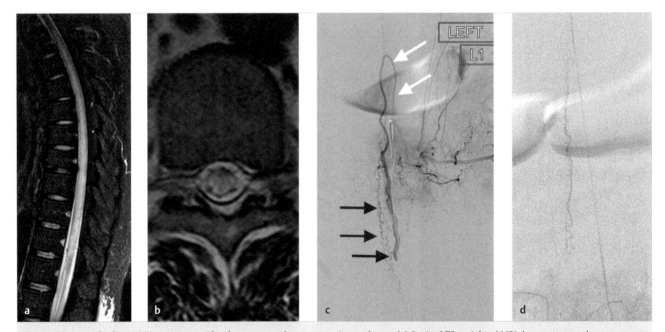

Fig. 11.15 Conus basket AVM in a patient with subacute onset lower extremity weakness. (**a**) Sagittal T2-weighted MRI demonstrates a long-segment myelopathy of the thoracic and lumbar spinal cord. There is a single vascular flow void at the ventral aspect of the conus. (**b**) Axial T2-weighted MRI demonstrates the cross sectional T2 hyperintensity along with a few flow voids along the dorsal aspect of the cord. (**c**) AP projection angiogram of the left L1 lumbar artery demonstrates a hypertrophied anterior spinal artery (*white arrows*) supplying a conus basket AVF with multiple dilated perimedullary draining veins (*black arrows*). (**d**) Example of a normal conus basket, which was mistaken for an AVM in a different patient. Note the normal size of the anterior spinal artery. The conus is richly vascularized due to anastomoses between the paired posterior spinal arteries and anterior spinal artery. Do not mistake this for an AVM!

11.3.5 What the Clinician Needs to Know

- Angioarchitecture and classification of the spinal vascular malformation
- The description of arterial feeders, level of the lesion, and effect of the lesion on the surrounding cord parenchyma
- Any associated imaging findings which point to an AVM-syndrome (i.e., HHT, *RASA*, neural tube defect, etc.)

11.3.6 High-yield Facts

- SEDAVFs often have similar imaging appearance of SDAVFs. However, spinal MRA will show marked engorgement of the epidural venous plexus at the level of the fistula.

- Ventral perimedullary AVFs are strongly associated with HHT and *RASA* mutations. The presence of such a lesion in a young child should prompt a genetic workup.
- Spinal vascular malformations which cause venous congestion almost always cause T2 changes in the conus, regardless of lesion location.

Further Reading

[1] Krings T. Vascular malformations of the spine and spinal cord* : anatomy, classification, treatment. Clin Neuroradiol. 2010; 20(1):5–24
[2] Lee YJ, Terbrugge KG, Saliou G, Krings T. Clinical features and outcomes of spinal cord arteriovenous malformations: comparison between nidus and fistulous types. Stroke. 2014; 45(9):2606–2612

11.4 Spinal Subarachnoid Hemorrhage

11.4.1 Clinical Case

A 76-year-old female with sudden onset back pain (▶ Fig. 11.16).

11.4.2 Description of Imaging Findings and Diagnosis

Diagnosis

Intrathecal hyperdensity on CT, focal area of enhancement along the posterolateral aspect of the spinal cord. No enlarged perimedullary flow voids. Findings consistent with spinal arterial aneurysm (▶ Fig. 11.16).

11.4.3 Background

Sulcal Subarachnoid Hemorrhage (sSAH) is very rare accounting for less than 1% of all subarachnoid hemorrhage (SAH). sSAH classically presents with sudden back pain or headache sometimes with accompanying neurological deficits including paraparesis, sensory disturbances, or sphincter weakness. Potential causes of sSAH include spinal arterial aneurysm, spinal vascular malformation, tumor, coagulopathy, trauma (such as an LP), and idiopathic. sSAH can be due to rupture of spinal arteries or radicular veins.

11.4.4 Imaging Findings

Understanding the anatomy of the spinal subarachnoid space is important to accurately characterize the imaging findings of sSAH. The spinal arachnoid mater is a connective tissue membrane closely attached to the dura mater and is also reflected off the spinal cord surface ensheathing blood vessels as they traverse the subarachnoid space. The intimate relationship between the arachnoid and dura is the main reason why sSAH often presents with concomitant spinal subdural hematoma. Oftentimes, the differentiation between a subdural and subarachnoid hematoma is difficult. However, a pure sSAH consists of blood isolated to the thecal sac while sSDH has a more semicircular or crescent-shaped appearance on cross-sectional imaging.

On CT, sSAH presents with high-density blood products in the thecal sac. On MRI, the appearance is somewhat variable. In the acute stage, sSAH is bright on T1 and T2-weighted images. However, in the subacute stage, it can be T2 dark and T1 bright. Because there is often a delay in the diagnosis of sSAH, the neuroradiologist should be cognizant of this fact. sSAH usually resolves spontaneously within 1 month. However, sometimes the blood products can form a focal hematoma which results in spinal cord compression and associated myelopathy.

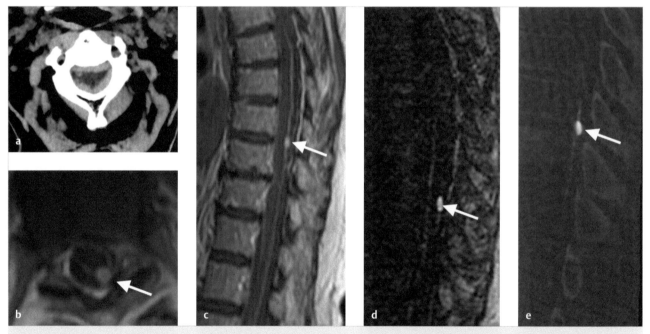

Fig. 11.16 Posterior spinal artery aneurysm in a 76-year-old patient with sSAH. (a) Axial cut from a head CT at the C2 level demonstrates dense subarachnoid blood surrounding the spinal cord consistent with a mixed sSAH and sSDH. This prompted a spinal MRI with IV contrast, which demonstrated a focus of enhancement along the dorsal aspect of the cord in the mid-thoracic spine (*arrows*) (b and c). Differential considerations were a spinal artery aneurysm versus hemangioblastoma or metastasis. (d) Spinal gadolinium bolus MRA demonstrated the aneurysm filling in the arterial phase-confirming the diagnosis (*arrow*). (e) Cone beam intraarterial CTA image performed in preparation for embolization demonstrates the aneurysm arising from the posterior spinal artery (*arrow*).

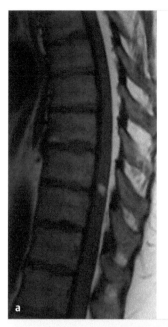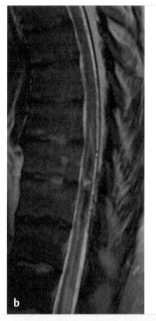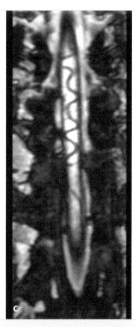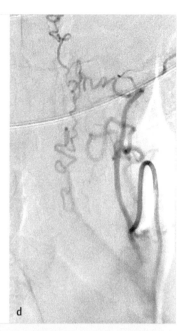

Fig. 11.17 Intramedullary hemorrhage from a spinal dural fistula. (**a**) Sagittal T1-weighted MRI demonstrates a focal area of T1 hyperintensity in the cord. (**b**) Sagittal T2-weighted MRI demonstrates an area of T2 hyperintensity surrounded by hemosiderin staining/T2 hypointensity and cord edema. (**c**) FIESTA image demonstrates dilatation and tortuosity of the coronal venous plexus on the dorsal aspect of the cord. (**d**) A spinal angiogram was performed which demonstrated a spinal dural fistula supplied by the left T4 intercostal artery. Bleeding from a spinal dural fistula is exceedingly rare.

Identifying the etiology of a sSAH is essential to avoiding recurrence. MR angiography is strongly recommended in all cases of sSAH in order to evaluate for the presence of a structural vascular cause such as a spinal arterial aneurysm or spinal vascular malformation. Spinal arterial aneurysms are a rare condition and are generally related to flow alterations in the setting of a spinal vascular malformation or aortic coarctation where there is an abnormal development of collaterals. Pure isolated spinal arterial aneurysms (i.e., those not associated with vascular malformations) are exceedingly rare. Morphologically, isolated spinal arterial aneurysms appear as fusiform dilatations, typically on the ascending portion of the radiculo-pial or radiculomedullary arteries. These lesions can be safely followed and can be resolved spontaneously. Conservative management is the management strategy of choice for anterior spinal artery aneurysms due to the high risk of paraplegia associated with surgical and endovascular interventions.

Non-AVM associated spinal arterial aneurysms have likely a dissecting origin as it is confirmed by histopathologic examination in most cases. Dissections are often the result of inherent vessel wall weakness, which can be promoted by autoimmune diseases, systemic infections, connective tissue disorders, or recreational drug abuse. Because these lesions have a dissecting etiology, patients with ruptured spinal arterial aneurysms can sometimes present with concomitant spinal cord infarct (described in section 11.1); however, this is exceedingly rare.

The other vascular cause of a sSAH is a ruptured spinal vascular malformation. Given their peripheral location, perimedullary AVFs are the most likely to result in sSAH while intramedullary AVMs will lead to hematomyelia. Identification of "weak-spots" in spinal vascular malformations is essential in guiding targeted therapy and altering the natural history of these lesions (▸ Fig. 11.17).

11.4.5 What the Clinician Needs to Know

- The presence of a structural cause of the sSAH
- The development of clot in the spinal subarachnoid space which could require evacuation in order to prevent compressive myelopathy
- Any cord signal abnormalities accompanying the sSAH

11.4.6 High-yield Facts

- Most sSAHs are secondary to trauma or iatrogenic causes.
- MR angiography is essential to ruling out a spinal arterial aneurysm or spinal vascular malformation. If MRA is negative and no cause is identified, conventional angiography should be considered.
- sSAH is hyperintense on T1/T2-weighted images in the acute phase and T2 hypointense and T1 hyperintense in the subacute phase.

Further Reading

[1] Onda K, Yoshida Y, Arai H, Terada T. Complex arteriovenous fistulas at C1 causing hematomyelia through aneurysmal rupture of a feeder from the anterior spinal artery. Acta Neurochir (Wien). 2012; 154(3):471–475

[2] Geibprasert S, Krings T, Apitzsch J, Reinges MH, Nolte KW, Hans FJ. Subarachnoid hemorrhage following posterior spinal artery aneurysm. A case report and review of the literature. Interv Neuroradiol. 2010; 16(2):183–190

11.5 Spinal Cord Cavernoma

11.5.1 Clinical Case

A 52-year-old male with subacute onset myelopathy (▶ Fig. 11.18).

11.5.2 Description of Imaging Findings and Diagnosis

Diagnosis

T2 hypointense T1 hyperintense intramedullary lesion with associated cord edema, consistent with a spinal cord cavernoma.

11.5.3 Background

Spinal cord cavernomas are relatively rare and make up less than 1% of all CNS cavernous malformations. These lesions can present with rapid or slowly progressive neurological decline. Acute episodes of neurological decline are usually due to acute macro-hemorrhages while the progressive myelopathic symptoms are due to microhemorrhages and ensuing gliosis. These lesions commonly present in the 3rd and 4th decades of life. They are most commonly found in the thoracic spinal cord. Spinal cord cavernomas are slightly more prevalent in patients with a family history of cavernoma (i.e., familial cavernomatosis). Thus, screening of the entire neuro-axis is probably useful in these patients.

11.5.4 Imaging Findings

The MRI appearance of spinal cord cavernomas is similar to that of brain cavernomas. These lesions have a popcorn appearance with heterogeneous T1 and T2 signal intensity due to presence of hemorrhage of various ages. On T2- and T2*-weighted imaging, these lesions have a rim of low signal. T2*-weighted images also show blooming. Internal enhancement patterns of these lesions are variable. The radiologist should be attuned to the effect of the cavernoma on the adjacent spinal cord parenchyma (i.e., T2 changes, cord atrophy, cord infarction, cord enlargement, etc.). The reason these cavernomas can impact the surrounding spinal cord is due to the fact that after hemorrhage, the microcirculation around the lesion can become thrombosed resulting in venous congestion.

Lesion location in relation to the spinal cord surface is essential to surgical management and in understanding natural history. T2-weighted sequences often demonstrate a T2 hypointense rim surrounding the lesion, which overestimates the true size of the cavernoma, T1-weighted scans depict better whether the lesion does reach the surface or not (▶ Fig. 11.19). Lesions which extend to the cord surface or are exophytic in appearance can be resected more easily than those which are surrounded by spinal cord parenchyma. In the latter cases, the surgeon has to make a myelotomy in the midline or over the dorsal root entry zone, which carries additional risk. Surface-located lesions can also result in sSAH which is why cavernoma is part of this differential.

11.5.5 What the Clinician Needs to Know

- The location of the cavernoma in relation to the cord surface
- Associated cord signal abnormalities such as intramedullary hemorrhage or cord edema

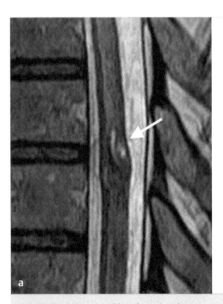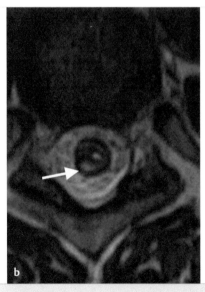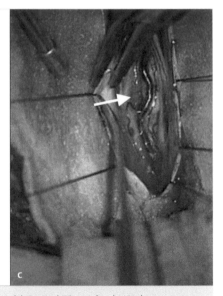

Fig. 11.18 A 52-year-old male with subacute onset myelopathy secondary to spinal cord cavernoma. (**a**) Sagittal T2-weighted MRI demonstrates a mixed T2 hyperintense and hypointense lesion, which appears to abut the cord surface (*arrow*). (**b**) Axial T2-weighted MRI demonstrates the cavernoma with surrounding hemosiderin staining (*arrow*). The cavernoma appears to be exophytic and appears to abut the cord surface. (**c**) Intraoperative photograph demonstrates the bluish tinged cavernoma at the cord surface (*arrow*), as expected by imaging.

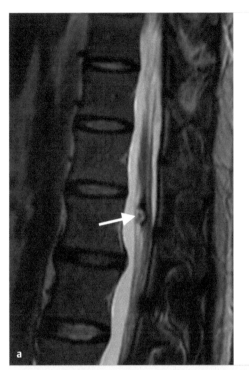
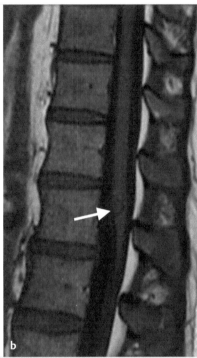
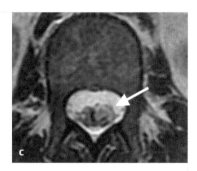
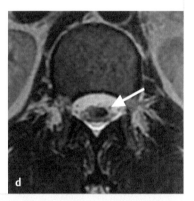

Fig. 11.19 Cavernoma of the conus. (**a**) Sagittal T2-weighted MRI demonstrates an exophytic cavernous malformation of the conus which is mixed T2 hyper and hypointense (*arrow*). There is hemosiderin staining at the poles of the cavernoma. (**b**) Sagittal T1-weighted MRI shows the cavernoma which abuts the cord surface (*arrow*). (**c**) and (**d**). Axial T2-weighted MRI shows the cord cavernoma which is T2 hypo and hyperintense with hemosiderin staining along its periphery (*arrow*).

11.5.6 High-yield Facts

- Spinal cord cavernomas, which abut the cord surface, are easier to resect surgically than those which do not.
- T2-weighted imaging can overestimate the size of a spinal cord cavernoma due to blooming artifact.

Further Reading

[1] Ogilvy CS, Louis DN, Ojemann RG. Intramedullary cavernous angiomas of the spinal cord: clinical presentation, pathological features, and surgical management. Neurosurgery. 1992; 31(2):219–229, discussion 229–230

[2] Weinzierl MR, Krings T, Korinth MC, Reinges MH, Gilsbach JM. MRI and intra-operative findings in cavernous haemangiomas of the spinal cord. Neuroradiology. 2004; 46(1):65–71

Index